AF760829

NEUROSCIENCE RESEARCH PROGRESS

Additional books in this series can be found on Nova's website under the Series tab.

Additional e-books in this series can be found on Nova's website under the e-book tab.

CELL BIOLOGY RESEARCH PROGRESS

Additional books in this series can be found on Nova's website under the Series tab.

Additional e-books in this series can be found on Nova's website under the e-book tab.

NEUROSCIENCE RESEARCH PROGRESS

GLIAL CELLS

EMBRYONIC DEVELOPMENT, TYPES/FUNCTIONS AND ROLE IN DIS

NEUROSCIENCE RESEARCH PROGRESS

GLIAL CELLS

EMBRYONIC DEVELOPMENT, TYPES/FUNCTIONS AND ROLE IN DISEASE

CHARANJIT KAUR
AND
ENG-ANG LING
EDITORS

NOVA BIOMEDICAL

New York

Copyright © 2013 by Nova Science Publishers, Inc.

All rights reserved. No part of this book may be reproduced, stored in a retrieval system or transmitted in any form or by any means: electronic, electrostatic, magnetic, tape, mechanical photocopying, recording or otherwise without the written permission of the Publisher.

For permission to use material from this book please contact us:
Telephone 631-231-7269; Fax 631-231-8175
Web Site: http://www.novapublishers.com

NOTICE TO THE READER

The Publisher has taken reasonable care in the preparation of this book, but makes no expressed or implied warranty of any kind and assumes no responsibility for any errors or omissions. No liability is assumed for incidental or consequential damages in connection with or arising out of information contained in this book. The Publisher shall not be liable for any special, consequential, or exemplary damages resulting, in whole or in part, from the readers' use of, or reliance upon, this material. Any parts of this book based on government reports are so indicated and copyright is claimed for those parts to the extent applicable to compilations of such works.

Independent verification should be sought for any data, advice or recommendations contained in this book. In addition, no responsibility is assumed by the publisher for any injury and/or damage to persons or property arising from any methods, products, instructions, ideas or otherwise contained in this publication.

This publication is designed to provide accurate and authoritative information with regard to the subject matter covered herein. It is sold with the clear understanding that the Publisher is not engaged in rendering legal or any other professional services. If legal or any other expert assistance is required, the services of a competent person should be sought. FROM A DECLARATION OF PARTICIPANTS JOINTLY ADOPTED BY A COMMITTEE OF THE AMERICAN BAR ASSOCIATION AND A COMMITTEE OF PUBLISHERS.

Additional color graphics may be available in the e-book version of this book.

Library of Congress Cataloging-in-Publication Data

ISBN: 978-1-62618-448-0

Library of Congress Control Number: 2013935073

Published by Nova Science Publishers, Inc. † New York

CONTENTS

PREFACE

Astrocytes, oligodendrocytes and microglia are the three types of glial cells in the brain. Research over the past years has provided evidence to their critical role in the proper development and functioning of the brain. Astrocytes and their processes are closely associated with neurons, synaptic terminals and the endothelial cells of the capillaries. They modulate synaptic function by uptake of neurotransmitters, release of neurotransmitter inhibitors and possibly by secretion of neurotransmitters into the synaptic cleft. The levels of some ions such as K+ ions in the extracellular space around the neurons are also regulated by astrocytes. Astrocyte processes in contact with the capillaries are important for the maintenance of proper function of the blood-brain barrier. Oligodendrocytes are involved in myelination of the axons and thus ensure their proper functioning. Microglia are the immunocompetent and phagocytic cells which act as sensors of brain pathology.

It is well documented that in neurological diseases glia can either have a protective or deleterious role. The glial cells especially the astrocytes and microglia may be detrimental to neurons in neurological diseases through production of nitric oxide, inflammatory cytokines and free radicals. They may also be involved in damaging the oligodendrocytes and axons through similar mechanisms. Oligodendrocytes are vulnerable to hypoxic ischemic injuries and damage to these cells leads to myelination deficits. However, the mechanisms that underlie these processes are not fully explored and further research is clearly desirable to gain an in-depth knowledge of the "cross talks" between glial cells, and between them and neurons to understand their role in the progression of damage to the nervous system in various insults. This may lead to the development of new therapeutic strategies for ameliorating the damage in brain insults.

This book should be of interest to neuroscientists and neurologists who can find the latest information on glial cells that will be useful in their continued effort in searching and designing potential therapeutic strategies for treatment of neurological diseases using these cells as drug targets.

Professor Charanjit Kaur
Professor Eng-Ang Ling

In: Glial Cells
Editors: Charanjit Kaur and Eng-Ang Ling

ISBN: 978-1-62618-448-0
© 2013 Nova Science Publishers, Inc.

Chapter 1

MACROLIAL CELLS: DEVELOPMENT, TYPES/FUNCTIONS AND ROLE IN DISEASE

Luciana Nogaroli[1] and Marcos R. Costa[2*]
[1]Institute of Biophysics Carlos Chagas Filho,
Federal University of Rio de Janeiro, Rio de Janeiro, Brazil
[2]Brain Institute, Federal University of Rio Grande do Norte, Natal, Brazil

ABSTRACT

During nervous system development, stem/progenitor cells generate a broad variety of neuronal and macroglial - astrocytes, oligodendrocytes and ependymal - cells. In the last decades, important progress has been made towards the identification of distinct types of neurons in the nervous system, as well as the cellular and molecular mechanisms controlling the generation of such diversity. In parallel, several works have contributed to identify a large variety of macroglial cells, which were raised to the rank of fundamental blocks for the normal function of the central nervous system. However, still little is known about the origin of different macroglial cells. In this review, we will discuss what has been known about the embryonic and early postnatal generation of astrocytes and oligodendrocytes in the cerebral cortex, with a special focus on the identification of distinct stem/progenitor populations that could support the generation of macroglial cell diversity. Next, we will touch upon the functions of macroglial cells in the mature cerebral cortex and discuss their possible implication to the onset of psychiatric and neurological diseases.

MACROGLIAL DIVERSITY IN THE CEREBRAL CORTEX

During development of the cerebral cortex, as throughout the nervous system, three main cell types have to be generated: neurons and the two major macroglial cell types, astrocytes

* Corresponding author: Marcos R. Costa, MD/PhD; Brain Institute – Federal University of Rio Grande do Norte; Av. Nascimento de Castro 2155, Lagoa Nova; Natal 59056-450, Brazil; Telephone/Fax: +55 84 3215-2709; e-mail: mrcosta@neuro.ufrn.br.

and oligodendrocytes. Each of these cell types comprises a great diversity of subtypes, based on their distinct morphology, chemical properties and functions (see e.g., Goldman and Vaysse, 1991, DeFelipe, 1993). This enormous diversity of cells is generated during a relatively short interval of time from progenitors located in the ventricular (VZ) and subventricular zone (SVZ) in both ventral and dorsal telencephalon (reviewed in Marin and Rubenstein, 2003, Gotz and Huttner, 2005, Miller and Gauthier, 2007, Pontious et al., 2008), as well as from progenitors in the dorsal marginal zone (MZ) (Costa et al., 2007, Breunig et al., 2012). In the mouse and rat cerebral cortex, birth dating experiments using the thymidine analogue Bromodeoxyuridine (5-bromo-2'-deoxyuridine, BrdU) have shown that most neurons are generated between the embryonic day (E) 12 and birth (around E20), whereas macroglial cells are mostly generated at late embryogenesis (E16 on) and first post natal weeks (Bayer et al., 1991, Cameron and Rakic, 1991). Recent studies have provided compelling evidence that some macroglial cells in the parenchyma of the cerebral cortex are generated from bipotent progenitors located in the dorsal telencephalon (Costa et al., 2009). These progenitors give rise to glutamatergic neurons and astroglial cells (Costa et al., 2009), likely contributing to the organization of neurons and astrocytes in discrete columns along the cerebral cortex (Magavi et al., 2012). However, other populations of progenitors in germinative niches of the ventral telencephalon and dorsal marginal zone, for instance, also contribute astrocytes and oligodendrocytes in the cerebral cortex (Kessaris et al., 2006, Costa et al., 2007, Breunig et al., 2012).

In the mature cerebral cortex, macroglial cells outnumber neurons and are involved in a myriad of processes, ranging from regulation of water balance and ion distribution to modulation of synaptic transmission (Wang and Bordey, 2008). However, despite their large numbers and wide range of functions, neuroscientists seeking to understand the mechanisms of brain functioning and diseases have mostly overlooked these cells. Evidence for this statement comes from the fact that classification of macroglial cells still relies greatly in morphological criteria and use of a few molecular markers.

Astrocytes, for instance, have been classically divided into two major subpopulations: fibrous astrocytes in the white matter and protoplasmic astrocytes in the gray matter (Miller and Raff, 1984). Fibrous astrocytes have long, thin processes, yielding a star-like appearance. Protoplasmic astrocytes have many branching processes, which contact and sheathe synapses, and usually one or two processes in contact with blood vessels. However, this classification is outdated in light of the great diversity of astrocytes revealed by more detailed morphological and biochemical analyses.

In fact, mature astrocytes can be identified by the expression of glial fibrillary acidic protein (GFAP), calcium-binding protein S100β, glutamate-aspartate transport (GLAST) and glutamate transport 1 (GLT-1), and additional markers have been recently suggested based on microarray gene expression profiles (Bachoo et al., 2004). Expressions of these markers, as well as astrocyte morphologies, vary considerably amongst cortical regions (Emsley and Macklis, 2006, Regan et al., 2007), suggesting that astrocyte subpopulations could be differently specified to display distinct biochemical/biophysical properties throughout discrete regions of the cerebral cortex (Emsley and Macklis, 2006).

A further degree of complexity is added by the differential expression of receptors for growth factors, chemokines, steroids and ion channels, bringing about an enormous diversity of astrocyte subpopulations, likely involved in specific functions (Wang and Bordey, 2008).

Similarly, oligodendrocytes are found in both gray and white matter of the central nervous system (CNS) and can be divided in two major morphofunctional classes: the myelinating oligodendrocytes and the NG2-expressing oligodendrocyte precursors (OPCs). Myelinating oligodendrocytes have been historically classified into types I to IV based on morphological characteristics including the number of primary and branching processes, the orientation of their processes, the shape and size of their somata and also the size of the axons they myelinate (Rio-Hortega, 1928, Bjartmar et al., 1994, Butt et al., 1995). Rio-Hortega's types I/II oligodendrocytes, which are morphological and biochemical indistinguishable, myelinate small-diameter axons (less than 2-4 μm) with a thin myelin sheath and multiple short internodes. These subtypes are found in spinal cord, cerebellum and forebrain, where type II is exclusively present in white matter, e.g. corpus callosum and optic nerve. Distinctively, types III/IV oligodendrocytes have larger cell bodies that lie near by the axon and myelinate large-diameter axons (larger than 4 μm) with a thick myelin sheath and restricted/single long internodes. They are found in the spinal cord, medulla oblongata, cerebral and cerebellar peduncles (Hildebrand et al., 1993).

Biochemically, oligodendrocytes can be identified at virtually all stages of development by the expression of the 2',3'-cyclic nucleotide 3'-phosphodiesterase (CNP; Braun et al., 1988) and the proteolipid protein 1 or its alternative splice form DM20 (Plp1; Spassky et al., 1998). On the other hand, platelet-derived growth factor receptor (PDGFR)α, polysialylated-neural cell adhesion molecule (PSA-NCAM) and NG2 label only OPCs, being devoid in mature cells (Hart et al., 1989, Fewou et al., 2007, Trotter et al., 2010). Immature oligodendrocytes can also be identified by monoclonal antibodies (O1 and O4) to oligodendrocyte cell surfaces (Sommer and Schachner, 1981), whereas more mature, myelinating cells, up regulate specific myelin proteins such as myelin basic protein (MBP; Sternberger et al., 1978) and myelin oligodendrocyte glycoprotein (MOG; Solly et al., 1996).

Transcription factors are also expressed at multiple stages of oligodendrocyte lineage specification and progressive phases of oligodendrocyte maturation including myelination. Sox10 is expressed by OPCs (Zhou et al., 2000), whereas Olig1 and Olig2 are present both in precursors and mature oligodendrocytes (Lu et al., 2000). It has also been reported that a subset of OPCs in the developing ventral forebrain expresses Mash1 (Lu et al., 2000). However, none of these transcription factors are restricted to the oligodendrocyte lineage. Olig2, for instance, is also associated with postnatal cortical astrocytes (Marshall et al., 2005), adult reactive astrocytes (Chen et al., 2008, Tatsumi et al., 2008) and motoneurons in the spinal cord (Mizuguchi et al., 2001, Novitch et al., 2001). Therefore, co-labeling with different markers is necessary to safely determine oligodendrocyte lineage commitment.

In the adult brain, besides myelinating oligodendrocytes, it has been identified a significant cell population of undifferentiated OPCs that is highly branched and express the integral membrane chondroitin sulfate proteoglycan NG2 (Levine and Card, 1987). Morphologically, they are similar to astrocytes, but they do not express GFAP, vimentin, or S100β protein, intracellular markers for astrocytes (Levine and Card, 1987). Instead, they co-label with PDGFRα (Nishiyama et al., 1996) and the transcription factor Olig2 (Ross et al., 2003), both expressed by cells of the oligodendrocyte lineage. Chondroitin sulfate proteoglycan NG2 is express by newborn OPCs in the germinative niches of the brain. As we will see later, NG2-expressing OPCs give rise to myelinating oligodendrocyte in the gray and white matter during development and in adulthood after demyelination (Dawson et al., 2000,

Reynolds et al., 2001). However, there is a subpopulation of newborn OPCs that does not differentiate into myelinating oligodendrocyte.

Several lines of evidence assign to NG2-expressing cells a role beyond just being a source of myelinating oligodendrocytes in the CNS. These cells are distributed throughout the cerebral cortex, in both gray and white matter, and have been reported to be the major proliferative cell type in the adult CNS (for a review see: Dawson et al., 2003, Psachoulia et al., 2009). Using cumulative BrdU labeling, Psachoulia and co-workers have identified two subpopulations of NG2-expressing OPCs in the cerebral cortex and corpus callosum, one proliferative and other quiescent, in a 1:1 ratio. The non-proliferative (quiescent) subpopulation becomes numerically stable in the cerebral cortex at the end of the first postnatal week and persists for the entire animal life (Psachoulia et al., 2009).

NG2-expressing OPCs are found associated with nodes of Ranvier, where they are suggested to be ideally situated to detect and respond to changes in axonal function during demyelination (Butt et al., 1999). However, the most intriguing feature of NG2-expressing cells is their ability to receive transient excitatory and inhibitory inputs (Bergles et al., 2000, Kukley et al., 2007, Karadottir et al., 2008) and the capacity to fire action potentials (Karadottir et al., 2008). These cells express voltage-gated sodium and potassium channels, generate action potentials when depolarized and are preferentially damaged in cerebral stroke and spinal cord injury, as they express more glutamate receptors, and receive increased spontaneous glutamatergic synaptic input (Karadottir et al., 2008).

Due to the heterogeneity of NG2-expressing cells, some authors attributed to these cells the identity of a fourth macroglial cell in the CNS, along with astrocytes, oligodendrocytes and ependymocytes. Over the years, they were also named as $NG2^+$ glial cells (Nishiyama et al., 1999), NG2 cells (Nishiyama, 2001), NG2-glia (Greenwood and Butt, 2003), synantocytes (Butt et al., 2005) and polydendrocytes (Nishiyama et al., 2009).

In sum, astrocytes and oligodendrocytes (including NG2-expressing cells) comprise a diverse population of cells, which can be distinguished by morphological, biochemical and biophysical criteria. In the next two topics we will discuss the origin of these two major macroglial cell types, as well as indicate some evidence for an early specification of both astrocytes and oligodendrocytes subtypes.

Origins of Astrocytes in the Cerebral Cortex

As discussed above, most macroglial cells in the rodent cerebral cortex are generated postnatally. In fact, during the first three weeks of postnatal development, the macroglial cell population, which contains predominantly astrocytes, expands 6–8-fold in the rodent brain (Bandeira et al., 2009).

Using injection of replicant-incompetent retrovirus, several works have shown that both white and gray matter cortical astrocytes are generated in the postnatal SVZ, from where they would migrate to populate the cerebral cortex (Levison et al., 1993, Levison and Goldman, 1993, Luskin and McDermott, 1994). These early works have also shown that astrocytes generated in the SVZ did not disperse long distances in the rostro-caudal axis (Levison et al., 1993) and that white and gray matter astrocytes, as well as oligodendrocytes (see below) are derived from separate macroglial progenitors (Luskin and McDermott, 1994).

Another source of astrocytes in the cerebral cortex is the direct transformation of radial glia cells into protoplasmic astrocytes (Schmechel and Rakic, 1979, Voigt, 1989, Alves et al., 2002, deAzevedo et al., 2003). During this process, radial glia cells lose their apical process and move towards the pial surface, eventually undergoing mitosis in the SVZ (Noctor et al., 2004). It is likely that these transforming cells represent at least a fraction of the macroglial progenitors labeled by retrovirus in the SVZ and studied in previous work, what could help to explain the little dispersion of clonally related astrocytes (Levison et al., 1993).

Accordingly, it has been recently shown that cortical progenitors labeled at early embryonic stages give rise to discrete columnar structures that contain both projection neurons and protoplasmic astrocytes (Magavi et al., 2012). Most columns of neurons contained multiple clusters of astrocytes, and the vast majority of labeled astrocytes was found within 50μm of a labeled neuronal column. The astrocyte to neuron ratio in a single developmental column was similar across the entire neocortex, indicating that column-associated astrocytes account for the majority of protoplasmic astrocytes in the neocortex. These data suggest that cortical protoplasmic astrocytes are generated in a spatially restricted manner from progenitors that also give rise to columns of pyramidal neurons.

Concurrently, it has also been shown that the vast majority of astrocytes in the postnatal cerebral cortex of mice is generated by local proliferation of differentiated astrocytes (Ge et al., 2012). These proliferative astrocytes are derived from cells in the neonatal SVZ, likely the very same cells studied in early works (Levison et al., 1993, Levison and Goldman, 1993, Luskin and McDermott, 1994). Taken together, these results suggest that astrocytes in the cerebral cortex are generated from radial glial cells that previously contribute neurons to a given cortical column (Costa et al., 2009, Magavi et al., 2012) and that expansion of cortical astrocytes is brought about by local proliferation (Ge et al., 2012) of macroglial progenitors derived from the neonatal SVZ (Levison et al., 1993, Levison and Goldman, 1993, Luskin and McDermott, 1994, Noctor et al., 2004, Ge et al., 2012). A schematic view of this process is illustrated in the Figure 1.

Notably, cortical excitatory neurons are spatially organized into individual cortical columns, which are involved in the processing of similar sensory stimuli (Mountcastle, 1997). It has been hypothesized that generation of neuronal cortical columns could be controlled by transcriptional codes expressed in progenitor cells at early development (Costa and Hedin-Pereira, 2010) and it is tempting to speculate that the columnar organization of astrocytes in the cerebral cortex (Magavi et al., 2012) could also reflect some degree of spatial specification in macroglial progenitors.

Consistent with this idea, it has been shown that spinal cord astrocytes are regionally specified in the spinal cord (Hochstim et al., 2008). In this work, the authors described three distinct subtypes of astrocytes in the spinal cord, which could be distinguished by the combinatorial expression of Reelin and Slit1 (Hochstim et al., 2008). These astrocyte subtypes originate from separate progenitor domains expressing the transcription factors Pax6 and Nkx6.1, suggesting that astrocyte diversification could be controlled by a premature transcriptional code.

An additional degree of specialization could be controlled by extrinsic signals in the region where astrocyte progenitors undergo cell division. In the embryonic and neonatal marginal zone (MZ)/layer 1, for example, a separate class of progenitors undergoes cell division and contributes with astrocytes, oligodendrocytes and neurons to the cerebral cortex (Costa et al., 2007, Breunig et al., 2012). MZ/layer 1 progenitors are derived from ventral and dorsal telencephalic ventricular zone, with a predominance of the latter at neonatal stage (Costa et al., 2007). Given the singular composition of the MZ/layer 1, it is possible that local proliferation in this region contribute to the generation of astrocyte diversification in the cerebral cortex (Costa et al., 2007).

Future experiments should help to clarify whether positionally and functionally distinct subtypes of astrocytes in the cerebral cortex develop from different sets of glial progenitors. These studies may also shed light in our understanding about the mechanisms subsidizing neurological and psychiatric diseases associated with astrocyte malfunction.

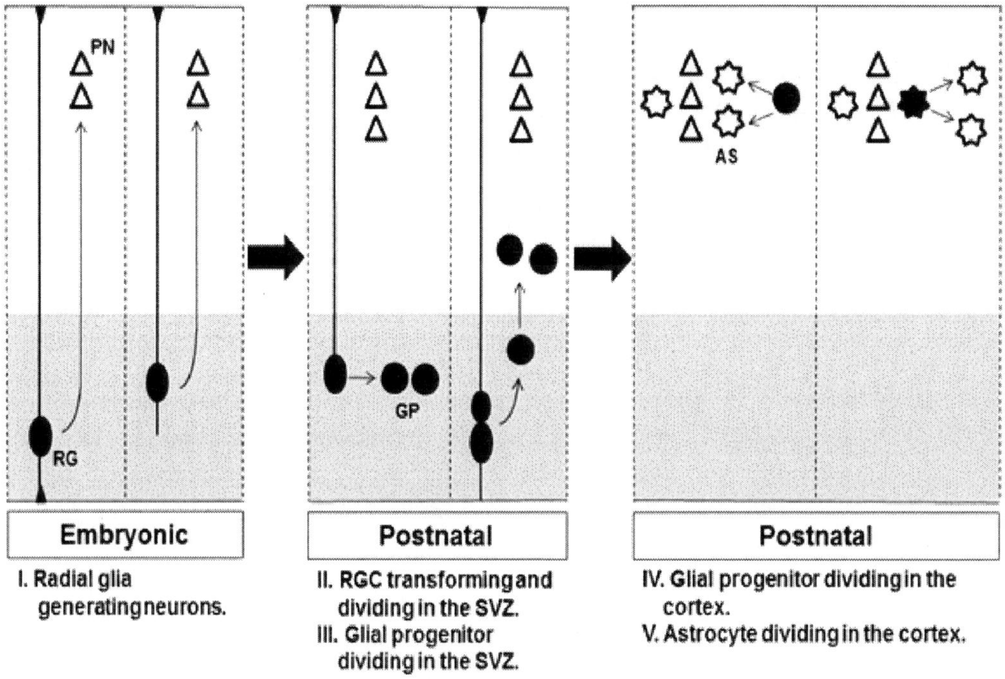

Figure 1. Origins of astrocytes in the cerebral cortex. (I) During early stages, radial glial cells (RGC) give rise to postmitotic neurons (PN) that migrate radially and settle in an individual cortical column. (II and III) Around birth, radial glial cells lose their apical processes and transform into parenchymal astrocytes. During transformation, RGC can undergo cell division in the SVZ. Similarly, glial progenitors (GP) derived from RGC also divide in the postnatal SVZ. (IV and V) GP and astrocytes (AS) proliferate locally in the cerebral cortex, amplifying the astrocytic population. Observe that developing astrocytes maintain the columnar organization of early generated neurons. Dashed lines indicate the boundaries of individual cortical columns. RG, radial glia; PN, postmitotic neuron; GP, glial progenitor; AS, astrocyte.

Origins of Oligodendrocytes in the Cerebral Cortex

Similar to astrocytes, it is warmly debated whether oligodendrocyte subtypes in the cortical parenchyma would be derived from a homogeneous population of OPCs or from separate classes of progenitors previously specified within the germinative niches of the developing telencephalon.

During development, OPCs originate from radial glia cells in restrict regions of the brain (Kriegstein and Alvarez-Buylla, 2009). Once generated, OPCs migrate tangentially and radially out of the germinative niche invading the cerebral cortex (Levison et al., 1993, Levison and Goldman, 1993, Luskin and McDermott, 1994, Suzuki and Goldman, 2003, Kessaris et al., 2006). For many years the origin of oligodendrocytes was a motif of debate. While some researchers defended a single origin from the ventral germinative zone of the neural tube (Pringle and Richardson, 1993), others favored the idea of multiple origins to the oligodendrocytes that populate the forebrain (for review see: Spassky et al., 1998). After a remarkable work of Richardson's group using Cre-lox fate mapping in transgenic mice, it became broadly accepted that oligodendrocytes arise from multiple sites of the telencephalic VZ in a spatiotemporal fashion (Kessaris et al., 2006).

Oligodendrocytes in the forebrain arise from three distinct regions along the dorsal-ventral axis generating successive waves of OPC that overlap in the developing cerebral cortex (Kessaris et al., 2006). To observe that, the authors took advantage of a regionally restricted expression of transcript factors within the germinative zones of the telencephalon (Brazel et al., 2003). Nkx2.1 is a transcript factor expressed by progenitor cells in the medial ganglionic eminence/ anterior entopeduncular area , whereas Gsh2 is expressed by progenitors in the lateral ganglionic eminence and caudal ganglionic eminence . Contrarily, progenitors in the germinative zone of the dorsal telencephalon (cortical VZ) express the transcription factor Emx1.

In the mouse forebrain, the first wave of oligodendrocytes originates at E11.5 from Nkx2.1-expressing cells located in the most ventral region, and migrates laterally and dorsally, reaching the cerebral cortex around E14.5-E16. This wave is followed by the second wave of Gsh2-lineage generated around E15. After E18, around birth, ventral waves start to decrease and the third wave of Emx1-derive cells takes place coming from the dorsal VZ. Surprisingly, by P10 Nkx2.1-lineage represents only 5-10% of the cortical oligodendrocytes/ progenitors in the cortex and by P30 it completely disappears. At this stage (P30) the cortical parenchyma is mostly populated by oligodendrocytes from the dorsal lineage with only a minor fraction derived from ventral Gsh2-expressing cells (Kessaris et al., 2006).

Oligodendrocyte progenitors derived from Gsh2- and Emx1-lineage likely proliferate in the postnatal SVZ (Figure 2), which is the major source of oligodendrocytes in the postnatal forebrain (Levison and Goldman, 1993, Luskin and McDermott, 1994, Brazel et al., 2003, Kessaris et al., 2006).

Using genetic fate mapping of NG2-expressing OPCs, it has also been demonstrated that early postnatal and adult NG2-expressing cells are able to differentiate into protoplasmic astrocytes in the gray matter of ventral forebrain, cerebellum and spinal cord, but not in fibrous astrocytes of white matter (Zhu et al., 2008a, Zhu et al., 2008b). Fate decision between astrocyte and oligodendrocyte lineages during postnatal development involves regulation of Olig2 and GFAP expression (Marshall et al., 2005, Zhu et al., 2012). In the early postnatal SVZ almost all GFAP-positive SVZ astrocytes co-label with Olig2 marker. Both markers are expressed in astrocytes and oligodendrocytes progenitor. However, during differentiation, protoplasmatic astrocytes sustain GFAP and lose Olig2 expression, whereas oligodendrocytes down regulate GFAP and maintain Olig2 expression (Zhu et al., 2008a). Specific deletion of Olig2 in NG2-expressing cells increased astrocytes at the expense of oligodendrocytes production (Marshall et al., 2005, Zhu et al., 2008a, Zhu et al., 2012).

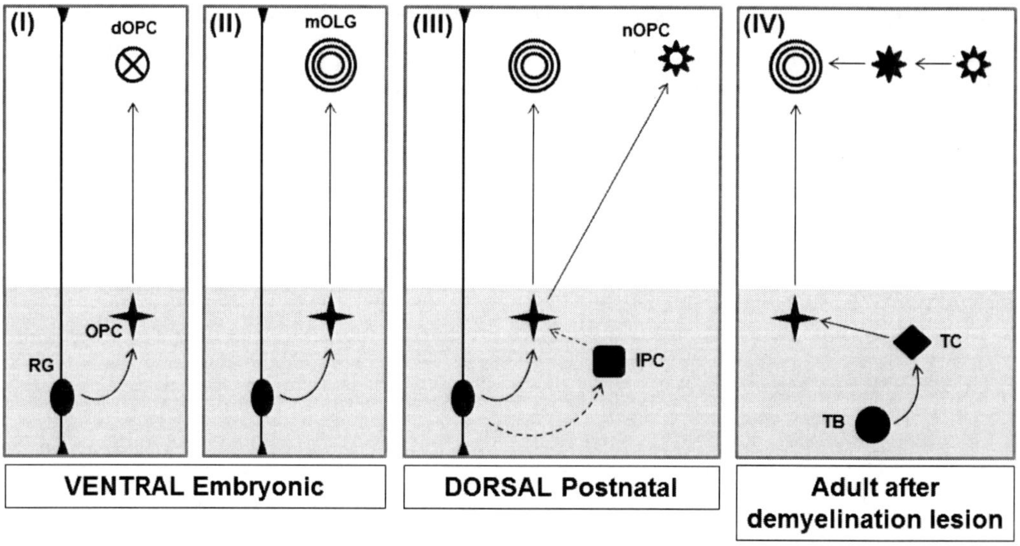

Figure 2. Origins of oligodendrocytes during development and in the adult cerebral cortex after demyelinate lesion. (I and II) Two waves of oligodendrocyte progenitor cells (OPC) to the cortical plate are derived from ventral radial glia (RG) during embryonic development. (I) First wave of OPCs disappears (dOPC) after birth and (II) the second wave generates myelinating oligodendrocytes (mOLG) in the cortical plate. (III) Third wave of OPCs generates mOLGs and non-proliferative NG2-expressing OPCs (nOPC). OPCs are formed directly from RG or from an intermediate progenitor (IPC). (IV) After demyelinating lesion mOPC are generated from the parenchymal nOPC that turn into proliferative nOPC and from type C cells (TC) and type B cells (TB) in the germinative niche. Ventricular/subventricular zones are represented in gray. Black filled figures represent mitotic cells. RG, radial glia; OPC, oligodendrocyte progenitor cell; dOPC, disappeared OPC; mOLG, myelinating oligodendrocyte; IPC, intermediate progenitor cell; nOPC, non-proliferative NG2-expressing OPC; TB, type B cell; TC, type C cell.

As discussed before, excitatory and inhibitory neurons are originated from progenitors in the dorsal and ventral domains of the telencephalon, respectively (Wonders and Anderson, 2006). Moreover, there are evidences for regionalization of astrocyte progenitors, at least in the spinal cord (Hochstim et al., 2008). Thus, it is likely that some patterning occurs amongst OPCs. Indeed, oligodendrocytes that myelinate different axonal tracts in the forebrain are generated from distinct progenitors (Kessaris et al., 2006). However, such regionalization may not result in functional specialization, as discussed below.

Individual waves of oligodendrocytes can be selectively eliminated from the brain using an inducible transgenic mouse line (Kessaris et al., 2006). In these animals, expression of the subunit A of the diphtheric toxin (DTA), under the control of Sox10 promoter and dependent of Cre-mediated recombination, leads to elimination of oligodendrocytes derived from specific lineages, i.e. Nkx2.1, Gsh2 or Emx1 (Kessaris et al., 2006). Following elimination of a single lineage, the number and distribution of oligodendrocytes (mature or progenitors) in the corpus callosum is virtually unaffected around P10. Similarly, myelination does not seem to be affected in the brain of adult animals. Based on this finding, the authors conclude that when oligodendrocytes derived from one source are eliminated, they can be successfully substituted by the other sources, suggesting that they are functionally redundant. Therefore, oligodendrocytes derived from distinct domains within the germinative niche would have similar functions or properties in the mature brain (Kessaris et al., 2006, Clarke et al., 2012)

However, the observation of distinct waves of oligodendrocytes under physiological conditions (Kessaris et al., 2006) could suggest that some degree of regional specification is important to generate oligodendrocytes with distinct properties. In fact, oligodendrocyte specification in different germinative niches seems to depend on exquisite signaling molecules, which are likely to generate oligodendrocytes with individual cellular properties (Rowitch and Kriegstein, 2010). In the forebrain, ventral derived population depends on sonic hedgehod (Shh) signaling (Tekki-Kessaris et al., 2001), whereas the dorsal source seems to be independent of Shh (Nery et al., 2001). Instead, dorsal lineage is regulated by fibroblast growth factor-2 (Furusho et al., 2011). On the other hand, PDGFRα signaling is required for both ventral and dorsal generation (Fruttiger et al., 1999, Spassky et al., 2001)

In sum, oligodendrocyte heterogeneity, i.e. type I/II, type III/IV and adult NG2-labeling progenitor, might reflect a combination of intrinsic programs during progenitor specification within the germinative zone and extrinsic factors when the progenitors reach their final destination in the cerebral cortex. Understand how this cellular diversity is regulated becomes an important step in order to manipulate endogenous neural stem cells for regenerative proposal when myelin is disrupted in the CNS.

Macroglial Cells And Brain Diseases

Macroglial cells are essential to maintain the normal functioning of the CNS and their dysfunction can be observed in many neurological diseases. In the last few decades, it has been appreciated that developmental alterations affecting either the generation or maturation of macroglial cells can be the cause of some neurological and psychiatric disorders (Rajkowska and Miguel-Hidalgo, 2007, Molofsky et al., 2012), rather than a consequence of these pathological conditions.

Astrocyte Functions and Diseases

Astrocytes regulate ion distribution and water balance in the CNS, as well as synthesize most proteins and adhesion molecules in the extracellular matrix, thus conveying structural support to other neural cells. They are also pivotal in the control of angiogenesis, blood-brain-barrier (formation and maintenance, glutamate and GABA uptake, detoxification and metabolic support (for a review see: Wang and Bordey, 2008). Besides these well-established functions of astrocytes for the homeostasis of the nervous system, it has been acknowledged in the last few years that astrocytes are not merely passive elements at synapses, but rather participate actively in synaptic transmission and plasticity.

Indeed, astrocytes in the hippocampus release the N-methyl-D-aspartate receptor co-agonist D-serine, which regulates long-term potentiation of synaptic transmission, suggesting that astrocytes could participate in mechanisms of learning and memory (Yang et al., 2003, Henneberger et al., 2010). Astrocytes also participate in synaptic formation during development (Eroglu and Barres, 2010) and maturation of dendritic spines in the adult brain

(Nishida and Okabe, 2007). Furthermore, astrocytes couple neuronal activity to vascular tone, contributing to an adequate oxygenation and energy supply of active cells (Zonta et al., 2003, Mulligan and MacVicar, 2004).

Given these pivotal roles of astrocytes for normal functioning of the CNS, it is not surprising that malfunctions of these cells could be associated with many neurological and psychiatric diseases. However, an important question to be addressed is whether such diseases would be caused by primary alterations in astrocytes or, even more sophisticatedly, in specific subtypes of astrocytes. The answer for this question is progressively emerging through the analyses of neurodevelopmental diseases caused by known genetic mutations.

For example, Rett syndrome is a disorder caused by the loss of the transcriptional repressor methyl-CpG-binding protein 2 (MeCP2) associated with autism, cognitive impairment and respiratory abnormalities (Chahrour and Zoghbi, 2007). MeCP2-deficient mice recapitulate several hallmarks of the human disease and have been largely used to study the pathological basis of neuronal dysfunction. Notably, co-culture of wild-type neurons with astrocytes isolated from MeCP2-deficient mice lead to abnormal development of neuronal dendrites, suggesting that astrocyte dysfunction has non-cell-autonomous effects on neuronal development, which could contribute to the defects observed in MeCP2-deficient mice (Ballas et al., 2009).

Altered dendrite morphology has also been observed in neurons grown on FMR1-deficient astrocytes (Jacobs and Doering, 2010). FMR1 mutation in humans causes the fragile X syndrome, a condition associated with mental retardation, autistic features, increased rates of epilepsy and motor abnormalities (Rooms and Kooy, 2011). Noteworthy, the tight association between fragile X syndrome and epilepsy may also indicate that astrocyte dysfunction is involved in the abnormal neuronal excitability observed in epileptic brains (Gomez-Gonzalo et al., 2010).

Other psychiatric diseases, such as schizophrenia and depression, have been related to neurodevelopmental abnormalities (Rubenstein, 2011). It remains to be studied whether primary dysfunction of astrocytes could also contribute to these conditions. A better understanding of astrocyte dysfunction in these diseases may contribute to the development of new treatment strategies.

Astrocyte dysfunction has been related to the onset of symptoms in Alzheimer's disease (AD), a neurodegenerative disorder that is clinically characterized by progressive memory loss and dysfunction of higher cognitive areas. In fact, astrocytes react to inflammatory signals observed at early stages of AD, and also contribute to inflammation through the release of cytokines and other pro-inflammatory mediators. Some of these modulators, such as interleukin-1β, can affect synaptic transmission directly by interfering with long-term potentiation (Murray and Lynch, 1998), what could help to explain some of the early cognitive deficits in AD. Moreover, astrocytes themselves undergo functional and structural changes in response to inflammation, contributing to synaptic malfunction, synaptic loss, and cognitive deficits (Olabarria et al., 2010). Therefore, astrocyte dysfunction can be associated with the etiology and progression of AD.

Oligodendrocyte Functions and Diseases

Myelination represents an important advantage in evolution since it enables the axon to conduct impulses at a high speed with additional saving of brain space and energy, which is particularly critical in the CNS (for review see: Hildebrand et al., 1993). Oligodendrocyte is the cellular component of the brain and spinal cord responsible for the production of myelin, a fatty insulation composed of modified plasma membrane that surrounds axons and promotes the rapid and efficient conduction of electrical impulses along myelinated axons, as well as contributes to maintain axonal integrity (Hildebrand et al., 1993, Nave, 2010). Myelination is essential for the normal functioning of the vertebrate CNS. When myelination fails or myelin is disrupted, as a result of injury, pathological degeneration, or genetic disorders, normal impulse conduction is compromised leading to severe functional deficits such as paralysis, sensory-motor dysfunction, cognitive impairment, mental retardation and death (Bradl and Lassmann, 2010).

In the CNS, myelin can be damaged by autoimmune disease (e.g. multiple sclerosis), inherited disorders affecting structural genes in myelin, (e.g. Charcot-Marie-Tooth disease), metabolic disorders (e.g. Krabbe's disease) and by infection, trauma, toxins, hormonal imbalance and asphyxia (e.g. periventricular leukomalacia) (for a review see: Fields, 2008). White matter defects have been recently associated with a wide range of psychiatric desorders, such as schizophrenia, bipolar disorder, major depression, anxiety and obsessive compulsive disorder, suggesting that oligodendrocytes might participate in some aspects of these diseases (reviewed in Rajkowska and Miguel-Hidalgo, 2007, Uranova et al., 2007, Fields, 2008).

Patients with chronic depression show reduction in gray matter volume and glial density in the prefrontal cortex and the hippocampus (Krishnan and Nestler, 2008) and decreased level of MBP in the anterior frontal cortex (Honer et al., 1999, Rajkowska and Miguel-Hidalgo, 2007). A recent study has shown that there is a correlation among oligodendrocyte gene variants, white matter tract integrity, and cognitive performance both in controls and patients with schizophrenia (Voineskos et al., 2012), further supporting the role of oligodendrocyte/white matter in schizophrenia.

Neuregulin 1 (NRG1) and its receptor, erbB4, are genetically linked with susceptibility to schizophrenia and bipolar disorder. In vivo studies using transgenic mice have shown that blockage of erbB signaling in oligodendrocytes lead to reduction in oligodendrocyte cell number and myelin thickness, as well as slower electrical conduction in CNS axons. These alterations in white matter cause increased levels of dopamine receptors and transporters and behavioral alterations consistent with neuropsychiatric disorders (Roy et al., 2007).

Another study corroborates the relationship between erbB signaling pathway, oligodendrocyte function and behavior alterations (Makinodan et al., 2012). Early social isolation results in adult behavioral and cognitive dysfunction that correlates with white matter alterations. Mice isolated for 2 weeks immediately after weaning have a reduction in the NRG1 expression by prefrontal cortex neurons resulting in reduced oligodendrocyte ErbB3 signaling, incomplete oligodendrocyte maturation and myelination (Makinodan et al., 2012). These alterations, which occur only during this critical period, are not recovered with reintroduction in a social environment. These findings indicate that social experience regulates prefrontal cortex myelination, which is essential for normal cognitive function.

It has been widely accepted that demyelination, in the adult brain, increases proliferation of OPCs in the adult SVZ (Nait-Oumesmar et al., 1999, Picard-Riera et al., 2002, Petratos et al., 2004, Menn et al., 2006, Aguirre and Gallo, 2007) and close to the lesion site (Gensert and Goldman, 1997, Fancy et al., 2004), involving both regions in the myelin repair (remyelination) process. This "activated" state seems to be triggered by factors derived from activated microglial cells, astrocytes and cerebrospinal fluid (Tiwari-Woodruff et al., 2004, Glezer et al., 2006, Rhodes et al., 2006). Indeed, it has been described an increase in mRNA levels for several growth factors in the SVZ, including HB-EGF, TGFα, VEGF, PDGF-A, PDGF-B and IGF-1 (Aguirre and Gallo, 2007). These growth factors might be involved in the regulation of proliferation, cell fate specification and/or progenitor cells migration.

Focal demyelination using lysolecthin up regulates proliferation in the adult SVZ increasing fourfold or more oligodendrogenesis comparing to normal condition/basal (Menn et al., 2006). Different from focal demyelination models, experimental autoimmune encephalomyelitis (EAE) models lead to multiples lesion plaques. In this case, proliferation is increased in all brain regions, but mainly within the lesions (Picard-Riera et al., 2002), most likely due to activation of local NG2-expression OPCs. It has been shown that quiescent NG2-expressing OPCs become proliferative in response to demyelination (Gensert and Goldman, 1997, Fancy et al., 2004).

Performing a lysolecthin demyelination followed by retrovirus injection in the SVZ, where dividing cells are labeled with green fluorescent protein (GFP), Menn and co-workers identified that new OPCs are derived from two sources of adult dividing cells: GFAP-expressing SVZ cells (i.e. type B cells) and non-GFAP dividing cells outside the SVZ (i.e. parenchymal NG2-expressing OPCs) (Menn et al., 2006). SVZ-derived OPCs are highly migratory compared to the parenchymal OPCs. In the SVZ, Olig2 expression is observed in a subpopulation of type B cells and a small population of type C cells, suggesting that OPC specification begins very early in the lineage (Menn et al., 2006).

After demyelination, migration of newborn SVZ-derived OPCs is increased (Picard-Riera et al., 2002) and, likewise proliferation, it is dependent of EGFR signaling (Aguirre and Gallo, 2007). Once in the demyelinated lesion sites, OPCs may form functional and transient glutamatergic synapses with naked axons (Etxeberria et al., 2010). These transitory synapses seem to be important for initial axon-OPC recognition and the subsequent capacity of OPCs to differentiate and become mature myelinating oligodendrocytes (Etxeberria et al., 2010).

In vitro studies using stem cell assays have shown that multiple regions of the human SVZ contained astrocyte-like cells that self-renewed and are multipotent giving rise to neurons, astrocytes and oligodendrocytes (Sanai et al., 2004). Interestingly, but not surprisingly, postmortem brains from multiple sclerosis patients show an increased proliferation in the SVZ associated with OPCs makers. OPCs were also detected in demyelinated lesions, where in active and chronic active lesions the number of OPCs was eightfold higher compared with chronic silent lesions. Periventricular lesions had 30 to 50% more OPCs than lesions remote from the ventricular wall. These findings indicate that, as in rodents, activation of gliogenesis in the SVZ occurs in multiple sclerosis (MS) patients and suggest the mobilization of SVZ-derived OPCs to periventricular lesions (Nait-Oumesmar et al., 2007).

Strikingly, it has also been described that some MS patients present autoantibodies to NG2 in the cerebralspinal fluid (Niehaus et al., 2000). These antibodies could interfere with remyelination by blocking OPCs migration or, more dramatically, being involved in the etiology of the disease by disrupting glial–neuronal signaling at synapses and paranodes (for a review see: Trotter, 2005). This finding may explain why MS patients do not successfully remyelinate as good as observed for animal models, despite the increased proliferation of OPCs (Nait-Oumesmar et al., 2007).

Understanding how OPCs heterogeneity is brought about will contribute to develop cell-based therapies for human neurological disorders taking advantage of endogenous source of glial progenitor cells (Goldman et al., 2008). Additionally, it is necessary to consider that adult OPCs accessible for remyelination may behave differently than OPCs originated during development. For example, adult OPCs have longer cell cycle time and slower rate of migration. Last but not least, transcription factors and extracellular signals required for generation of oligodendrocytes are likely to be different in developing and mature brains (Bradl and Lassmann, 2010).

Conclusion

In this chapter, we pointed out some evidences suggesting that precise developmental programs could contribute to generate the vast diversity of astrocytes and oligodendrocytes in the cerebral cortex. Future studies should help to clarify whether alterations in the normal generation and/or specification of these macroglial cells could lead to the onset of neurological and psychiatric diseases. In another direction, understanding the developmental programs and roles of individual subpopulations of macroglial cells will likely contribute to the development of new cell-based therapies to treat brain disorders.

References

Aguirre A, Gallo V (2007) Reduced EGFR signaling in progenitor cells of the adult subventricular zone attenuates oligodendrogenesis after demyelination. *Neuron Glia Biol* 3:209-220.

Alves JA, Barone P, Engelender S, Froes MM, Menezes JR (2002) Initial stages of radial glia astrocytic transformation in the early postnatal anterior subventricular zone. *J Neurobiol* 52:251-265.

Bachoo RM, Kim RS, Ligon KL, Maher EA, Brennan C, Billings N, Chan S, Li C, Rowitch DH, Wong WH, DePinho RA (2004) Molecular diversity of astrocytes with implications for neurological disorders. *Proc Natl Acad Sci U S A* 101:8384-8389.

Ballas N, Lioy DT, Grunseich C, Mandel G (2009) Non-cell autonomous influence of MeCP2-deficient glia on neuronal dendritic morphology. *Nat Neurosci* 12:311-317.

Bandeira F, Lent R, Herculano-Houzel S (2009) Changing numbers of neuronal and non-neuronal cells underlie postnatal brain growth in the rat. *Proc Natl Acad Sci U S A* 106:14108-14113.

Bayer SA, Altman J, Russo RJ, Dai XF, Simmons JA (1991) Cell migration in the rat embryonic neocortex. *J Comp Neurol* 307:499-516.

Bergles DE, Roberts JD, Somogyi P, Jahr CE (2000) Glutamatergic synapses on oligodendrocyte precursor cells in the hippocampus. *Nature* 405:187-191.

Bjartmar C, Hildebrand C, Loinder K (1994) Morphological heterogeneity of rat oligodendrocytes: electron microscopic studies on serial sections. *Glia* 11:235-244.

Bradl M, Lassmann H (2010) Oligodendrocytes: biology and pathology. *Acta neuropathologica* 119:37-53.

Braun PE, Sandillon F, Edwards A, Matthieu JM, Privat A (1988) Immunocytochemical localization by electron microscopy of 2'3'-cyclic nucleotide 3'-phosphodiesterase in developing oligodendrocytes of normal and mutant brain. *J Neurosci* 8:3057-3066.

Brazel CY, Romanko MJ, Rothstein RP, Levison SW (2003) Roles of the mammalian subventricular zone in brain development. *Prog Neurobiol* 69:49-69.

Breunig JJ, Gate D, Levy R, Rodriguez J, Jr., Kim GB, Danielpour M, Svendsen CN, Town T (2012) Rapid genetic targeting of pial surface neural progenitors and immature neurons by neonatal electroporation. *Neural Dev* 7:26.

Butt AM, Duncan A, Hornby MF, Kirvell SL, Hunter A, Levine JM, Berry M (1999) Cells expressing the NG2 antigen contact nodes of Ranvier in adult CNS white matter. *Glia* 26:84-91.

Butt AM, Hamilton N, Hubbard P, Pugh M, Ibrahim M (2005) Synantocytes: the fifth element. *Journal of anatomy* 207:695-706.

Butt AM, Ibrahim M, Ruge FM, Berry M (1995) Biochemical subtypes of oligodendrocyte in the anterior medullary velum of the rat as revealed by the monoclonal antibody Rip. *Glia* 14:185-197.

Cameron RS, Rakic P (1991) Glial cell lineage in the cerebral cortex: a review and synthesis. *Glia* 4:124-137.

Chahrour M, Zoghbi HY (2007) The story of Rett syndrome: from clinic to neurobiology. *Neuron* 56:422-437.

Chen Y, Miles DK, Hoang T, Shi J, Hurlock E, Kernie SG, Lu QR (2008) The basic helix-loop-helix transcription factor olig2 is critical for reactive astrocyte proliferation after cortical injury. *J Neurosci* 28:10983-10989.

Clarke LE, Young KM, Hamilton NB, Li H, Richardson WD, Attwell D (2012) Properties and fate of oligodendrocyte progenitor cells in the corpus callosum, motor cortex, and piriform cortex of the mouse. *J Neurosci* 32:8173-8185.

Costa MR, Bucholz O, Schroeder T, Gotz M (2009) Late origin of glia-restricted progenitors in the developing mouse cerebral cortex. *Cereb Cortex 19 Suppl* 1:i135-143.

Costa MR, Hedin-Pereira C (2010) Does cell lineage in the developing cerebral cortex contribute to its columnar organization? *Front Neuroanat* 4:26.

Costa MR, Kessaris N, Richardson WD, Gotz M, Hedin-Pereira C (2007) The marginal zone/layer I as a novel niche for neurogenesis and gliogenesis in developing cerebral cortex. *J Neurosci* 27:11376-11388.

Dawson MR, Levine JM, Reynolds R (2000) NG2-expressing cells in the central nervous system: are they oligodendroglial progenitors? *Journal of neuroscience research* 61:471-479.

Dawson MR, Polito A, Levine JM, Reynolds R (2003) NG2-expressing glial progenitor cells: an abundant and widespread population of cycling cells in the adult rat CNS. *Molecular and cellular neurosciences* 24:476-488.

deAzevedo LC, Fallet C, Moura-Neto V, Daumas-Duport C, Hedin-Pereira C, Lent R (2003) Cortical radial glial cells in human fetuses: depth-correlated transformation into astrocytes. *J Neurobiol* 55:288-298.

DeFelipe J (1993) Neocortical neuronal diversity: chemical heterogeneity revealed by colocalization studies of classic neurotransmitters, neuropeptides, calcium-binding proteins, and cell surface molecules. *Cereb Cortex 3*:273-289.

Emsley JG, Macklis JD (2006) Astroglial heterogeneity closely reflects the neuronal-defined anatomy of the adult murine CNS. *Neuron Glia Biol* 2:175-186.

Eroglu C, Barres BA (2010) Regulation of synaptic connectivity by glia. *Nature* 468:223-231.

Etxeberria A, Mangin JM, Aguirre A, Gallo V (2010) Adult born SVZ progenitors receive transient synapses during remyelination in corpus callosum. *Nat Neurosci* 13:287-289.

Fancy SP, Zhao C, Franklin RJ (2004) Increased expression of Nkx2.2 and Olig2 identifies reactive oligodendrocyte progenitor cells responding to demyelination in the adult CNS. *Molecular and cellular neurosciences* 27:247-254.

Fewou SN, Ramakrishnan H, Bussow H, Gieselmann V, Eckhardt M (2007) Down-regulation of polysialic acid is required for efficient myelin formation. *The Journal of biological chemistry* 282:16700-16711.

Fields RD (2008) White matter in learning, cognition and psychiatric disorders. *Trends in neurosciences* 31:361-370.

Fruttiger M, Karlsson L, Hall AC, Abramsson A, Calver AR, Bostrom H, Willetts K, Bertold CH, Heath JK, Betsholtz C, Richardson WD (1999) Defective oligodendrocyte development and severe hypomyelination in PDGF-A knockout mice. *Development* 126:457-467.

Furusho M, Kaga Y, Ishii A, Hebert JM, Bansal R (2011) Fibroblast growth factor signaling is required for the generation of oligodendrocyte progenitors from the embryonic forebrain. *J Neurosci* 31:5055-5066.

Ge WP, Miyawaki A, Gage FH, Jan YN, Jan LY (2012) Local generation of glia is a major astrocyte source in postnatal cortex. *Nature* 484:376-380.

Gensert JM, Goldman JE (1997) Endogenous progenitors remyelinate demyelinated axons in the adult CNS. *Neuron* 19:197-203.

Glezer I, Lapointe A, Rivest S (2006) Innate immunity triggers oligodendrocyte progenitor reactivity and confines damages to brain injuries. *FASEB journal:* official publication of the Federation of American Societies for Experimental Biology 20:750-752.

Goldman JE, Vaysse PJ (1991) Tracing glial cell lineages in the mammalian forebrain. *Glia* 4:149-156.

Goldman SA, Schanz S, Windrem MS (2008) Stem cell-based strategies for treating pediatric disorders of myelin. *Human molecular genetics* 17:R76-83.

Gomez-Gonzalo M, Losi G, Chiavegato A, Zonta M, Cammarota M, Brondi M, Vetri F, Uva L, Pozzan T, de Curtis M, Ratto GM, Carmignoto G (2010) An excitatory loop with astrocytes contributes to drive neurons to seizure threshold. *PLoS Biol* 8:e1000352.

Gotz M, Huttner WB (2005) The cell biology of neurogenesis. *Nat Rev Mol Cell Biol* 6:777-788.

Greenwood K, Butt AM (2003) Evidence that perinatal and adult NG2-glia are not conventional oligodendrocyte progenitors and do not depend on axons for their survival. *Molecular and cellular neurosciences* 23:544-558.

Hart IK, Richardson WD, Bolsover SR, Raff MC (1989) PDGF and intracellular signaling in the timing of oligodendrocyte differentiation. *The Journal of cell biology* 109:3411-3417.

Henneberger C, Papouin T, Oliet SH, Rusakov DA (2010) Long-term potentiation depends on release of D-serine from astrocytes. *Nature* 463:232-236.

Hildebrand C, Remahl S, Persson H, Bjartmar C (1993) Myelinated nerve fibres in the CNS. *Prog Neurobiol* 40:319-384.

Hochstim C, Deneen B, Lukaszewicz A, Zhou Q, Anderson DJ (2008) Identification of positionally distinct astrocyte subtypes whose identities are specified by a homeodomain code. *Cell* 133:510-522.

Honer WG, Falkai P, Chen C, Arango V, Mann JJ, Dwork AJ (1999) Synaptic and plasticity-associated proteins in anterior frontal cortex in severe mental illness. *Neuroscience* 91:1247-1255.

Jacobs S, Doering LC (2010) Astrocytes prevent abnormal neuronal development in the fragile x mouse. *J Neurosci* 30:4508-4514.

Karadottir R, Hamilton NB, Bakiri Y, Attwell D (2008) Spiking and nonspiking classes of oligodendrocyte precursor glia in CNS white matter. *Nat Neurosci* 11:450-456.

Kessaris N, Fogarty M, Iannarelli P, Grist M, Wegner M, Richardson WD (2006) Competing waves of oligodendrocytes in the forebrain and postnatal elimination of an embryonic lineage. *Nat Neurosci* 9:173-179.

Kriegstein A, Alvarez-Buylla A (2009) The glial nature of embryonic and adult neural stem cells. *Annu Rev Neurosci* 32:149-184.

Krishnan V, Nestler EJ (2008) The molecular neurobiology of depression. *Nature* 455:894-902.

Kukley M, Capetillo-Zarate E, Dietrich D (2007) Vesicular glutamate release from axons in white matter. *Nat Neurosci* 10:311-320.

Levine JM, Card JP (1987) Light and electron microscopic localization of a cell surface antigen (NG2) in the rat cerebellum: association with smooth protoplasmic astrocytes. *J Neurosci* 7:2711-2720.

Levison SW, Chuang C, Abramson BJ, Goldman JE (1993) The migrational patterns and developmental fates of glial precursors in the rat subventricular zone are temporally regulated. *Development* 119:611-622.

Levison SW, Goldman JE (1993) Both oligodendrocytes and astrocytes develop from progenitors in the subventricular zone of postnatal rat forebrain. *Neuron* 10:201-212.

Lu QR, Yuk D, Alberta JA, Zhu Z, Pawlitzky I, Chan J, McMahon AP, Stiles CD, Rowitch DH (2000) Sonic hedgehog--regulated oligodendrocyte lineage genes encoding bHLH proteins in the mammalian central nervous system. *Neuron* 25:317-329.

Luskin MB, McDermott K (1994) Divergent lineages for oligodendrocytes and astrocytes originating in the neonatal forebrain subventricular zone. *Glia* 11:211-226.

Magavi S, Friedmann D, Banks G, Stolfi A, Lois C (2012) Coincident generation of pyramidal neurons and protoplasmic astrocytes in neocortical columns. *J Neurosci* 32:4762-4772.

Makinodan M, Rosen KM, Ito S, Corfas G (2012) A critical period for social experience-dependent oligodendrocyte maturation and myelination. *Science* 337:1357-1360.

Marin O, Rubenstein JL (2003) Cell migration in the forebrain. *Annu Rev Neurosci* 26:441-483.

Marshall CA, Novitch BG, Goldman JE (2005) Olig2 directs astrocyte and oligodendrocyte formation in postnatal subventricular zone cells. *J Neurosci* 25:7289-7298.

Menn B, Garcia-Verdugo JM, Yaschine C, Gonzalez-Perez O, Rowitch D, Alvarez-Buylla A (2006) Origin of oligodendrocytes in the subventricular zone of the adult brain. *J Neurosci* 26:7907-7918.

Miller FD, Gauthier AS (2007) Timing is everything: making neurons versus glia in the developing cortex. *Neuron* 54:357-369.

Miller RH, Raff MC (1984) Fibrous and protoplasmic astrocytes are biochemically and developmentally distinct. *J Neurosci* 4:585-592.

Mizuguchi R, Sugimori M, Takebayashi H, Kosako H, Nagao M, Yoshida S, Nabeshima Y, Shimamura K, Nakafuku M (2001) Combinatorial roles of olig2 and neurogenin2 in the coordinated induction of pan-neuronal and subtype-specific properties of motoneurons. *Neuron* 31:757-771.

Molofsky AV, Krencik R, Ullian EM, Tsai HH, Deneen B, Richardson WD, Barres BA, Rowitch DH (2012) Astrocytes and disease: a neurodevelopmental perspective. *Genes Dev* 26:891-907.

Mountcastle VB (1997) The columnar organization of the neocortex. *Brain* 120 (Pt 4):701-722.

Mulligan SJ, MacVicar BA (2004) Calcium transients in astrocyte endfeet cause cerebrovascular constrictions. *Nature* 431:195-199.

Murray CA, Lynch MA (1998) Evidence that increased hippocampal expression of the cytokine interleukin-1 beta is a common trigger for age- and stress-induced impairments in long-term potentiation. *J Neurosci* 18:2974-2981.

Nait-Oumesmar B, Decker L, Lachapelle F, Avellana-Adalid V, Bachelin C, Baron-Van Evercooren A (1999) Progenitor cells of the adult mouse subventricular zone proliferate, migrate and differentiate into oligodendrocytes after demyelination. *The European journal of neuroscience* 11:4357-4366.

Nait-Oumesmar B, Picard-Riera N, Kerninon C, Decker L, Seilhean D, Hoglinger GU, Hirsch EC, Reynolds R, Baron-Van Evercooren A (2007) Activation of the subventricular zone in multiple sclerosis: evidence for early glial progenitors. *Proc Natl Acad Sci U S A* 104:4694-4699.

Nave KA (2010) Myelination and support of axonal integrity by glia. *Nature* 468:244-252.

Nery S, Wichterle H, Fishell G (2001) Sonic hedgehog contributes to oligodendrocyte specification in the mammalian forebrain. *Development* 128:527-540.

Niehaus A, Shi J, Grzenkowski M, Diers-Fenger M, Archelos J, Hartung HP, Toyka K, Bruck W, Trotter J (2000) Patients with active relapsing-remitting multiple sclerosis synthesize antibodies recognizing oligodendrocyte progenitor cell surface protein: implications for remyelination. *Annals of neurology* 48:362-371.

Nishida H, Okabe S (2007) Direct astrocytic contacts regulate local maturation of dendritic spines. *J Neurosci* 27:331-340.

Nishiyama A (2001) NG2 cells in the brain: a novel glial cell population. *Human cell* 14:77-82.

Nishiyama A, Chang A, Trapp BD (1999) NG2+ glial cells: a novel glial cell population in the adult brain. *Journal of neuropathology and experimental neurology* 58:1113-1124.

Nishiyama A, Komitova M, Suzuki R, Zhu X (2009) Polydendrocytes (NG2 cells): multifunctional cells with lineage plasticity. *Nature reviews Neuroscience* 10:9-22.

Nishiyama A, Lin XH, Giese N, Heldin CH, Stallcup WB (1996) Co-localization of NG2 proteoglycan and PDGF alpha-receptor on O2A progenitor cells in the developing rat brain. *Journal of neuroscience research* 43:299-314.

Noctor SC, Martinez-Cerdeno V, Ivic L, Kriegstein AR (2004) Cortical neurons arise in symmetric and asymmetric division zones and migrate through specific phases. *Nat Neurosci* 7:136-144.

Novitch BG, Chen AI, Jessell TM (2001) Coordinate regulation of motor neuron subtype identity and pan-neuronal properties by the bHLH repressor Olig2. *Neuron* 31:773-789.

Olabarria M, Noristani HN, Verkhratsky A, Rodriguez JJ (2010) Concomitant astroglial atrophy and astrogliosis in a triple transgenic animal model of Alzheimer's disease. *Glia* 58:831-838.

Petratos S, Gonzales MF, Azari MF, Marriott M, Minichiello RA, Shipham KA, Profyris C, Nicolaou A, Boyle K, Cheema SS, Kilpatrick TJ (2004) Expression of the low-affinity neurotrophin receptor, p75(NTR), is upregulated by oligodendroglial progenitors adjacent to the subventricular zone in response to demyelination. *Glia* 48:64-75.

Picard-Riera N, Decker L, Delarasse C, Goude K, Nait-Oumesmar B, Liblau R, Pham-Dinh D, Evercooren AB (2002) Experimental autoimmune encephalomyelitis mobilizes neural progenitors from the subventricular zone to undergo oligodendrogenesis in adult mice. *Proc Natl Acad Sci U S A* 99:13211-13216.

Pontious A, Kowalczyk T, Englund C, Hevner RF (2008) Role of intermediate progenitor cells in cerebral cortex development. *Dev Neurosci* 30:24-32.

Pringle NP, Richardson WD (1993) A singularity of PDGF alpha-receptor expression in the dorsoventral axis of the neural tube may define the origin of the oligodendrocyte lineage. *Development* 117:525-533.

Psachoulia K, Jamen F, Young KM, Richardson WD (2009) Cell cycle dynamics of NG2 cells in the postnatal and ageing brain. *Neuron Glia Biol* 5:57-67.

Rajkowska G, Miguel-Hidalgo JJ (2007) Gliogenesis and glial pathology in depression. *CNS and neurological disorders drug targets* 6:219-233.

Regan MR, Huang YH, Kim YS, Dykes-Hoberg MI, Jin L, Watkins AM, Bergles DE, Rothstein JD (2007) Variations in promoter activity reveal a differential expression and physiology of glutamate transporters by glia in the developing and mature CNS. *J Neurosci* 27:6607-6619.

Reynolds R, Cenci di Bello I, Dawson M, Levine J (2001) The response of adult oligodendrocyte progenitors to demyelination in EAE. *Progress in brain research* 132:165-174.

Rhodes KE, Raivich G, Fawcett JW (2006) The injury response of oligodendrocyte precursor cells is induced by platelets, macrophages and inflammation-associated cytokines. *Neuroscience* 140:87-100.

Rio-Hortega P (1928) Tercera aportación al conocimiento morfologica e interpretacion funcional de la oligodendroglia. *Mem Real Soc Esp Hist Nat Madrid* 14:122.

Rooms L, Kooy RF (2011) Advances in understanding fragile X syndrome and related disorders. *Curr Opin Pediatr* 23:601-606.

Ross SE, Greenberg ME, Stiles CD (2003) Basic Helix-Loop-Helix Factors in Cortical Development. *Neuron* 39:13-25.

Rowitch DH, Kriegstein AR (2010) Developmental genetics of vertebrate glial-cell specification. *Nature* 468:214-222.

Roy K, Murtie JC, El-Khodor BF, Edgar N, Sardi SP, Hooks BM, Benoit-Marand M, Chen C, Moore H, O'Donnell P, Brunner D, Corfas G (2007) Loss of erbB signaling in oligodendrocytes alters myelin and dopaminergic function, a potential mechanism for neuropsychiatric disorders. *Proc Natl Acad Sci U S A* 104:8131-8136.

Rubenstein JL (2011) Annual Research Review: Development of the cerebral cortex: implications for neurodevelopmental disorders. *J Child Psychol Psychiatry* 52:339-355.

Sanai N, Tramontin AD, Quinones-Hinojosa A, Barbaro NM, Gupta N, Kunwar S, Lawton MT, McDermott MW, Parsa AT, Manuel-Garcia Verdugo J, Berger MS, Alvarez-Buylla A (2004) Unique astrocyte ribbon in adult human brain contains neural stem cells but lacks chain migration. *Nature* 427:740-744.

Schmechel DE, Rakic P (1979) A Golgi study of radial glial cells in developing monkey telencephalon: morphogenesis and transformation into astrocytes. *Anat Embryol* (Berl) 156:115-152.

Solly SK, Thomas JL, Monge M, Demerens C, Lubetzki C, Gardinier MV, Matthieu JM, Zalc B (1996) Myelin/oligodendrocyte glycoprotein (MOG) expression is associated with myelin deposition. *Glia* 18:39-48.

Sommer I, Schachner M (1981) Monoclonal antibodies (O1 to O4) to oligodendrocyte cell surfaces: an immunocytological study in the central nervous system. *Developmental biology* 83:311-327.

Spassky N, Goujet-Zalc C, Parmantier E, Olivier C, Martinez S, Ivanova A, Ikenaka K, Macklin W, Cerruti I, Zalc B, Thomas JL (1998) Multiple restricted origin of oligodendrocytes. *J Neurosci* 18:8331-8343.

Spassky N, Heydon K, Mangatal A, Jankovski A, Olivier C, Queraud-Lesaux F, Goujet-Zalc C, Thomas JL, Zalc B (2001) Sonic hedgehog-dependent emergence of oligodendrocytes in the telencephalon: evidence for a source of oligodendrocytes in the olfactory bulb that is independent of PDGFRalpha signaling. *Development* 128:4993-5004.

Sternberger NH, Itoyama Y, Kies MW, Webster HD (1978) Myelin basic protein demonstrated immunocytochemically in oligodendroglia prior to myelin sheath formation. *Proc Natl Acad Sci U S A* 75:2521-2524.

Suzuki SO, Goldman JE (2003) Multiple cell populations in the early postnatal subventricular zone take distinct migratory pathways: a dynamic study of glial and neuronal progenitor migration. *J Neurosci* 23:4240-4250.

Tatsumi K, Takebayashi H, Manabe T, Tanaka KF, Makinodan M, Yamauchi T, Makinodan E, Matsuyoshi H, Okuda H, Ikenaka K, Wanaka A (2008) Genetic fate mapping of Olig2 progenitors in the injured adult cerebral cortex reveals preferential differentiation into astrocytes. *Journal of neuroscience research* 86:3494-3502.

Tekki-Kessaris N, Woodruff R, Hall AC, Gaffield W, Kimura S, Stiles CD, Rowitch DH, Richardson WD (2001) Hedgehog-dependent oligodendrocyte lineage specification in the telencephalon. *Development* 128:2545-2554.

Tiwari-Woodruff SK, Myers LW, Bronstein JM (2004) Cerebrospinal fluid immunoglobulin G promotes oligodendrocyte progenitor cell migration. *Journal of neuroscience research* 77:363-366.

Trotter J (2005) NG2-positive cells in CNS function and the pathological role of antibodies against NG2 in demyelinating diseases. *Journal of the neurological sciences* 233:37-42.

Trotter J, Karram K, Nishiyama A (2010) NG2 cells: Properties, progeny and origin. *Brain research reviews* 63:72-82.

Uranova NA, Vostrikov VM, Vikhreva OV, Zimina IS, Kolomeets NS, Orlovskaya DD (2007) The role of oligodendrocyte pathology in schizophrenia. The international journal of neuropsychopharmacology / *official scientific journal of the Collegium Internationale Neuropsychopharmacologicum* 10:537-545.

Voigt T (1989) Development of glial cells in the cerebral wall of ferrets: direct tracing of their transformation from radial glia into astrocytes. *J Comp Neurol* 289:74-88.

Voineskos AN, Felsky D, Kovacevic N, Tiwari AK, Zai C, Chakravarty MM, Lobaugh NJ, Shenton ME, Rajji TK, Miranda D, Pollock BG, Mulsant BH, McIntosh AR, Kennedy JL (2012) Oligodendrocyte Genes, White Matter Tract Integrity, and Cognition in Schizophrenia. *Cereb Cortex.*

Wang DD, Bordey A (2008) The astrocyte odyssey. *Prog Neurobiol* 86:342-367.

Wonders CP, Anderson SA (2006) The origin and specification of cortical interneurons. *Nature reviews Neuroscience* 7:687-696.

Yang Y, Ge W, Chen Y, Zhang Z, Shen W, Wu C, Poo M, Duan S (2003) Contribution of astrocytes to hippocampal long-term potentiation through release of D-serine. *Proc Natl Acad Sci U S A* 100:15194-15199.

Zhou Q, Wang S, Anderson DJ (2000) Identification of a novel family of oligodendrocyte lineage-specific basic helix-loop-helix transcription factors. *Neuron* 25:331-343.

Zhu X, Bergles DE, Nishiyama A (2008a) NG2 cells generate both oligodendrocytes and gray matter astrocytes. *Development* 135:145-157.

Zhu X, Hill RA, Nishiyama A (2008b) NG2 cells generate oligodendrocytes and gray matter astrocytes in the spinal cord. *Neuron Glia Biol* 4:19-26.

Zhu X, Zuo H, Maher BJ, Serwanski DR, LoTurco JJ, Lu QR, Nishiyama A (2012) Olig2-dependent developmental fate switch of NG2 cells. *Development* 139:2299-2307.

Zonta M, Angulo MC, Gobbo S, Rosengarten B, Hossmann KA, Pozzan T, Carmignoto G (2003) Neuron-to-astrocyte signaling is central to the dynamic control of brain microcirculation. *Nat Neurosci* 6:43-50.

In: Glial Cells
Editors: Charanjit Kaur and Eng-Ang Ling

ISBN: 978-1-62618-448-0
© 2013 Nova Science Publishers, Inc.

Chapter 2

ROLE OF GLIAL CELLS IN PERIVENTRICULAR WHITE MATTER DAMAGE IN HYPOXIC NEONATAL BRAINS

Gurugirijha Rathnasamy, Madhuvika Murugan, Eng-Ang Ling and Charanjit Kaur *

Department of Anatomy, Yong Loo Lin School of Medicine,
National University of Singapore, Singapore

ABSTRACT

Periventricular white matter (PWM) damage (PWMD) is a common form of brain injury found in survivors of preterm birth and, is the major determinant of neurological morbidity in premature infants. Among various factors predisposing to PWMD hypoxia-ischemia remains as the major contributing factor. Hallmark events of PWMD include death of oligodendrocytes, degeneration of axons, hypomyelination, microglial activation and astrogliosis. Activation of microglia and astrocytes in the developing PWM, in response to hypoxic insults, results in excess production of glutamate, free radicals, cytokines along with vascular changes such as increased permeability which are implicated in the pathogenesis of PWMD. In addition, deficiency of antioxidant enzymes in oligodendrocyte progenitor cells renders them highly susceptible to hypoxic damage. The death of oligodendrocytes in hypoxic PWM may result in myelination disturbances.

Though the multi-factorial pathogenesis of PWMD is not fully understood, the cross talk between the glial cells reviewed in this chapter could shed some light on the mechanisms mediating oligodendrocyte death in hypoxic PWM.

* Corresponding author - Professor Charanjit Kaur; Email: antkaurc@nus.edu.sg. Fax: 65-67787643; Phone: 65-65163209.

1. Introduction

Periventricular white matter (PWM) damage (PWMD), also known as the periventricular leukomalacia (PVL) remains as the predominant cause of morbidity in premature infants (Back 2006; Back and Rivkees 2004; Ferriero 2004; Volpe 2000). Advancements in medical sciences have led to the increased survival of premature infants, yet they suffer long-term neurological impairments (Wilson-Costello et al. 2005; World Health Organization; March of Dimes; The Partnership for Maternal NCHStC 2012). PWMD is particularly evident in premature infants born between 23 and 37 weeks of gestation and with low birth weight <1500g (Folkerth 2006; Follett et al. 2004; Johnston 1997; McQuillen and Ferriero 2004; Rezaie and Dean 2002; Volpe 2003).

Various factors such as infection, inflammation, vascular changes, hypoxia, bradycardia, pre-eclampsia, and genetic factors have been suggested to predispose the immature brains to PWMD. Among the above mentioned factors reduced supply of oxygen to the brain, or hypoxia remains as a major contributing factor to PWMD in premature neonates (Alvarez-Diaz et al. 2007; Baud et al. 2004a; Huang and Castillo 2008). PWMD is either focal characterized by localized cellular loss and subsequent cyst formation, or diffuse characterized by reactive microglia and astrocytes and associated injury to the glial cells (Volpe 2003), particularly the oligodendrocyte progenitors (Deng et al. 2008). The extreme vulnerability of PWM to hypoxic insult is due to the lack of blood vessel anastomoses and extensive occurrence of oligodendrocyte progenitors (Folkerth 2006). Damage to the oligodendrocyte progenitors results in delayed or disrupted myelination (Huang et al. 2009; Tzarouchi et al. 2009) leading to neurodevelopmental deficits such as cerebral palsy, impaired vision, hearing impairments, cognitive deficits and mental retardation (Back and Rivkees 2004; Inder et al. 2003; Iwata et al. 2004; Nosarti et al. 2004; Vannucci and Vannucci 2005). Besides the above, the pathological events in hypoxic PWMD include axonal swelling (Volpe 2009), astrogliosis and activation of microglia.

The pathogenesis of PWMD is multifaceted and not completely understood. Lack of antioxidant enzymes in the oligodendrocytes render them highly susceptible to hypoxia mediated injury. Additionally, factors such as reduced cerebral blood flow autoregulation (Berger et al. 2002), enhanced expression of factors such as nitric oxide synthases and vascular endothelial growth factor (Kaur et al. 2006a), glutamate toxicity (Volpe 2001), impaired intracellular calcium turnover, release of inflammatory cytokines, iron accumulation (Adcock et al. 1996; Palmer et al. 1999) and overproduction of free-radicals (Amato and Donati 2000) have been proposed to mediate white matter damage. Both experimental and clinical studies have traced the origin of these factors to activated microglia and astrocytes in the developing white matter (Haynes et al. 2003; Kaur et al. 2006a; Murugan et al. 2011; Rathnasamy et al. 2011; Sivakumar et al. 2010; Volpe 2003). Activated glia and their response to hypoxia are thought to play an important role in damaging axons and oligodendrocytes in hypoxic PWM. Though studies in the past two decades have unravelled mechanisms by which activated microglia and astrocytes mediate damage of oligodendrocytes and axons, there are various molecular mechanisms yet to be investigated. While a clear understanding of the pathogenesis of PWMD is still lacking, the present available information on glial-mediated injury to PWM in response to hypoxic insults, as reviewed in this chapter, would be of help to those who seek to identify therapeutic possibilities for PWMD.

2. Composition of Periventricular White Matter

The PWM region peripheral to the lateral ventricles is composed of axons, blood vessels and the glial cells (microglia, astrocytes and oligodendrocytes). Though in developing brain the axons are generally unmyelinated, through the course of development the axons are wrapped by myelin sheaths that are extensions of oligodendroglial processes. The myelin sheath enables saltatory conduction and results in faster transmission of neural signals.

Oligodendrocytes are the myelin forming cells in the central nervous system (CNS), originating from the neuroepithelial cells of the ventricular zone during early embryonic life (Thomas et al. 2000). Oligodendrocytes express phenotypically different markers during development. On the basis of this, they are classified into early oligodendrocyte progenitors (A2B5+), late oligodendrocyte progenitors (PDGFα+, O4+, NG2+), immature oligodendrocytes (CC1+, O1+) and mature oligodendrocytes (MBP+). During the high risk periods of PWMD, the premyelinating or the immature oligodendrocytes dominate the white matter region (Back et al. 2002). Since these oligodendrocytes lack certain antioxidant enzymes when compared to mature oligodendrocytes, they are highly vulnerable to hypoxic damage.

Astrocytes are star shaped glial cells essential for maintanence of extracellular ion balance, blood brain barrier (BBB) integrity and glutamate homeostasis (Abbott 2002; Anderson and Swanson 2000; Simard and Nedergaard 2004). Like oligodendrocytes, astrocytes also originate from the ventricular zone. Additionally radial glial cells originating from subventricular zones also act as source for astrocytes (Liu et al. 2006). Among the two different types of astrocytes (protoplasmic and fibrous) it is the fibrous type that is visualized in PWM (Miller and Raff 1984). Upon injury the astrocytes become reactive and exhibit characteristic features such as cellular hyperplasia, hypertrophy, increased expression of glial fibrillary acidic protein (GFAP) (Zhu et al. 2004), swelling of end-feet enveloping capillaries forming the BBB and increased proliferation (Sullivan et al. 2010). Prolonged astrocytosis could also lead to release of cytokines that are toxic to oligodendrocytes.

Microglia are the resident immune cells of the brain and are present in abundance in the developing PWM (Ling and Wong 1993). The origin of microglia has been debated extensively, the most widely accepted theory being the hematopoietic origin of microglia (Kaur et al. 2001; Ling et al. 1991). Microglial precursors invade the developing brain from the blood stream (Imamoto and Leblond 1978; Ling et al. 1980) and increase in numbers with maturation of the brain. In the developing brain, microglia exhibit amoeboid phenotype and they are abundant in the developing white matter. Amoeboid microglial cells (AMCs) have been implicated in rebuilding the histo-architecture of white matter during development by involving in phagocytosis of cellular debris/apoptotic cells, synaptic pruning and myelination. In the course of development, AMCs transform into ramified microglia cells (RMCs), the resting form of microglial cells. Microglia being highly sensitive to changes in micro-environment of the brain, become activated under pathological conditions and may cause damage to oligodendrocytes.

The PWM is scarcely vascularised (Ballabh et al. 2005; Miyawaki et al. 1998) and the basal blood flow to the PWM is approximately 20 % less than that supplied to the grey matter in the developing brain (Borch and Greisen 1998). PWM is suggested to be supplied by the short and long penetrating arteries, which lack anastomoses (Nakamura et al. 1994; Takashima and Tanaka 1978) and form a vascular end zone (Nakamura et al. 1994; Takashima and Tanaka 1978) which increases the susceptibility of PWM to hypoxic damage. Besides the above, the blood vessel density in the PWM was found to be transiently low between 28-36 weeks of gestation but increased at later gestational ages. Under ischemic conditions the blood flow to PWM was reduced by ~ 50% in comparison to grey matter (Back et al. 2006). The reduced cerebral blood flow to the PWM along with other factors further contributes to PWMD (Back 2006; Nakamura et al. 1994).

3. Pathology of Periventricular White Matter Damage

The pathological consequences in the developing PWM in response to hypoxic-ischemic insults range from necrosis to myelination deficits. Oligodendroglial damage, axonal swelling, microglial activation and astrocytosis are the pathological hallmarks of PWMD (Ness et al. 2001; Obonai and Takashima 1998; Skoff et al. 2001). A common finding in hypoxic PWM is the presence of apoptotic and necrotic cells (Deng et al. 2008; Kaur and You 2000). With the help of specific markers, these apoptotic and necrotic cells were identified to be oligodendrocytes (Deng et al. 2008). In addition, glioblasts known to be oligodendrocyte precursors displayed ballooning of nuclear envelope associated with splitting of inner and outer nuclear membrane (Kaur and Ling 2009). Oligodendrocytes are known to be actively involved in myelination of axons in the developing brain, the process of myelination in humans beginning during the midgestation period. Oligodendrocyte precursors are known to dominate the PWM during 23-32 weeks of gestation in the human brain (Pang et al. 2000). Hence, a hypoxic-ischemic injury during this gestational period, which causes apoptosis of oligodendrocytes results in delayed/disrupted myelin formation; leading to severe neurobehavioral anomalies that last through childhood and adulthood (Volpe 2003). In accordance with this, decreased myelin basic protein expression has been demonstrated in hypoxic-ischemic PWM in animal models (Biran et al. 2006; Kaur et al. 2006a; Liu et al. 2002). The cystic cavities found during the later stages of PWM injury are usually accompanied by impaired or delayed myelination (Cai et al. 2001; Jelinski et al. 1999; Kurumatani et al. 1998).

Along with the apoptotic oligodendrocytes, the axons involved in the transmission of neural information across and within the cerebral hemispheres were found to be swollen and degenerating (Kaur et al. 2006a). In neonatal brains, the number of degenerating axons was reported to be enhanced following hypoxia (Kaur et al. 2006a). The damaged axons were found to be deficient in axoplasm and, if myelinated, had distorted myelin sheath (Kaur et al. 2006a). Recent studies reported that the axon-glial synapses in the white matter of developing rats, were profoundly damaged following hypoxic-ischemic insults (Shen et al. 2012).

The presence of activated microglia has been detected in the PWM of children with signs of periventricular leukomalacia (Deguchi et al. 1996; Haynes et al. 2003; Kadhim et al. 2001) and in asphyxiated animal foetuses (Mallard et al. 2003). In view of the preponderance of microglial cells in the developing PWM (Billiards et al. 2006), activation of microglia is implicated in the pathogenesis of PWMD. Activation of microglia induces the production of a repertoire of cytotoxic factors which are implicated in oligodendrocyte progenitor death. In hypoxic PWM, activated microglia were found to actively phagocytose the apoptotic and necrotic cells and the degenerating axons (Kaur and Ling 2009).

Cerebral white matter astrocytosis is another characteristic feature of PWMD (Hirayama et al. 2001). Though astrocytosis could favour the repair of PWM, excess astrocytosis results in damage to the axons and oligodendrocytes (Zawadzka and Kaminska 2003), either by producing pro-inflammatory cytokines (Deng et al. 2010) or by inhibiting axonal re-growth (Di Giovanni et al. 2005). The astrocytes along with the extracellular matrix form the glial scar at the site of lesion (Di Giovanni et al. 2005). Vascular endothelial growth factor (VEGF), an angiogenic growth factor, known to induce vasculogenesis is also described as vascular permeability enhancing factor (Croll et al. 2004). Ment et al. (1997) demonstrated the up-regulated expression of VEGF in astrocytes in white matter at the vicinity of foci of necrosis. Following hypoxic insult, the up-regulation of VEGF expression in astrocytes in PWM was suggested to have a critical role in edema formation by enhancing vascular leakage (Kaur et al. 2006a).

The pathogenesis of PWMD is further contributed by factors such as, circulatory disturbances, edema, hemorrhage and consequent coagulation necrosis (Nakamura et al. 1994). PWMD is often accompanied by germinal matrix hemorrhage (Folkerth 2005) and intraventricular hemorrhage (Okoshi et al. 2001). In response to hypoxic insults, vacuoles were observed in ependymal cells lining the lateral ventricles along with widening of intercellular spaces (Kaur and Ling 2009). These structural changes were speculated to favour extravsation of cerebro-spinal fluid into the PWM, thereby enhancing edema formation (Kaur and Ling 2009). Studies have also reported the widening of perivascular spaces and consequent edema formation in PWM (Kadhim et al. 2003; Kaur et al. 2006a; Sridhar et al. 2001).. The vulnerability of PWM to hypoxic injury is attributed to the hypovascularisation of this region (Folkerth 2006).

4. MICROGLIA

Microglia, the resident immune cells present ubiquitously in the brain, were first described by del Rio-Hortega. Microglia with amoeboid shape, called the AMCs dominate the perinatal PWM (Ling and Wong 1993). Although the functions of AMCs in the developing brain are deemed beneficial, their activation leads to bystander injury to other CNS cells. Activated microglia are known to release toxic factors such as glutamate, nitric oxide, cytokines and free radicals which have been shown to be toxic to the oligodendrocytes (Mitrovic et al. 1994; Zajicek et al. 1992). Experimental studies carried out in our laboratory, in the past decade, have furthered our understanding on the role of microglia in mediating oligodendrocyte damage in PWMD. Evidences supporting microglial contribution to the development of lesions in the PWM are discussed here.

4.1. Microglia, Glutamate and Periventricular White Matter Damage

Excessive accumulation of glutamate in response to hypoxic-ischemic insults has been reported by both experimental and clinical studies on PVL. Following hypoxic-ischemic insults, in immature rat brains, the glutamate content was found to be elevated when measured by means of microdialysis (Benveniste et al. 1984; Silverstein et al. 1991). Further support to this was the clinical demonstration of elevated glutamate levels in perinatal infants who suffered hypoxic-ischemia (Hagberg 1992). Consistent with this, a recent study in our laboratory demonstrated a drastic increase in glutamate content in the hypoxic PWM (Sivakumar et al. 2010) which was suggested to mediate the pathogenesis of PWMD (Fern and Moller 2000). Increase in glutamate concentrations was thought to be from multiple sources including release of glutamate from damaged axons (Kukley et al. 2007) and dysregulation of glutamate transporters (Fern and Moller 2000). In addition, activated hypoxic microglia are implicated in enhanced release of glutamate (Sivakumar et al. 2010). Excess glutamate in turn activates the metabotropic and ionotropic glutamate receptors [alpha-amino-3- hydroxy-5-methyl-4-isoxazole propionic acid receptors (AMPAR), kinate receptors and N-methyl-D-aspartate receptors (NMDAR)] expressed on the glial cells. Alleviation of white matter injury in response to treatment with glutamate receptor antagonist (Follett et al. 2000, 2004) suggested that, activation of glutamate receptors mediated oligodendrocyte death (Deng et al. 2003; McDonald et al. 1998; Yoshioka et al. 1995).

Noda et al. (2000) first demonstrated the existence of AMPAR and kainate receptors in primary rat microglia. This study reported the protein and mRNA expression of AMPA receptors (GluR1 to GluR4) and kainate receptors (GluR5 and GluR7) in microglial cells. Studies on rodents with transient forebrain ischemia demonstrated the expression of NR1 subunit of NMDAR (Gottlieb and Matute 1997; Matute et al. 1997). Consistent with this we demonstrated the expression of AMPAR (GluR1-4) and NMDAR subunits (NR1, NR2A-D) in microglia of hypoxic PWM (Kaur et al. 2006b; Murugan et al. 2011; Sivakumar et al. 2010). Activation of these glutamate receptors was demonstrated to induce Ca^{2+} influx into the microglial cells (Murugan et al. 2011; Noda et al. 2000). Though the molecular mechanism through which they mediate PWMD is yet to be elucidated completely, the increased intracellular Ca^{2+} was reported to be a prerequisite for nitric oxide (NO) and cytokine release by microglia (Farber and Kettenmann 2006).

Recently, glutamate receptor-induced NO production in hypoxic microglia was demonstrated. As mentioned above, the activation of NMDAR resulted in increased intracellular Ca^{2+} influx in microglia. Furthermore, the activation of functional NMDAR induced enhanced production of inducible nitric oxide synthase (iNOS) in hypoxic microglia. The simultaneous expression of iNOS and NR1 in the microglia of hypoxic PWM in neonatal rats lends support to the NMDAR mediated iNOS expression (Kaur et al. 2006a; You and Kaur 2000). It was suggested that the up-regulation of iNOS by NMDAR was mediated via the nuclear factor-κB (NF-κB) signalling pathway (Murugan et al. 2011) as there was a significant decrease in iNOS expression by hypoxia exposed microglial cells treated with BAY, an inhibitor of NF-κB. iNOS produced by activated microglia is known to induce tissue injury through production of NO. Death of oligodendrocytes was more pronounced in oligdendroglial cultures treated with conditioned medium from hypoxic microglia. However, on treatment with NMDAR antagonist MK801, BAY and iNOS inhibitor 1400W, the observed apoptosis of oligodendrocyte was reduced. These results collectively imply an active role of functional NMDAR in causing oligodendrocyte death through iNOS mediated NO production via activation of NF-κB (Murugan et al. 2011). In the light of above findings, it was suggested that activation of microglial NMDAR by extracellular glutamate results in exacerbation of PWMD (Murugan et al. 2011).

Activation of AMPA and NMDA receptors on microglial cells is further implicated in the production of pro-inflammatory cytokines (Murugan et al. 2011; Noda et al. 2000). Supporting this is the demonstration of increased secretion of pro-inflammatory cytokines by hypoxic microglia on treatment with glutamate (Sivakumar et al. 2010). When compared to hypoxic microglia, there was a significant increase in tumor necrosis factor (TNF)-α and interleukin (IL)-1β levels secreted by microglial cells treated with glutamate (Sivakumar et al. 2010). Also, there was a significant decrease in TNF-α and IL-1β production in hypoxic microglia treated with MK801 (Murugan et al. 2011). In addition an increased release of glutamate by hypoxic microglia into the culture medium suggested that they could contribute to enhanced extracellular glutamate levels detected in hypoxic PWMD (Sivakumar et al. 2010). Taken together, it may be speculated that the enhanced glutamate release by hypoxic microglia could initiate a vicious cycle by augmenting the production of TNF-α and IL-1β through activation of microglial glutamate receptors.

Besides the above, glutamate could exacerbate the PWMD by suppressing the release of insulin like growth factor (IGF-I and IGF-II) from hypoxic microglia. IGF-I and IGF-II, known to play a significant role in tissue repair following hypoxic-ischemic insults (Guan et al. 2003), were shown to be produced by activated microglia in response to hypoxia (Sivakumar et al. 2010). Interestingly, addition of glutamate to the hypoxic microglial cells *in vitro* resulted in reduced production of IGF-I and IGF-II (Sivakumar et al. 2010). The masking effect exhibited by extracellular glutamate on the production of growth factors may favour excess glutamate mediated pro-inflammatory cytokine production by microglia. This was evident from the results of our studies which demonstrated the increased secretion of glutamate, TNF-α, and IL-1β on silencing IGF-I in hypoxic microglia (Sivakumar et al. 2010). Considering the fact that IGF-I protects developing oligodendrocytes from glutamate mediated injury (Ness et al. 2004; Ness and Wood 2002), the reduction in growth factor secretion by microglia in the presence of extracellular glutamate would conceivably result in damage to the oligodendrocytes.

4.2. Microglia, Inflammation and Periventricular White Matter Damage

A series of experimental and clinical studies suggest that inflammation plays a major role in PWMD (Deng et al. 2008; Kadhim et al. 2002). Hypoxic insults have been reported to trigger the production of inflammatory chemokines and cytokines (Carloni et al. 2006; Guo and Bhat 2006). In the inflamed brain, microglia serve as the predominant source of cytokines (Hanisch et al. 2001; Kaur et al. 2007), with astrocytes being the secondary source. Consistent with this we have shown the enhanced expression of TNF-α and IL-1β in microglia of hypoxic PWM (Deng et al. 2008). Activation of mitogen activated protein kinases and/or translocation of NF-κB into the nucleus mediated the production of TNF-α and IL-1β in hypoxic microglia (Deng et al. 2008; Murugan et al. 2011). Cytokine production in microglia was either favoured by hypoxia induced NMDAR activation or iron accumulation in microglia (Murugan et al. 2011; Rathnasamy et al. 2011). In addition, the expression of ion channels such as Kv1.1 and Kv1.2 and heparan sulphate glycosaminoglycan-containing cell surface proteins such as syndecan-2 on hypoxic microglia promotes release of inflammatory cytokines and chemokines (Kaur et al. 2009; Li et al. 2008; Wu et al. 2009). TNF-α exerts its action by binding to its receptors TNFR1 and TNFR2. While TNFR1 activation elicits caspase mediated apoptosis (Nakazawa et al. 2006), binding of TNF-α to TNFR2 has been suggested to promote cell growth and proliferation (Fontaine et al. 2002). In hypoxic PWM, oligodendrocytes were reported to express TNFR1 (Deng et al. 2008). Moreover, incubation of oligodendrocytes with conditioned medium from hypoxic microglia resulted in a significant increase in cleaved caspase-3 labelling, which was inhibited on neutralizing the medium with anti-TNF-α antibody (Rathnasamy et al. 2011). These results confirmed that TNF-α could induce oligodendrocyte death in hypoxic PWM through caspase mediated pathway. Along with oligodendrocytes, the axons of hypoxic PWM also expressed TNFR1 and this was coupled with reduced myelin basic protein expression (Deng et al. 2010) suggesting hypomyelination. IL-1β acts through binding to type I and type II IL-1R. In hypoxic PWM, IL-1R1 expression was found to be significantly increased on the oligodendrocytes (Deng et al. 2008). Though IL-1β was reported to be non-toxic to oligodendrocytes it reduced the proliferation rate of late oligodendrocyte progenitors (Vela et al. 2002). It is speculated that the high levels of IL-1β in the hypoxic PWM may impede the recovery by inhibiting the proliferation of oligodendrocyte progenitors.

Besides the above, hypoxic microglia may exacerbate PWMD by influencing cytokine production by astrocytes. This was shown to be mediated by the increased expression of macrophage colony stimulating factor (M-CSF/CSF-1) in microglia of hypoxic PWM (Deng et al. 2010). M-CSF is deemed to be an important mediator of inflammation (Hao et al. 2002) and it exerts its actions by binding to its receptor CSF-1R (Murphy et al. 2000). The simultaneous increase in M-CSF expression in microglia and CSF-1R expression in astrocytes in hypoxic PWM suggests that the cytokine and its receptor could orchestrate astrocyte reaction. Very interestingly, incubating astrocyte cultures with conditioned medium from hypoxic microglia showed that cytokine production in astrocytes was augmented (Deng et al. 2010). The results implied a cross talk between microglia and astrocytes in hypoxic PWM and that their interaction via M-CSF could aggravate the PWMD by enhancing inflammatory response (Deng et al. 2010).

Chemokines are another set of immunoregulatory molecules secreted by microglia during inflammation. They are small peptides (8-14 kDa) capable of mediating infiltration of leukocytes to the vicinity of inflammation. Chemokines are divided into four major families (CXC, CC, C and CX_3C) based on their cysteine motif (Pan et al. 1997; Vaddi et al. 1997). Microglial cells express chemokines such as monocyte chemoattractant protein 1 (MCP1), macrophage inflammatory protein-1α (MIP-1α), MIP-1β, MIP-2, CCL6 and RANTES (Cowell and Silverstein 2003; Deng et al. 2009; Kanno et al. 2005; Sunnemark et al. 2003). MCP-1 promotes migration of activated microglial cells and leukocytes to the inflammatory sites in the CNS (Lu et al. 1998; Yan et al. 2007) by binding to its receptor CCR2. It was reported that microglia in hypoxic PWM served as the primary source of MCP-1 in the neonatal brain (Deng et al. 2009). Coupled with this was an increase in their number which was attributed to the migration of microglia from the neighbouring areas or via invasion of the monocytes into the hypoxic brain (Deng et al. 2009). Migration of microglia to foci of lesion is also facilitated by the expression of CXCR4, a receptor for stromal cell-derived factor-1α which is produced during brain injuries including hypoxia (Wang et al. 2008).

These chemokines can also regulate migration of monocytes and lymphocytes to the site of damage (Ambrosini and Aloisi 2004; Cross and Woodroofe 1999).

4.3. Microglia, Iron and Periventricular White Matter Damage

The requirement for iron in developing brain is high as iron dependant enzymes form an integral part of energy metabolism, neurotransmitter synthesis and myelin formation (Beard and Connor 2003; Connor and Menzies 1996), yet excess iron could lead to tissue injury by promoting oxidative damage via reactive oxygen species (ROS). Hypoxic-ischemic injury has been demonstrated to favour iron accumulation in the brain of neonatal rodents (Adcock et al. 1996). Similar to other tissues, in response to hypoxic insult, the PWM is also known to drastically accumulate iron (Rathnasamy et al. 2011) which is implicated in the pathogenesis of PWMD. The increased iron in hypoxic PWM of neonatal rats, was localized in microglia (Rathnasamy et al. 2011) and was previously suggested as a measure taken by microglia to sequester the surplus iron in order to prevent oxidative damage (Kaur and Ling 1999).

Adding to this is the demonstration of increased expression of proteins involved in iron acquisition such as the iron regulatory proteins and transferrin receptor (Kaur and Ling 1999; Rathnasamy et al. 2011). Studies in hypoxic-ischemic animal models reported that increased accumulation of iron in microglia occurred when oligodendrocyte development was compromised (Connor and Menzies 1990). In accordance with this several studies suggested the presence of iron positive microglial cells in the vicinity of the lesion (Berg et al. 2001; Gorter et al. 2005; Mehlhase et al. 2005). Hypoxia induced iron accumulation in microglia resulted in increased secretion of pro-inflammatory cytokines TNF-α and IL-1β (Rathnasamy et al. 2011). This finding has put forward the role of iron in mediating cytokine production in hypoxic microglia. In addition, increased iron within microglia resulted in increased ROS production.

The cytotoxic factors released by iron positive hypoxic microglia resulted in apoptosis of oligodendrocytes through glutathione depletion, increased lipid peroxidation, increased caspase-3 labelling and reduced proliferation (Rathnasamy et al. 2011) thereby leading to PWMD.

4.4. Microglia, Nitric Oxide and Periventricular White Matter Damage

The pleiotropic role of NO from being a vascular dilator to a potent neurotoxin has been well documented. The specific function of NO depends on the cellular source of NO which executes various functions by interacting with guanylate cyclase, cytochrome P450, cyclooxygenase, and hemoglobin. The detrimental effect of NO is pronounced when NO combines with free radicals such as superoxides to produce highly reactive peroxynitrite, which is implicated in DNA strand breaks, lipid peroxidation and protein nitration. NO is released from L-arginine, on its enzymatic conversion to L- citrulline, which is catalysed by family of NO synthase (NOS) (Marletta 1993). NOS family comprises neuronal NOS (nNOS), endothelial NOS (eNOS) and iNOS. While nNOS and eNOS are calcium dependant (Vincent et al. 1998), iNOS is calcium independant and NO produced by iNOS is well known to modulate immune activities and cytotoxic functions (Brown and Bal-Price 2003). In the developing white matter of postnatal rats, expression of iNOS is hardly detected; on the other hand, when the rats were subjected to hypoxic exposure the expression of iNOS in hypoxic PWM was increased (Kaur et al. 2006a). As activated microglia expressing iNOS serve as a major source of NO under pathological conditions (Murphy et al. 1993), the iNOS positive microglia in the hypoxic PWM were considered to be the main cellular source of increased production of NO (Kaur et al. 2006a). This is supported by our recent demonstration of increased iNOS mediated NO production by hypoxic microglia (Murugan et al. 2011). Earlier *in vitro* studies have proposed a role for NO in mediating oligodendrocyte damage (Merrill et al. 1993). The high levels of NO released, could result in oligodendrocyte cell death by inhibiting mitochondrial respiration (Baud et al. 2004b). Besides the above, the synergistic activation of iNOS and phagocyte NADPH oxidase (PHOX) in activated microglia could result in generation of peroxynitrite, an extremely potent oxidising agent (Brown 2007) implicated in the pathogenesis of PWMD by being harmful to the immature oligodendrocytes (Haynes et al. 2005).

4.5. Microglia, Oxidative Stress and Periventricular White Matter Damage

A common sequel associated with hypoxia is the increased production of free radicals or ROS. The free radicals such as hydroxyl radical (OH), hydrogen peroxide (H_2O_2), singlet oxygen ($1O_2$), hypochlorus acid (HOCl), peroxynitrite anion (ONOO-) and peroxynitrous acid (ONOOH) are produced by the multisubunit PHOX composed of P22 phox, P47 phox, P67 phox and gp91 phox (Bedard and Krause 2007). The free radicals are unstable molecules capable of initiating oxidative damage by causing oxidation of lipids, DNA and proteins (Rahman 2003). Under physiological conditions the above mentioned free radicals are neutralized by endogenous anti-oxidant defence system. Oxidative stress occurs when this neutralisation is vanquished with excessive production of ROS leading to cellular damage via lipid peroxidation, protein modification, and DNA strand breaks. The immature brain is at a greater risk of free radical mediated damage owing to the imbalance in antioxidant and oxidant generating system (Buonocore et al. 2001; Welin et al. 2005). Following hypoxic-ischemic insults, antioxidant enzymes such as glutathione have been reported to be decreased in the brain of neonatal rats (Wallin et al. 2000). Associated with this, studies have demonstrated increased ROS production in the developing white matter (Welin et al. 2005) and microglia have been implicated in their generation (Colton et al. 1996). In accordance with this, enhanced ROS production in microglia of PWM was reported in neonatal rats subjected to hypoxia (Kaur et al. 2009; Rathnasamy et al. 2011). Expression of mRNAs and proteins of all subunits of PHOX has been demonstrated in microglia (Green et al. 2001; Infanger et al. 2006; Lavigne et al. 2001; Sankarapandi et al. 1998; Zekry et al. 2003). Activation of PHOX in microglia enables increased ROS production (Huo et al. 2011; Lavigne et al. 2001). Among the subunits of PHOX, gp91phox and p47phox are essential for ROS production in microglia as deficiency in one of these subunits attenuated superoxide production (Lavigne et al. 2001; Qin et al. 2004).

ROS produced by activated microglia is known to damage myelin sheath (van der Goes et al. 1998) and immature oligodendrocytes (Haynes et al. 2005) by enabling lipid peroxidation (Griot et al. 1990). In oligodendrocytes subjected to hypoxia there was increased lipid peroxidation associated with depletion in glutathione content (Rathnasamy et al. 2011).

The ability of edaravone, an antioxidant drug, to inhibit ROS production by microglia in hypoxic PWM suggests that there is a lack of antioxidant enzymes in the neonatal PWM (Kaur et al., 2009). The depletion in glutathione content and reduced antioxidant enzymes in the hypoxic PWM render the oligodendrocyte progenitors selectively vulnerable to hypoxia induced microglial-ROS mediated damage (Volpe, 2001).

5. Astrocytes

As explained earlier, activation of astrocytes is another characteristic feature of PWMD (Haynes et al. 2003) and is associated with hypertrophy of astrocytes. In injuries, such as hypoxia, astrocytes in the injured area undergo active proliferation termed reactive astrocytosis (Miller and Gauthier 2007; Ridet et al. 1997) and display increased activity of various lysosomic and oxidative enzymes (Chao et al. 1996; Schwab and Bartholdi 1996). The reactive astrocytes could isolate the injured area of the brain by forming a glial scar (Smith et al. 1986) thereby impeding the axonal regeneration. Though the mechanisms by which astrocytes could result in PWMD is yet unclear, they are considered to be involved in damage of immature oligodendrocytes through production of inflammatory cytokines, free radicals and by altering the glutamate levels (Back 2006; Rezaie and Dean 2002).

5.1. Astrocytes, Dysregulated Glutamate Homeostasis and Perventricular White Matter Damage

The astrocytes express Na+ dependent glutamate transporters, which are primarily responsible for the maintenance of glutamate homeostasis in the brain (Robinson and Dowd 1997). As mentioned earlier, enhanced glutamate levels following hypoxia-ischemia have been implicated in the pathogenesis of hypoxic PWMD. Glutamate uptake being an energy-dependent process, energy compromising events such as hypoxia, reverse the function of glutamate transporters, further augmenting astroglial glutamate release (Allen et al. 2004; Danbolt 2001; Malarkey and Parpura 2008; O'Shea 2002). Chronic perinatal hypoxia was shown to alter the uptake of glutamate by astrocytic glutamate transporters via the Janus kinase (JAK) / Signal transducer and activator of transcription (STAT) pathway, contributing to the increased levels of extracellular glutamate in hypoxic PWM (Raymond et al. 2011). Activation of the JAK/ STAT pathway in astrocytes is important for cellular differentiation and is thought to regulate the transformation of immature nestin-expressing astrocytes to mature GFAP-expressing astrocytes (Gautron et al. 2006; Sriram et al. 2004). In addition, JAK/STAT signaling is also involved in the process of astrogliosis and scar formation in different CNS pathologies (Herrmann et al. 2008; Justicia et al. 2000). In line with the above findings, another study demonstrated a role for JAK/STAT signaling in altering the uptake of glutamate by astrocytes, indicating that this pathway plays a pathological role in PWMD (Raymond et al. 2011).

As mentioned earlier, damaged axons and activated microglia contribute to increased glutamate in the PWM under hypoxic conditions (Barger et al. 2007; Domercq et al. 1999; Kukley et al. 2007; Li and Stys 2000; Sivakumar et al. 2010; Stys 1998). Excess glutamate has been shown to be toxic to oligodendrocytes *in vivo* and *in vitro* by receptor-independent (Back et al. 1998; Oka et al. 1993; Yoshioka et al. 1996) and receptor-mediated mechanisms (Matute et al. 1997; McDonald et al. 1998; Pitt et al. 2000; Yoshioka et al. 1996; Yoshioka et al. 1995) resulting in PWMD. These findings strongly suggest that impaired astrocyte ability to clear glutamate after hypoxia would result in accumulation of glutamate in the extracellular space, which in turn leads to excitotoxic death of oligodendrocyte progenitors and/or delayed myelination (Steinhauser and Gallo 1996; Yoshioka et al. 1996). Taken together, dysregulation of glutamate homeostasis in white matter astrocytes is considered to be one of the major contributing factors underlying oligodendrocyte pathology following hypoxic injury.

5.2. Astrocytes, Glutamate receptors and Periventricular White Matter Damage

Excess glutamate is known to cause excitotoxic damage to the developing PWM; however, the effect of glutamate on astrocytes under hypoxic conditions has not been well defined. As mentioned previously, excess glutamate accumulation following hypoxia in the PWM may mediate damage via receptor-dependent and/or receptor independent mechanisms (Oka et al. 1993; Yoshioka et al. 1996; Yoshioka et al. 1995). Apart from acting directly on oligodendrocyte glutamate receptors, glutamate may also activate the glutamate receptors expressed on astrocytes. Hypoxia induced changes in the expression of astrocytic glutamate receptors may shed light on glutamate-mediated regulation of astrocyte function. Astrocytes are known to express functional glutamate receptors both inotropic and metabotropic (Backus et al. 1989; MacVicar et al. 1988). The expression of NMDAR, an ionotropic glutamate receptor, was demonstrated in astrocytes following transient forebrain ischemia (Gottlieb and Matute 1997). It was later reported that both transient global forebrain ischemia *in vivo* and anoxia *in vitro* resulted in the specific expression of NR2B subunits in astrocytes and their colocalization with NR1 subunits suggested that they were functional (Krebs et al. 2003). Activation of glutamate receptors in astrocytes triggers a complex Ca^{2+}-signaling machinery. The potential consequences of Ca^{2+} signaling in astrocytes includes the stimulation of NOS, activation of second-messenger systems that are linked to gene expression including those for cytoskeletal elements and effects on other ion channels, such as an increased activation of Ca^{2+}-dependent K+ channels (Barres et al. 1990; Quandt and MacVicar 1986).

In addition to the excitatory mechanisms, glutamate was shown to mediate a reduction in the glutathione levels in astrocytes (Chen and Swanson 2003). Glutathione is an essential antioxidant and its decrease has been reported to render the immature PWM particularly sensitive to oxidative stress (Miller et al. 2009). Glutamate treatment caused an additional increase in the mRNA and protein expression of VEGF, a mediator of vascular permeability, in astrocyte cultures exposed to hypoxia (Liu et al. 2010). This increment in the expression of VEGF was attributed to the adaptive changes occurring in the glutamate receptors in astrocytes as a result of hypoxia (Liu et al. 2010). The effect of upregulated VEGF expression in hypoxic PWMD is discussed in subsection 5.4.

5.3. Astrocytes, Inflammation and Periventricular White Matter Damage

Although microglia are the primary source of cytokine production, astrocytes also contribute to the secretion of cytokines in the brain (Lieberman et al. 1989; van Neerven et al. 2010). Astrocyte-derived inflammatory cytokines such as TNF-α and IL-1β have been shown to promote death of oligodendrocytes in the PWM of hypoxic neonatal rats (Deng et al. 2010). An increased level of interferon-γ was reported to be detected in the gliotic white matter of infants diagnosed with PVL (Folkerth et al. 2004). Enhanced levels of TNF-α and IL-6 were also observed in white matter lesions of PVL brains (Deguchi et al. 1997; Kadhim et al. 2001; Yoon et al. 1997). In hypoxic PWMD, it has been shown that microglial cytokines orchestrate astrocytic responses. For instance, microglial CSF-1 acts via astroglial CSF-1 receptor activating the synthesis of TNF-α and IL-1β by the latter cell type (Deng et al. 2011). A recent study showed that hypoxia-induced production of astrocytic TNF-α and IL-1β was mediated by the activation of NMDAR, an ionotropic glutamate receptor (unpublished data). The cytokines secreted by astrocytes could also act in a similar manner as that of microglial cytokines on oligodendrocytes and axons expressing TNF-1R and IL-1R, leading to delayed myelination in hypoxic PWMD (Akassoglou et al. 1998; Deng et al. 2010).

5.4. Astrocytes, Vascular factors and Periventricular White Matter Damage

The BBB is a selective barrier made up of tight junctions between the endothelial cells of the capillaries (Balabanov et al. 1999; Balabanov and Dore-Duffy 1998). In addition to the tight junctions, the BBB is supported by the astrocytic end-feet and its integrity is essential for the maintenance of ionic homeostasis in the brain (Brown et al. 2004).

Though the BBB is functional at the early stages of fetal development (Mollgard and Saunders 1986; Saunders et al. 1991), it may be weakened by hypoxic-ischemic insults resulting in an increased vascular permeability (Abbott 2000; de Vries et al. 1997). Hypoxia-induced increased vascular permeability may be due to increase in production of VEGF/NO by astrocytes. VEGF has been characterized as an inducer of vascular permeability promoting the leakage of plasma proteins from blood vessels (Fischer et al. 1999). Similarly, NO is also known to be a potent vasodilator and has been implicated in the regulation of BBB permeability (Janigro et al. 1994). Increase in VEGF and NO production has been observed in the PWM of neonatal rats in response to hypoxia (Kaur et al. 2006a).

The hypoxia-induced increased VEGF expression was localized specifically in astrocytes in the PWM (Kaur et al. 2006a) and this was attributed to the activation of glutamate receptors in them (Liu et al. 2010). In astrocyte cultures, addition of TNF-α and IL-1β promoted the production of NO (Chao et al. 1995). Enhanced production of VEGF and NO by astrocytes has been reported to contribute to altered vascular permeability in hypoxic PWM (Kaur et al. 2010). Concomitantly, a large number of degenerating axons were observed in the vicinity of the blood vessels in the PWM of neonatal rats subjected to hypoxia suggesting that increased leakage of serum-derived substances may be involved in axonal degeneration, a characteristic feature of PWMD (Kaur et al. 2006a).

5.5. Astrocytes, Edema Formation and Periventricular White Matter Damage

Astrocytic swelling and edema formation are pathological features commonly associated with hypoxic PWMD. The initial astroglial response to hypoxia-ischemia is their prominent swelling (Garcia et al. 1977; Petito et al. 1982). Following hypoxic insults, the astrocytic swelling which initiates in the end-feet surrounding the capillaries spreads to the entire cell as observed in the neonatal hypoxic brain (Kaur and Ling 2008). It has been suggested that the BBB breakdown following hypoxic injury may result in an increase in intracranial pressure (Klatzo et al. 1980).

Astrocytic swelling following focal cerebral ischemia occurs as an osmotic consequence of increased glutamate, K+ ions, and lactate and in an attempt to buffer the accumulation of these molecules in the extracellular space (Aschner 1998; Landis 1994). Aquaporin-4 (AQ4), a member of aquaporin family of integral membrane proteins localized in astrocytic end-feet, is required for the maintenance of water homeostasis, and is the primary influx route for water during brain edema formation (Thrane et al. 2011). Upregulated expression of AQ4 in astrocytes has been reported to be associated with edema formation in the white matter of rat and human brain (Skjolding et al. 2013). Similar increase in expression of AQ4 in astrocytes was reported following neonatal hypoxic-ischemic insults (Fu et al. 2007). Hence it is suggested that prolonged activation of astrocytes accompanied by upregulated expression of AQ4 might cause brain edema (Fu et al. 2007), astrocytosis (Leviton and Gilles 1974) and thereby worsen the prognosis of premature infants suffering from PWMD (Ferrari et al. 2010). However, swollen astrocytes also release taurine, an inhibitory amino acid, which is known to possess antioxidant properties and has been reported to be neuroprotective in hypoxia-ischemia (Kimelberg et al. 1990; Klatzo et al. 1980).

5.6. Astrocytes, Gap Junctions and Periventricular White Matter Damage

Astrocytes are known to contribute to the cellular and molecular mechanisms associated with oligodendrocyte damage in white matter injury observed following hypoxia. In the brain parenchyma, astrocytes interact with adjacent cells through hemi channels known as gap junctions. The gap junctions are specialized intercellular connections that aid in the homeostatic regulation of extracellular pH, K^+, and glutamate levels by astrocytes (Anderson and Swanson 2000; Ransom et al. 2003; Ransom et al. 2000). The astrocytes form the largest gap junctions coupled cell network in the brain. Gap junctions have been identified to be abundantly expressed in astrocytes in the developing white matter (Nagy et al. 1999; Pastor et al. 1998). Apart from gap junctions formed between astrocytes, gap junctions have also been identified between oligodendrocytes and astrocytes (Kamasawa et al. 2005; Massa and Mugnaini 1982; Nagy et al. 2001; Rash et al. 2001). The expression of functional gap junctions between astrocytes and oligodendrocytes in the developing PWM was reported (Maglione et al. 2010) and it was shown that these gap junctions allow calcium signaling across astrocytes and oligodendrocytes (Parys et al. 2010) that is essential for glial survival and development (Magnotti et al. 2011). Under hypoxic-ischemic conditions, the gap junctions have been reported to remain open and thereby aid in propagating calcium signals across cells resulting in spreading of excitotoxic lesions (Cotrina et al. 1998). In a traumatic injury model, damage to the white matter was found to be associated to the expression of gap junctions (Theriault et al. 1997), suggesting that astrocyte-oligodendrocyte gap junctions may be involved in spreading of calcium signals in hypoxia-induced damage to PWM.

6. OLIGODENDROCYTES

The chronic myelination disturbance found in PWMD suggests that the oligodendrocytes are the main target cells in hypoxic-ischemic injuries of PWM (Back et al. 2002). Back et al. (2002) suggested that the vulnerability of oligodendrocytes to hypoxic-ischemic injuries depends on their stage of maturation. In both humans and rodents, during the high risk periods of PWMD, it was the late oligodendrocyte progenitors which dominated the white matter (Back et al. 2001). These late oligodendrocyte progenitor cells were reported to be highly susceptible to both intrinsic and extrinsic sources of oxidative stress associated with reduction in glutathione content (Back et al. 1998). Experimental studies carried out in fetal sheep of 0.65 gestational age, revealed that of the frontal PWM, the medial PWM was highly prone to damage compared to the lateral PWM. This was explained by the abundance of oligodendrocyte progenitors in the medial PWM while differentiated or matured oligodendrocytes were preponderant in the lateral PWM (Back et al. 2002). Thus the damage to oligodendrocytes in response to hypoxic-ischemic insults was suggested to be maturation-dependent (Back et al. 2002). Although the underlying causes for late oligodendrocyte progenitors being vulnerable to hypoxic-ischemic insults are not fully clear, oligodendrocyte death has been attributed primarily to glutamate mediated excitotoxicity, oxidative stress and mitochondrial impairment.

6.1. Oligodendrocytes, Glutamate Excitotoxicity and Periventricular White Matter Damage

As described earlier there are evidences which point to the susceptibility of oligodendrocytes to glutamate mediated excitotoxicity. Oka et al. (1993) were the first to demonstrate the death of oligodendrocytes on exposing them to glutamate. This was later supported by the demonstration of glutamate receptors on oligodendrocytes. Throughout a wide range of developmental stages, oligodendrocytes express functional AMPAR, kainate receptors (Matute et al. 2007) and NMDAR (Bakiri et al. 2009; Karadottir et al. 2005; Micu et al. 2006; Salter and Fern 2005). In accordance with this, the oligodendrocyte progenitors in PWM of human fetal brains between 23-32 weeks of gestation were shown to express AMPAR (Follett et al. 2004). Deng et al. (2004) demonstrated the expression of all three groups of metabotropic glutamate receptors in oligodendrocytes, which were developmentally regulated. Prolonged activation of AMPAR, kainate receptors and NMDAR leads to death of oligodendrocytes both *in vitro* and *in vivo* (Li and Stys 2000; Matute et al. 1997; McDonald et al. 1998; Yoshioka et al. 1996). The toxicity is attributed to the increased Ca^{2+} accumulation within the oligodendrocytes (Sanchez-Gomez and Matute 1999). The increased intracellular Ca^{2+} within oligodendrocytes results in mitochondrial Ca^{2+} accumulation and subsequent mitochondrial membrane depolarisation (Sanchez-Gomez et al. 2003). This is further accompanied by release of pro-apoptotic factors and activation of caspase (Sanchez-Gomez et al., 2003). AMPAR induced excitotoxicity of oligodendrocytes could also be mediated via a caspase independent pathway, wherein the apoptosis-inducing factor released from mitochondria causes death of oligodendrocytes through Poly [ADP-ribose] polymerase 1 (Sanchez-Gomez et al., 2003).

In addition to glutamate receptors, glutamate transporters also play a significant role in excitotoxicity of oligodendrocytes. Pitt et al. (2003) reported that the oligodendrocytes of subcortical white matter primarily express glutamate aspartate transporters (GLAST; also named as excitatory amino acid transporters or EAAT). They demonstrated the expression of EAAT-1 and EAAT-2 in human fetal oligodendrocytes *in vitro*. Owing to the expression of these glutamate transporters on oligodendrocytes, these cells were suggested to play a major role in maintaining glutamate concentrations in the white matter (Pitt et al., 2003). Yet under conditions of neuroinflammation the enhanced production of cytokines such as TNF-α could result in reduced expression of glutamate transporters in the oligodendrocytes (Pitt et al., 2003) which could be implicated in the increase of glutamate levels in hypoxic PWM. Domercq et al. (2005) showed that the inhibition of glutamate uptake by oligodendrocytes resulted in excitotoxicity of oligodendrocytes which was mediated by AMPAR and kainate receptors. Futhermore, in animal models, inhibition of glutamate transporter function, resulted in severe demyelination with associated loss of oligodendrocytes (Domercq et al. 2005). It could be speculated that the integrity of PWM depends on the balance between glutamate uptake and glutamate release. Perturbations in glutamate uptake could also result from lack of glutaminase, an enzyme that catalyses the conversion of glutamate from glutamine, in microglia (Werner et al. 2001) and/or by reduction in glutamate transporters in oligodendrocytes as a consequence of prolonged exposure to pro-inflammatory cytokines (Takahashi et al. 2003). Furthermore, glutamate could indirectly induce death of oligodendrocytes by enabling release of toxic factors from other glial cells. For example, activation of NMDAR in microglia resulted in enhanced secretion of TNF-α and IL-1β following hypoxia (Murugan et al. 2011). The secreted pro-inflammatory cytokines resulted in oligodendrocyte death by inducing cleavage of caspase-3 and reduced the proliferation of oligodendrocytes (Rathnasamy et al. 2011). TNF-α thus produced has been reported to result in destruction of myelin and axons (Merrill and Benveniste 1996). Collectively these results suggest that glutamate either directly or indirectly results in oligodendrocyte cell death which could be implicated in PWMD associated hypomyelination.

6.2. Oligodendrocytes, Oxidative Stress and Periventricular White Matter Damage

Oxidative stress due to free radicals has been reported to disrupt oligodendrocyte maturation resulting in paucity of mature myelinating oligodendrocytes (French et al. 2009).The susceptibility of oligodendrocytes to oxidative stress was attributed to their high requirement of oxygen for their metabolic processes, high concentrations of unsaturated fatty acids, reduced antioxidant enzymes and free radical scavengers (Back et al. 1998; Baud et al. 2004b; Fern and Moller 2000; Halliwell 1992). Late oligodendrocyte progenitors were at high risk of oxidative damage when incubated with glutathione-depleting agents such as buthionine sulfoximine (BSO) and diethylmaleate (Back et al. 1998) suggesting a role of glutathione in oxidative stress. Depletion of glutathione in these oligodendrocyte progenitors was followed by ROS accumulation as measured by the oxidation of a redox sensitive probe dihydrorhodamine 123 (Back et al., 1998). Additionally, lipid peroxidation products such as E_2-isoprostanes were found to be highly toxic to the oligodendrocyte progenitors (Brault et al. 2004). The evidence for oxidative stress in causing PWMD comes from autopsy studies on early human PWMD, which reported elevated concentrations of F_2-isoprostane, a stable lipid peroxidation marker for oxidative damage, with associated oligodendrocyte progenitor depletion (Back et al. 2005). Further, treatment with antioxidants such as α-tocopherol, idebenone, and glutathione monoethylester prevented the oligodendrocyte progenitor death (Back et al., 1998).

Besides oligodendrocyte cell death, recent studies unravelled the alternative mechanisms by which oxidative stress could lead to myelination deficits in PWMD. French et al. (2009) demonstrated that oxidative stress led to maturation arrest in oligodendrocyte progenitors. Associated with this, is the down-regulation of genes such as sonic hedgehog, Sox10, histone deacetylase 3, Olig1 and Olig2 known to promote oligodendrocyte differentiation at various stages of maturation (Ligon et al. 2006; Nery et al. 2001; Shen et al. 2005; Stolt et al. 2002; Zhou and Anderson 2002). In addition, genes involved in inhibition of differentiation (ID) such as ID2 and ID4 were up-regulated in oligodendrocytes exposed to BSO (French et al., 2009). ROS has been further demonstrated to cause an increase in histone acetylase activity (Ito et al. 2001) known to negatively influence the fate of oligodendrocytes from neural stem cells. Oligodendrocyte maturation could also be inhibited by increased expression of bone morphogenetic protein 4 in the PWM (Reid et al. 2012).

6.3. Oligodendrocyte apoptosis and Periventricular White Matter Damage

The death of oligodendrocytes is a hallmark feature of PWMD. Several studies have reported the apoptosis of oligodendrocytes in response to hypoxic insult (Deng et al. 2008; Kaur and Ling 2009; Murugan et al. 2011). The demonstration of swollen mitochondria in oligodendrocyte progenitors challenged with free radicals led to the hypothesis of mitochondrial lesion mediated apoptosis of oligodendrocytes (Back et al., 1998). Excitotoxic damage of oligodendrocytes is also considered to be mediated via mitochondrial pathway. The overactivation of ionotropic glutamate receptors on the oligodendrocytes results in increased accumulation of Ca^{2+} which leads to mitochondrial membrane depolarization and caspase dependent or independent oligodendrocyte death (Sánchez-Gómez, 2003).

Ca^{2+} mediated mitochondrial disruption is also favoured by calcium induced calcium release (CICR) from endoplasmic reticulum (ER) through ryanodine receptors (RyR) (Ruiz et al. 2010). The close association between the membranes of ER and mitochondria has been previously demonstrated. Immuno-electron microscopy studies revealed the increased concentration of RyR channels at the ER subdomains aligned closely with mitochondria. This coupling enables the transfer of Ca^{2+} into the inner membrane of mitochondria [reviewed in (Hajnoczky et al. 2000)].

Mitochondrial calcium accumulation is suggested to result in reduced transmembrane potential as well as ROS generation (Lenaz et al. 2002). The depolarisation of mitochondrial membrane is associated with release of cytochrome c into the cytoplasm of oligodendrocytes

(Sanchez-Gomez et al. 2003).The released cytochrome c could induce caspase cascade by interacting with apoptotic protease activating factor 1 (Li et al. 1997). Supporting this is our demonstration of hypoxia induced increased expression of caspase-3, an apoptosis marker (Armstrong et al. 1996; Wang et al. 1996), in oligodendrocyte cell lines (Kaur et al. 2010).

Taking into account the free radical mediated damage and excitotoxicity of oligodendrocytes in hypoxic PWM, it could be suggested that the above explained mitochondrial apoptotic pathway could further exacerbate hypoxia induced oligodendrocyte death in PWM.

CONCLUSION

Hypoxic insult to the immature brain during the mid-gestation period has a predilection for PWM which was attributed to the extreme vulnerability of oligodendrocyte progenitors dominating the white matter region during this period. Toxic factors produced by activated microglia and astrocytes in response to hypoxic insults, further exacerbated the PWMD by inducing oligodendrocyte apoptosis. In view of the complex interplay of etiological factors and glial cells in PWMD, in-depth investigations are essential for a thorough understanding. Thus, studies exploring the interaction between activated glial cells and oligodendrocyte progenitors would help to better define the mechanisms *in vivo*. Translational studies confirming and re-evaluating the proposed molecular mechanisms would be desirable for identification of alternative therapeutic strategies to ameliorate PWMD.

REFERENCES

Abbott NJ. 2000. Inflammatory mediators and modulation of blood-brain barrier permeability. *Cell Mol Neurobiol* 20:131-47.

Abbott NJ. 2002. Astrocyte-endothelial interactions and blood-brain barrier permeability. *J Anat* 200:629-38.

Adcock LM, Yamashita Y, Goddard-Finegold J, Smith CV. 1996. Cerebral hypoxia-ischemia increases microsomal iron in newborn piglets. *Metab Brain Dis* 11:359-67.

Akassoglou K, Bauer J, Kassiotis G, Pasparakis M, Lassmann H, Kollias G, Probert L. 1998. Oligodendrocyte apoptosis and primary demyelination induced by local TNF/p55TNF receptor signaling in the central nervous system of transgenic mice: models for multiple sclerosis with primary oligodendrogliopathy. *Am J Pathol* 153:801-13.

Allen NJ, Karadottir R, Attwell D. 2004. Reversal or reduction of glutamate and GABA transport in CNS pathology and therapy. *Pflugers Arch* 449:132-42.

Alvarez-Diaz A, Hilario E, de Cerio FG, Valls-i-Soler A, Alvarez-Diaz FJ. 2007. Hypoxic-ischemic injury in the immature brain - Key vascular and cellular players. *Neonatology* 92:227-235.

Amato M, Donati F. 2000. Update on perinatal hypoxic insult: mechanism, diagnosis and interventions. *Eur J Paediatr Neurol* 4:203-9.

Ambrosini E, Aloisi F. 2004. Chemokines and glial cells: a complex network in the central nervous system. *Neurochem Res* 29:1017-38.

Anderson CM, Swanson RA. 2000. Astrocyte glutamate transport: review of properties, regulation, and physiological functions. *Glia* 32:1-14.

Armstrong RC, Aja T, Xiang J, Gaur S, Krebs JF, Hoang K, Bai X, Korsmeyer SJ, Karanewsky DS, Fritz LC and others. 1996. Fas-induced activation of the cell death-related protease CPP32 Is inhibited by Bcl-2 and by ICE family protease inhibitors. *J Biol Chem* 271:16850-5.

Aschner M. 1998. Immune and inflammatory responses in the CNS: modulation by astrocytes. *Toxicol Lett* 102-103:283-7.

Back SA, Craig A, Kayton RJ, Luo NL, Meshul CK, Allcock N, Fern R. 2007. Hypoxia-ischemia preferentially triggers glutamate depletion from oligodendroglia and axons in perinatal cerebral white matter. *J Cereb Blood Flow Metab* 27:334-47.

Back SA, Gan X, Li Y, Rosenberg PA, Volpe JJ. 1998. Maturation-dependent vulnerability of oligodendrocytes to oxidative stress-induced death caused by glutathione depletion. *J Neurosci* 18:6241-53.

Back SA, Han BH, Luo NL, Chricton CA, Xanthoudakis S, Tam J, Arvin KL, Holtzman DM. 2002. Selective vulnerability of late oligodendrocyte progenitors to hypoxia-ischemia. *J Neurosci* 22:455-63.

Back SA, Luo NL, Borenstein NS, Levine JM, Volpe JJ, Kinney HC. 2001. Late oligodendrocyte progenitors coincide with the developmental window of vulnerability for human perinatal white matter injury. *J Neurosci* 21:1302-12.

Back SA, Luo NL, Mallinson RA, O'Malley JP, Wallen LD, Frei B, Morrow JD, Petito CK, Roberts CT, Jr., Murdoch GH and others. 2005. Selective vulnerability of preterm white matter to oxidative damage defined by F2-isoprostanes. *Ann Neurol* 58:108-20.

Back SA, Riddle A, Hohimer AR. 2006. Role of instrumented fetal sheep preparations in defining the pathogenesis of human periventricular white-matter injury. *J Child Neurol* 21:582-9.

Back SA, Rivkees SA. 2004. Emerging concepts in periventricular white matter injury. *Semin Perinatol* 28:405-14.

Back SA. 2006. Perinatal white matter injury: the changing spectrum of pathology and emerging insights into pathogenetic mechanisms. *Ment Retard Dev Disabil Res Rev* 12:129-40.

Backus KH, Kettenmann H, Schachner M. 1989. Pharmacological characterization of the glutamate receptor in cultured astrocytes. *J Neurosci Res* 22:274-82.

Bakiri Y, Burzomato V, Frugier G, Hamilton NB, Karadottir R, Attwell D. 2009. Glutamatergic signaling in the brain's white matter. *Neuroscience* 158:266-74.

Balabanov R, Beaumont T, Dore-Duffy P. 1999. Role of central nervous system microvascular pericytes in activation of antigen-primed splenic T-lymphocytes. *J Neurosci Res* 55:578-87.

Balabanov R, Dore-Duffy P. 1998. Role of the CNS microvascular pericyte in the blood-brain barrier. *J Neurosci Res* 53:637-44.

Ballabh P, Hu F, Kumarasiri M, Braun A, Nedergaard M. 2005. Development of tight junction molecules in blood vessels of germinal matrix, cerebral cortex, and white matter. *Pediatr Res* 58:791-8.

Barger SW, Goodwin ME, Porter MM, Beggs ML. 2007. Glutamate release from activated microglia requires the oxidative burst and lipid peroxidation. *J Neurochem* 101:1205-13.

Barres BA, Koroshetz WJ, Chun LL, Corey DP. 1990. Ion channel expression by white matter glia: the type-1 astrocyte. *Neuron* 5:527-44.

Baud O, Daire JL, Dalmaz Y, Fontaine RH, Krueger RC, Sebag G, Evrard P, Gressens P, Verney C. 2004a. Gestational hypoxia induces white matter damage in neonatal rats: a new model of periventricular leukomalacia. *Brain Pathol* 14:1-10.

Baud O, Li JR, Zhang YM, Neve RL, Volpe JJ, Rosenberg PA. 2004b. Nitric oxide-induced cell death in developing oligodendrocytes is associated with mitochondrial dysfunction and apoptosis-inducing factor translocation. *European Journal of Neuroscience* 20:1713-1726.

Beard JL, Connor JR. 2003. Iron status and neural functioning. *Annu Rev Nutr* 23:41-58.

Bedard K, Krause KH. 2007. The NOX family of ROS-generating NADPH oxidases: physiology and pathophysiology. *Physiol Rev* 87:245-313.

Benveniste H, Drejer J, Schousboe A, Diemer NH. 1984. Elevation of the extracellular concentrations of glutamate and aspartate in rat hippocampus during transient cerebral ischemia monitored by intracerebral microdialysis. *J Neurochem* 43:1369-74.

Berg D, Gerlach M, Youdim MBH, Double KL, Zecca L, Riederer P, Becker G. 2001. Brain iron pathways and their relevance to Parkinson's disease. *Journal of neurochemistry* 79:225-236.

Berger R, Garnier Y, Jensen A. 2002. Perinatal brain damage: underlying mechanisms and neuroprotective strategies. *J Soc Gynecol Investig* 9:319-28..

Billiards SS, Haynes RL, Folkerth RD, Trachtenberg FL, Liu LG, Volpe JJ, Kinney HC. 2006. Development of microglia in the cerebral white matter of the human fetus and infant. *Journal of Comparative Neurology* 497:199-208.

Biran V, Joly LM, Heron A, Vernet A, Vega C, Mariani J, Renolleau S, Charriaut-Marlangue C. 2006. Glial activation in white matter following ischemia in the neonatal P7 rat brain. *Exp Neurol* 199:103-12.

Borch K, Greisen G. 1998. Blood flow distribution in the normal human preterm brain. *Pediatr Res* 43:28-33.

Brault S, Martinez-Bermudez AK, Roberts J, 2nd, Cui QL, Fragoso G, Hemdan S, Liu HN, Gobeil F, Jr., Quiniou C, Kermorvant-Duchemin E and others. 2004. Cytotoxicity of the E(2)-isoprostane 15-E(2t)-IsoP on oligodendrocyte progenitors. *Free Radic Biol Med* 37:358-66.

Brown GC, Bal-Price A. 2003. Inflammatory neurodegeneration mediated by nitric oxide, glutamate, and mitochondria. *Mol Neurobiol* 27:325-55.

Brown GC. 2007. Mechanisms of inflammatory neurodegeneration: iNOS and NADPH oxidase. *Biochem Soc Trans* 35:1119-21.

Brown RC, Mark KS, Egleton RD, Davis TP. 2004. Protection against hypoxia-induced blood-brain barrier disruption: changes in intracellular calcium. *Am J Physiol Cell Physiol* 286:C1045-52.

Buonocore G, Perrone S, Bracci R. 2001. Free radicals and brain damage in the newborn. *Biol Neonate* 79:180-6.

Cai Z, Pang Y, Xiao F, Rhodes PG. 2001. Chronic ischemia preferentially causes white matter injury in the neonatal rat brain. *Brain Res* 898:126-35.

Carloni S, Mazzoni E, Cimino M, De Simoni MG, Perego C, Scopa C, Balduini W. 2006. Simvastatin reduces caspase-3 activation and inflammatory markers induced by hypoxia-ischemia in the newborn rat. *Neurobiol Dis* 21:119-26.

Chao CC, Hu S, Ehrlich L, Peterson PK. 1995. Interleukin-1 and tumor necrosis factor-alpha synergistically mediate neurotoxicity: involvement of nitric oxide and of N-methyl-D-aspartate receptors. *Brain Behav Immun* 9:355-65.

Chao CC, Hu S, Peterson PK. 1996. Glia: the not so innocent bystanders. *Journal of Neurovirology* 2:234-9.

Chen Y, Swanson RA. 2003. Astrocytes and brain injury. *J Cereb Blood Flow Metab* 23:137-49.

Colton C, Wilt S, Gilbert D, Chernyshev O, Snell J, Dubois-Dalcq M. 1996. Species differences in the generation of reactive oxygen species by microglia. *Mol Chem Neuropathol* 28:15-20.

Connor JR, Menzies SL. 1990. Altered cellular distribution of iron in the central nervous system of myelin deficient rats. *Neuroscience* 34:265-71.

Connor JR, Menzies SL. 1996. Relationship of iron to oligodendrocytes and myelination. *Glia* 17:83-93.

Cotrina ML, Kang J, Lin JH, Bueno E, Hansen TW, He L, Liu Y, Nedergaard M. 1998. Astrocytic gap junctions remain open during ischemic conditions. *J Neurosci* 18:2520-37.

Cowell RM, Silverstein FS. 2003. Developmental changes in the expression of chemokine receptor CCR1 in the rat cerebellum. *J Comp Neurol* 457:7-23.

Croll SD, Goodman JH, Scharfman HE. 2004. Vascular endothelial growth factor (VEGF) in seizures: a double-edged sword. *Adv Exp Med Biol* 548:57-68.

Cross AK, Woodroofe MN. 1999. Chemokines induce migration and changes in actin polymerization in adult rat brain microglia and a human fetal microglial cell line in vitro. *J Neurosci Res* 55:17-23.

Danbolt NC. 2001. Glutamate uptake. *Prog Neurobiol* 65:1-105.

de Vries HE, Kuiper J, de Boer AG, Van Berkel TJ, Breimer DD. 1997. The blood-brain barrier in neuroinflammatory diseases. *Pharmacol Rev* 49:143-55.

Deguchi K, Mizuguchi M, Takashima S. 1996. Immunohistochemical expression of tumor necrosis factor alpha in neonatal leukomalacia. *Pediatr Neurol* 14:13-6.

Deguchi K, Oguchi K, Takashima S. 1997. Characteristic neuropathology of leukomalacia in extremely low birth weight infants. *Pediatr Neurol* 16:296-300.

Deng W, Rosenberg PA, Volpe JJ, Jensen FE. 2003. Calcium-permeable AMPA/kainate receptors mediate toxicity and preconditioning by oxygen-glucose deprivation in oligodendrocyte precursors. *Proc Natl Acad Sci USA* 100:6801-6.

Deng W, Wang H, Rosenberg PA, Volpe JJ, Jensen FE. 2004. Role of metabotropic glutamate receptors in oligodendrocyte excitotoxicity and oxidative stress. *Proc Natl Acad Sci U S A* 101:7751-6.

Deng Y, Lu J, Sivakumar V, Ling EA, Kaur C. 2008. Amoeboid microglia in the periventricular white matter induce oligodendrocyte damage through expression of proinflammatory cytokines via MAP kinase signaling pathway in hypoxic neonatal rats. *Brain Pathol* 18:387-400.

Deng YY, Lu J, Ling EA, Kaur C. 2009. Monocyte chemoattractant protein-1 (MCP-1) produced via NF-kappaB signaling pathway mediates migration of amoeboid microglia in the periventricular white matter in hypoxic neonatal rats. *Glia* 57:604-21.

Deng YY, Lu J, Ling EA, Kaur C. 2010. Microglia-derived macrophage colony stimulating factor promotes generation of proinflammatory cytokines by astrocytes in the periventricular white matter in the hypoxic neonatal brain. *Brain Pathol* 20:909-25.

Deng YY, Lu J, Ling EA, Kaur C. 2011. Role of microglia in the process of inflammation in the hypoxic developing brain. *Front Bio*sci (Schol Ed) 3:884-900.

Di Giovanni S, Faden AI, Yakovlev A, Duke-Cohan JS, Finn T, Thouin M, Knoblach S, De Biase A, Bregman BS, Hoffman EP. 2005. Neuronal plasticity after spinal cord injury: identification of a gene cluster driving neurite outgrowth. *FASEB J* 19:153-4.

Domercq M, Etxebarria E, Perez-Samartin A, Matute C. 2005. Excitotoxic oligodendrocyte death and axonal damage induced by glutamate transporter inhibition. *Glia* 52:36-46.

Domercq M, Sanchez-Gomez MV, Areso P, Matute C. 1999. Expression of glutamate transporters in rat optic nerve oligodendrocytes. *Eur J Neurosci* 11:2226-36.

Farber K, Kettenmann H. 2006. Functional role of calcium signals for microglial function. *Glia* 54:656-665.

Fern R, Moller T. 2000. Rapid ischemic cell death in immature oligodendrocytes: a fatal glutamate release feedback loop. *J Neurosci* 20:34-42.

Ferrari DC, Nesic O, Perez-Polo JR. 2010. Perspectives on neonatal hypoxia/ischemia-induced edema formation. *Neurochem Res* 35:1957-65.

Ferriero DM. 2004. Neonatal brain injury. *N Engl J Med* 351:1985-95.

Fischer S, Renz D, Wiesnet M, Schaper W, Karliczek GF. 1999. Hypothermia abolishes hypoxia-induced hyperpermeability in brain microvessel endothelial cells. *Brain Res Mol Brain Res* 74:135-44.

Folkerth RD, Keefe RJ, Haynes RL, Trachtenberg FL, Volpe JJ, Kinney HC. 2004. Interferon-gamma expression in periventricular leukomalacia in the human brain. *Brain Pathol* 14:265-74.

Folkerth RD. 2005. Neuropathologic substrate of cerebral palsy. *J Child Neurol* 20:940-9.

Folkerth RD. 2006. Periventricular leukomalacia: overview and recent findings. *Pediatr Dev Pathol* 9:3-13.

Follett PL, Deng W, Dai W, Talos DM, Massillon LJ, Rosenberg PA, Volpe JJ, Jensen FE. 2004. Glutamate receptor-mediated oligodendrocyte toxicity in periventricular leukomalacia: a protective role for topiramate. *J Neurosci* 24:4412-20.

Follett PL, Rosenberg PA, Volpe JJ, Jensen FE. 2000. NBQX attenuates excitotoxic injury in developing white matter. *J Neurosci* 20:9235-41.

Fontaine V, Mohand-Said S, Hanoteau N, Fuchs C, Pfizenmaier K, Eisel U. 2002. Neurodegenerative and neuroprotective effects of tumor Necrosis factor (TNF) in retinal ischemia: opposite roles of TNF receptor 1 and TNF receptor 2. *J Neurosci* 22:RC216.

French HM, Reid M, Mamontov P, Simmons RA, Grinspan JB. 2009. Oxidative stress disrupts oligodendrocyte maturation. *J Neurosci Res* 87:3076-87.

Fu X, Li Q, Feng Z, Mu D. 2007. The roles of aquaporin-4 in brain edema following neonatal hypoxia ischemia and reoxygenation in a cultured rat astrocyte model. *Glia* 55:935-41.

Garcia JH, Kalimo H, Kamijyo Y, Trump BF. 1977. Cellular events during partial cerebral ischemia. I. Electron microscopy of feline cerebral cortex after middle-cerebral-artery occlusion. *Virchows Arch B Cell Pathol* 25:191-206.

Gautron L, De Smedt-Peyrusse V, Laye S. 2006. Characterization of STAT3-expressing cells in the postnatal rat brain. *Brain Res* 1098:26-32.

Gorter JA, Mesquita ARM, van Vliet EA, da Silva FHL, Aronica E. 2005. Increased expression of ferritin, an iron-storage protein, in specific regions of the parahippocampal cortex of epileptic rats. *Epilepsia* 46:1371-1379.

Gottlieb M, Matute C. 1997. Expression of ionotropic glutamate receptor subunits in glial cells of the hippocampal CA1 area following transient forebrain ischemia. *J Cereb Blood Flow Metab* 17:290-300.

Green SP, Cairns B, Rae J, Errett-Baroncini C, Hongo JA, Erickson RW, Curnutte JT. 2001. Induction of gp91-phox, a component of the phagocyte NADPH oxidase, in microglial cells during central nervous system inflammation. *J Cereb Blood Flow Metab* 21:374-84.

Griot C, Vandevelde M, Richard A, Peterhans E, Stocker R. 1990. Selective degeneration of oligodendrocytes mediated by reactive oxygen species. *Free Radic Res Commun* 11:181-93.

Guan J, Bennet L, Gluckman PD, Gunn AJ. 2003. Insulin-like growth factor-1 and post-ischemic brain injury. *Prog Neurobiol* 70:443-62.

Guo G, Bhat NR. 2006. Hypoxia/reoxygenation differentially modulates NF-kappaB activation and iNOS expression in astrocytes and microglia. *Antioxid Redox Signal* 8:911-8.

Hagberg H. 1992. Hypoxic-Ischemic Damage in the Neonatal Brain - Excitatory Amino-Acids. *Developmental Pharmacology and Therapeutics* 18:139-144.

Hajnoczky G, Csordas G, Krishnamurthy R, Szalai G. 2000. Mitochondrial calcium signaling driven by the IP3 receptor. *J Bioenerg Biomembr* 32:15-25.

Halliwell B. 1992. Reactive oxygen species and the central nervous system. *Journal of neurochemistry* 59:1609-23.

Hanisch UK, Prinz M, Angstwurm K, Hausler KG, Kann O, Kettenmann H, Weber JR. 2001. The protein tyrosine kinase inhibitor AG126 prevents the massive microglial cytokine induction by pneumococcal cell walls. *Eur J Immunol* 31:2104-15.

Hao AJ, Dheen ST, Ling EA. 2002. Expression of macrophage colony-stimulating factor and its receptor in microglia activation is linked to teratogen-induced neuronal damage. *Neuroscience* 112:889-900.

Haynes RL, Baud O, Li J, Kinney HC, Volpe JJ, Folkerth DR. 2005. Oxidative and nitrative injury in periventricular leukomalacia: a review. *Brain Pathol* 15:225-33.

Haynes RL, Folkerth RD, Keefe RJ, Sung I, Swzeda LI, Rosenberg PA, Volpe JJ, Kinney HC. 2003. Nitrosative and oxidative injury to premyelinating oligodendrocytes in periventricular leukomalacia. *J Neuropathol Exp Neurol* 62:441-50.

Herrmann JE, Imura T, Song B, Qi J, Ao Y, Nguyen TK, Korsak RA, Takeda K, Akira S, Sofroniew MV. 2008. STAT3 is a critical regulator of astrogliosis and scar formation after spinal cord injury. *J Neurosci* 28:7231-43.

Hirayama A, Okoshi Y, Hachiya Y, Ozawa Y, Ito M, Kida Y, Imai Y, Kohsaka S, Takashima S. 2001. Early immunohistochemical detection of axonal damage and glial activation in extremely immature brains with periventricular leukomalacia. *Clin Neuropathol* 20:87-91.

Huang BY, Castillo M. 2008. Hypoxic-ischemic brain injury: imaging findings from birth to adulthood. *Radiographics* 28:417-39; quiz 617.

Huang Z, Liu J, Cheung PY, Chen C. 2009. Long-term cognitive impairment and myelination deficiency in a rat model of perinatal hypoxic-ischemic brain injury. *Brain Res* 1301:100-9.

Huo Y, Rangarajan P, Ling EA, Dheen ST. 2011. Dexamethasone inhibits the Nox-dependent ROS production via suppression of MKP-1-dependent MAPK pathways in activated microglia. *BMC Neurosci* 12:49.

Imamoto K, Leblond CP. 1978. Radioautographic investigation of gliogenesis in the corpus callosum of young rats. II. Origin of microglial cells. *The Journal of comparative neurology* 180:139-63.

Inder TE, Wells SJ, Mogridge NB, Spencer C, Volpe JJ. 2003. Defining the nature of the cerebral abnormalities in the premature infant: a qualitative magnetic resonance imaging study. *J Pediatr* 143:171-9.

Infanger DW, Sharma RV, Davisson RL. 2006. NADPH oxidases of the brain: distribution, regulation, and function. *Antioxid Redox Signal* 8:1583-96.

Ito K, Jazrawi E, Cosio B, Barnes PJ, Adcock IM. 2001. p65-activated histone acetyltransferase activity is repressed by glucocorticoids: mifepristone fails to recruit HDAC2 to the p65-HAT complex. *J Biol Chem* 276:30208-15.

Iwata O, Iwata S, Tamura M, Nakamura T, Hirabayashi S, Fueki N, Kondou Y, Hizume E, Kihara H. 2004. Periventricular low intensities on fluid attenuated inversion recovery imaging in the newborn infant: relationships to the clinical data and long-term outcome. *Pediatr Int* 46:150-7.

Janigro D, West GA, Nguyen TS, Winn HR. 1994. Regulation of blood-brain barrier endothelial cells by nitric oxide. *Circ Res* 75:528-38.

Jelinski SE, Yager JY, Juurlink BH. 1999. Preferential injury of oligodendroblasts by a short hypoxic-ischemic insult. *Brain Res* 815:150-3.

Johnston MV. 1997. Hypoxic and ischemic disorders of infants and children. Lecture for 38th meeting of Japanese Society of Child Neurology, Tokyo, Japan, July 1996. *Brain Dev* 19:235-9.

Justicia C, Gabriel C, Planas AM. 2000. Activation of the JAK/STAT pathway following transient focal cerebral ischemia: signaling through Jak1 and Stat3 in astrocytes. *Glia* 30:253-70.

Kadhim H, Tabarki B, De Prez C, Rona AM, Sebire G. 2002. Interleukin-2 in the pathogenesis of perinatal white matter damage. *Neurology* 58:1125-8.

Kadhim H, Tabarki B, De Prez C, Sebire G. 2003. Cytokine immunoreactivity in cortical and subcortical neurons in periventricular leukomalacia: are cytokines implicated in neuronal dysfunction in cerebral palsy? *Acta Neuropathol* 105:209-16.

Kadhim H, Tabarki B, Verellen G, De Prez C, Rona AM, Sebire G. 2001. Inflammatory cytokines in the pathogenesis of periventricular leukomalacia. *Neurology* 56:1278-84.

Kamasawa N, Sik A, Morita M, Yasumura T, Davidson KG, Nagy JI, Rash JE. 2005. Connexin-47 and connexin-32 in gap junctions of oligodendrocyte somata, myelin sheaths, paranodal loops and Schmidt-Lanterman incisures: implications for ionic homeostasis and potassium siphoning. *Neuroscience* 136:65-86.

Kanno M, Suzuki S, Fujiwara T, Yokoyama A, Sakamoto A, Takahashi H, Imai Y, Tanaka J. 2005. Functional expression of CCL6 by rat microglia: a possible role of CCL6 in cell-cell communication. *J Neuroimmunol* 167:72-80.

Karadottir R, Cavelier P, Bergersen LH, Attwell D. 2005. NMDA receptors are expressed in oligodendrocytes and activated in ischaemia. *Nature* 438:1162-6.

Kaur C, Dheen ST, Ling EA. 2007. From blood to brain: amoeboid microglial cell, a nascent macrophage and its functions in developing brain. *Acta Pharmacol Sin* 28:1087-96.

Kaur C, Hao AJ, Wu CH, Ling EA. 2001. Origin of microglia. *Microsc Res Tech* 54:2-9.

Kaur C, Ling EA. 1999. Increased expression of transferrin receptors and iron in amoeboid microglial cells in postnatal rats following an exposure to hypoxia. *Neurosci Lett* 262:183-6.

Kaur C, Ling EA. 2008. Blood brain barrier in hypoxic-ischemic conditions. *Curr Neurovasc Res* 5:71-81.

Kaur C, Ling EA. 2009. Periventricular white matter damage in the hypoxic neonatal brain: Role of microglial cells. *Progress in Neurobiology* 87:264-280.

Kaur C, Sivakumar V, Ang LS, Sundaresan A. 2006a. Hypoxic damage to the periventricular white matter in neonatal brain: role of vascular endothelial growth factor, nitric oxide and excitotoxicity. *J Neurochem* 98:1200-16.

Kaur C, Sivakumar V, Dheen ST, Ling EA. 2006b. Insulin-like growth factor I and II expression and modulation in amoeboid microglial cells by lipopolysaccharide and retinoic acid. *Neuroscience* 138:1233-44.

Kaur C, Sivakumar V, Ling EA. 2010. Melatonin protects periventricular white matter from damage due to hypoxia. *J Pineal Res* 48:185-93.

Kaur C, Sivakumar V, Yip GW, Ling EA. 2009. Expression of syndecan-2 in the amoeboid microglial cells and its involvement in inflammation in the hypoxic developing brain. *Glia* 57:336-49.

Kaur C, You Y. 2000. Ultrastructure and function of the amoeboid microglial cells in the periventricular white matter in postnatal rat brain following a hypoxic exposure. *Neuroscience letters* 290:17-20.

Kimelberg HK, Goderie SK, Higman S, Pang S, Waniewski RA. 1990. Swelling-induced release of glutamate, aspartate, and taurine from astrocyte cultures. *J Neurosci* 10:1583-91.

Klatzo I, Chui E, Fujiwara K, Spatz M. 1980. Resolution of vasogenic brain edema. *Adv Neurol* 28:359-73.

Krebs C, Fernandes HB, Sheldon C, Raymond LA, Baimbridge KG. 2003. Functional NMDA receptor subtype 2B is expressed in astrocytes after ischemia in vivo and anoxia in vitro. *J Neurosci* 23:3364-72.

Kukley M, Capetillo-Zarate E, Dietrich D. 2007. Vesicular glutamate release from axons in white matter. *Nat Neurosci* 10:311-20.

Kurumatani T, Kudo T, Ikura Y, Takeda M. 1998. White matter changes in the gerbil brain under chronic cerebral hypoperfusion. *Stroke* 29:1058-62.

Landis DM. 1994. The early reactions of non-neuronal cells to brain injury. *Annu Rev Neurosci* 17:133-51.

Lavigne MC, Malech HL, Holland SM, Leto TL. 2001. Genetic requirement of p47phox for superoxide production by murine microglia. *FASEB J* 15:285-7.

Lenaz G, Bovina C, D'Aurelio M, Fato R, Formiggini G, Genova ML, Giuliano G, Merlo Pich M, Paolucci U, Parenti Castelli G and others. 2002. Role of mitochondria in oxidative stress and aging. *Ann N Y Acad Sci* 959:199-213.

Leviton A, Gilles FH. 1974. Astrocytosis without globules in infant cerebral white matter. An epidemiologic study. *J Neurol Sci* 22:329-40.

Li F, Lu J, Wu CY, Kaur C, Sivakumar V, Sun J, Li S, Ling EA. 2008. Expression of Kv1.2 in microglia and its putative roles in modulating production of proinflammatory cytokines and reactive oxygen species. *J Neurochem* 106:2093-105.

Li P, Nijhawan D, Budihardjo I, Srinivasula SM, Ahmad M, Alnemri ES, Wang X. 1997. Cytochrome c and dATP-dependent formation of Apaf-1/caspase-9 complex initiates an apoptotic protease cascade. *Cell* 91:479-89.

Li S, Stys PK. 2000. Mechanisms of ionotropic glutamate receptor-mediated excitotoxicity in isolated spinal cord white matter. *J Neurosci* 20:1190-8.

Lieberman AP, Pitha PM, Shin HS, Shin ML. 1989. Production of tumor necrosis factor and other cytokines by astrocytes stimulated with lipopolysaccharide or a neurotropic virus. *Proc Natl Acad Sci U S A* 86:6348-52.

Ligon KL, Kesari S, Kitada M, Sun T, Arnett HA, Alberta JA, Anderson DJ, Stiles CD, Rowitch DH. 2006. Development of NG2 neural progenitor cells requires Olig gene function. *Proc Natl Acad Sci U S A* 103:7853-8.

Ling EA, Kaur C, Wong WC. 1991. Expression of major histocompatibility complex and leukocyte common antigens in amoeboid microglia in postnatal rats. *J Anat* 177:117-26.

Ling EA, Penney D, Leblond CP. 1980. Use of carbon labeling to demonstrate the role of blood monocytes as precursors of the 'ameboid cells' present in the corpus callosum of postnatal rats. *J Comp Neurol* 193:631-57.

Ling EA, Wong WC. 1993. The origin and nature of ramified and amoeboid microglia: a historical review and current concepts. *Glia* 7:9-18.

Liu CX, Liu Y, Shi W, Chen XL, Xiao XL, Zhao LY, Tian YM, Zhang JF. 2010. [Effect of glutamate on vascular endothelial growth factor mRNA and protein expressions in hypoxic rat astrocytes in vitro]. *Nan Fang Yi Ke Da Xue Xue Bao* 30:435-8.

Liu X, Bolteus AJ, Balkin DM, Henschel O, Bordey A. 2006. GFAP-expressing cells in the postnatal subventricular zone display a unique glial phenotype intermediate between radial glia and astrocytes. *Glia* 54:394-410.

Liu Y, Silverstein FS, Skoff R, Barks JD. 2002. Hypoxic-ischemic oligodendroglial injury in neonatal rat brain. *Pediatr Res* 51:25-33.

Lu B, Rutledge BJ, Gu L, Fiorillo J, Lukacs NW, Kunkel SL, North R, Gerard C, Rollins BJ. 1998. Abnormalities in monocyte recruitment and cytokine expression in monocyte chemoattractant protein 1-deficient mice. *J Exp Med* 187:601-8.

MacVicar BA, Baker K, Crichton SA. 1988. Kainic acid evokes a potassium efflux from astrocytes. *Neuroscience* 25:721-5.

Maglione M, Tress O, Haas B, Karram K, Trotter J, Willecke K, Kettenmann H. 2010. Oligodendrocytes in mouse corpus callosum are coupled via gap junction channels formed by connexin47 and connexin32. *Glia* 58:1104-17.

Magnotti LM, Goodenough DA, Paul DL. 2011. Deletion of oligodendrocyte Cx32 and astrocyte Cx43 causes white matter vacuolation, astrocyte loss and early mortality. *Glia* 59:1064-74.

Malarkey EB, Parpura V. 2008. Mechanisms of glutamate release from astrocytes. *Neurochem Int* 52:142-54.

Mallard C, Welin AK, Peebles D, Hagberg H, Kjellmer I. 2003. White matter injury following systemic endotoxemia or asphyxia in the fetal sheep. *Neurochem Res* 28:215-23.

Marletta MA. 1993. Nitric oxide synthase: function and mechanism. *Adv Exp Med Biol* 338:281-4.

Massa PT, Mugnaini E. 1982. Cell junctions and intramembrane particles of astrocytes and oligodendrocytes: a freeze-fracture study. *Neuroscience* 7:523-38.

Matute C, Alberdi E, Domercq M, Sanchez-Gomez MV, Perez-Samartin A, Rodriguez-Antiguedad A, Perez-Cerda F. 2007. Excitotoxic damage to white matter. *J Anat* 210:693-702.

Matute C, Sanchez-Gomez MV, Martinez-Millan L, Miledi R. 1997. Glutamate receptor-mediated toxicity in optic nerve oligodendrocytes. *Proc Natl Acad Sci U S A* 94:8830-5.

McDonald JW, Althomsons SP, Hyrc KL, Choi DW, Goldberg MP. 1998. Oligodendrocytes from forebrain are highly vulnerable to AMPA/kainate receptor-mediated excitotoxicity. *Nat Med* 4:291-7.

McQuillen PS, Ferriero DM. 2004. Selective vulnerability in the developing central nervous system. *Pediatric Neurology* 30:227-235.

Mehlhase J, Sandig G, Pantopoulos K, Grune T. 2005. Oxidation-induced ferritin turnover in microglial cells: role of proteasome. *Free Radical Biology and Medicine* 38:276-285.

Ment LR, Stewart WB, Fronc R, Seashore C, Mahooti S, Scaramuzzino D, Madri JA. 1997. Vascular endothelial growth factor mediates reactive angiogenesis in the postnatal developing brain. *Brain Res Dev Brain Res* 100:52-61.

Merrill JE, Benveniste EN. 1996. Cytokines in inflammatory brain lesions: helpful and harmful. *Trends Neurosci* 19:331-8.

Merrill JE, Ignarro LJ, Sherman MP, Melinek J, Lane TE. 1993. Microglial cell cytotoxicity of oligodendrocytes is mediated through nitric oxide. *J Immunol* 151:2132-41.

Micu I, Jiang Q, Coderre E, Ridsdale A, Zhang L, Woulfe J, Yin X, Trapp BD, McRory JE, Rehak R and others. 2006. NMDA receptors mediate calcium accumulation in myelin during chemical ischaemia. *Nature* 439:988-92.

Miller FD, Gauthier AS. 2007. Timing is everything: making neurons versus glia in the developing cortex. *Neuron* 54:357-69.

Miller RH, Raff MC. 1984. Fibrous and protoplasmic astrocytes are biochemically and developmentally distinct. *J Neurosci* 4:585-92.

Miller VM, Lawrence DA, Mondal TK, Seegal RF. 2009. Reduced glutathione is highly expressed in white matter and neurons in the unperturbed mouse brain--implications for oxidative stress associated with neurodegeneration. *Brain Res* 1276:22-30.

Mitrovic B, Ignarro LJ, Montestruque S, Smoll A, Merrill JE. 1994. Nitric-Oxide as a Potential Pathological Mechanism in Demyelination - Its Differential-Effects on Primary Glial-Cells in-Vitro. *Neuroscience* 61:575-585.

Miyawaki T, Matsui K, Takashima S. 1998. Developmental characteristics of vessel density in the human fetal and infant brains. *Early Hum Dev* 53:65-72.

Mollgard K, Saunders NR. 1986. The development of the human blood-brain and blood-CSF barriers. *Neuropathol Appl Neurobiol* 12:337-58.

Murphy GM, Jr., Zhao F, Yang L, Cordell B. 2000. Expression of macrophage colony-stimulating factor receptor is increased in the AbetaPP(V717F) transgenic mouse model of Alzheimer's disease. *Am J Pathol* 157:895-904.

Murphy S, Simmons ML, Agullo L, Garcia A, Feinstein DL, Galea E, Reis DJ, Minc-Golomb D, Schwartz JP. 1993. Synthesis of nitric oxide in CNS glial cells. *Trends Neurosci* 16:323-8.

Murugan M, Sivakumar V, Lu J, Ling EA, Kaur C. 2011. Expression of N-methyl D-aspartate receptor subunits in amoeboid microglia mediates production of nitric oxide via NF-kappaB signaling pathway and oligodendrocyte cell death in hypoxic postnatal rats. *Glia* 59:521-39.

Nagy JI, Li X, Rempel J, Stelmack G, Patel D, Staines WA, Yasumura T, Rash JE. 2001. Connexin26 in adult rodent central nervous system: demonstration at astrocytic gap junctions and colocalization with connexin30 and connexin43. *J Comp Neurol* 441:302-23.

Nagy JI, Patel D, Ochalski PA, Stelmack GL. 1999. Connexin30 in rodent, cat and human brain: selective expression in gray matter astrocytes, co-localization with connexin43 at gap junctions and late developmental appearance. N*euroscience* 88:447-68.

Nakamura Y, Okudera T, Hashimoto T. 1994. Vascular architecture in white matter of neonates: its relationship to periventricular leukomalacia. *J Neuropathol Exp Neurol* 53:582-9.

Nakazawa T, Nakazawa C, Matsubara A, Noda K, Hisatomi T, She H, Michaud N, Hafezi-Moghadam A, Miller JW, Benowitz LI. 2006. Tumor necrosis factor-alpha mediates oligodendrocyte death and delayed retinal ganglion cell loss in a mouse model of glaucoma. *J Neurosci* 26:12633-41.

Nery S, Wichterle H, Fishell G. 2001. Sonic hedgehog contributes to oligodendrocyte specification in the mammalian forebrain. *Development* 128:527-40.

Ness JK, Romanko MJ, Rothstein RP, Wood TL, Levison SW. 2001. Perinatal hypoxia-ischemia induces apoptotic and excitotoxic death of periventricular white matter oligodendrocyte progenitors. *Developmental Neuroscience* 23:203-208.

Ness JK, Scaduto RC, Jr., Wood TL. 2004. IGF-I prevents glutamate-mediated bax translocation and cytochrome C release in O4+ oligodendrocyte progenitors. *Glia* 46:183-94.

Ness JK, Wood TL. 2002. Insulin-like growth factor I, but not neurotrophin-3, sustains Akt activation and provides long-term protection of immature oligodendrocytes from glutamate-mediated apoptosis. *Mol Cell Neurosci* 20:476-88.

Noda M, Nakanishi H, Nabekura J, Akaike N. 2000. AMPA-kainate subtypes of glutamate receptor in rat cerebral microglia. *J Neurosci* 20:251-8.

Nosarti C, Rushe TM, Woodruff PW, Stewart AL, Rifkin L, Murray RM. 2004. Corpus callosum size and very preterm birth: relationship to neuropsychological outcome. *Brain* 127:2080-9.

Obonai T, Takashima S. 1998. In utero brain lesions in SIDS. Pediatric Neurology 19:23-25.

Oka A, Belliveau MJ, Rosenberg PA, Volpe JJ. 1993. Vulnerability of oligodendroglia to glutamate: pharmacology, mechanisms, and prevention. *J Neurosci* 13:1441-53.

Okoshi Y, Itoh M, Takashima S. 2001. Characteristic neuropathology and plasticity in periventricular leukomalacia. *Pediatr Neurol* 25:221-6.

O'Shea RD. 2002. Roles and regulation of glutamate transporters in the central nervous system. *Clin Exp Pharmacol Physiol* 29:1018-23.

Palmer C, Menzies SL, Roberts RL, Pavlick G, Connor JR. 1999. Changes in iron histochemistry after hypoxic-ischemic brain injury in the neonatal rat. *J Neurosci Res* 56:60-71.

Pan Y, Lloyd C, Zhou H, Dolich S, Deeds J, Gonzalo JA, Vath J, Gosselin M, Ma J, Dussault B and others. 1997. Neurotactin, a membrane-anchored chemokine upregulated in brain inflammation. *Nature* 387:611-7.

Pang Y, Cai Z, Rhodes PG. 2000. Effects of lipopolysaccharide on oligodendrocyte progenitor cells are mediated by astrocytes and microglia. *J Neurosci Res* 62:510-20.

Parys B, Cote A, Gallo V, De Koninck P, Sik A. 2010. Intercellular calcium signaling between astrocytes and oligodendrocytes via gap junctions in culture. *Neuroscience* 167:1032-43.

Pastor A, Kremer M, Moller T, Kettenmann H, Dermietzel R. 1998. Dye coupling between spinal cord oligodendrocytes: differences in coupling efficiency between gray and white matter. *Glia* 24:108-20.

Petito CK, Pulsinelli WA, Jacobson G, Plum F. 1982. Edema and vascular permeability in cerebral ischemia: comparison between ischemic neuronal damage and infarction. *J Neuropathol Exp Neurol* 41:423-36.

Pitt D, Nagelmeier IE, Wilson HC, Raine CS. 2003. Glutamate uptake by oligodendrocytes: Implications for excitotoxicity in multiple sclerosis. *Neurology* 61:1113-20.

Pitt D, Werner P, Raine CS. 2000. Glutamate excitotoxicity in a model of multiple sclerosis. *Nat Med* 6:67-70.

Qin L, Liu Y, Wang T, Wei SJ, Block ML, Wilson B, Liu B, Hong JS. 2004. NADPH oxidase mediates lipopolysaccharide-induced neurotoxicity and proinflammatory gene expression in activated microglia. *J Biol Chem* 279:1415-21.

Quandt FN, MacVicar BA. 1986. Calcium activated potassium channels in cultured astrocytes. *Neuroscience* 19:29-41.

Rahman I. 2003. Oxidative stress, chromatin remodeling and gene transcription in inflammation and chronic lung diseases. *J Biochem Mol Biol* 36:95-109.

Ransom CB, Liu X, Sontheimer H. 2003. Current transients associated with BK channels in human glioma cells. *J Membr Biol* 193:201-13.

Ransom CB, Ransom BR, Sontheimer H. 2000. Activity-dependent extracellular K+ accumulation in rat optic nerve: the role of glial and axonal Na+ pumps. *J Physiol* 522 Pt 3:427-42.

Rash JE, Yasumura T, Davidson KG, Furman CS, Dudek FE, Nagy JI. 2001. Identification of cells expressing Cx43, Cx30, Cx26, Cx32 and Cx36 in gap junctions of rat brain and spinal cord. *Cell Commun Adhes* 8:315-20.

Rathnasamy G, Ling EA, Kaur C. 2011. Iron and iron regulatory proteins in amoeboid microglial cells are linked to oligodendrocyte death in hypoxic neonatal rat periventricular white matter through production of proinflammatory cytokines and reactive oxygen/nitrogen species. *J Neurosci* 31:17982-95.

Raymond M, Li P, Mangin JM, Huntsman M, Gallo V. 2011. Chronic perinatal hypoxia reduces glutamate-aspartate transporter function in astrocytes through the Janus kinase/signal transducer and activator of transcription pathway. *J Neurosci* 31:17864-71.

Reid MV, Murray KA, Marsh ED, Golden JA, Simmons RA, Grinspan JB. 2012. Delayed myelination in an intrauterine growth retardation model is mediated by oxidative stress upregulating bone morphogenetic protein 4. *J Neuropathol Exp Neurol* 71:640-53.

Rezaie P, Dean A. 2002. Periventricular leukomalacia, inflammation and white matter lesions within the developing nervous system. *Neuropathology* 22:106-132.

Ridet JL, Malhotra SK, Privat A, Gage FH. 1997. Reactive astrocytes: cellular and molecular cues to biological function. *Trends Neurosci* 20:570-7.

Robinson MB, Dowd LA. 1997. Heterogeneity and functional properties of subtypes of sodium-dependent glutamate transporters in the mammalian central nervous system. *Adv Pharmacol* 37:69-115.

Ruiz A, Matute C, Alberdi E. 2010. Intracellular Ca2+ release through ryanodine receptors contributes to AMPA receptor-mediated mitochondrial dysfunction and ER stress in oligodendrocytes. *Cell Death Dis* 1:e54.

Salter MG, Fern R. 2005. NMDA receptors are expressed in developing oligodendrocyte processes and mediate injury. *Nature* 438:1167-71.

Sanchez-Gomez MV, Alberdi E, Ibarretxe G, Torre I, Matute C. 2003. Caspase-dependent and caspase-*independent oligodendrocyte death mediated by AMPA and kainate receptors. J Neurosci* 23:9519-28.

Sanchez-Gomez MV, Matute C. 1999. AMPA and kainate receptors each mediate excitotoxicity in oligodendroglial cultures. *Neurobiol Dis* 6:475-85.

Sankarapandi S, Zweier JL, Mukherjee G, Quinn MT, Huso DL. 1998. Measurement and characterization of superoxide generation in microglial cells: evidence for an NADPH oxidase-dependent pathway. *Arch Biochem Biophys* 353:312-21.

Saunders NR, Dziegielewska KM, Mollgard K. 1991. The importance of the blood-brain barrier in fetuses and embryos. *Trends Neurosci* 14:14-5.

Schwab ME, Bartholdi D. 1996. Degeneration and regeneration of axons in the lesioned spinal cord. *Physiol Rev* 76:319-70.

Shen S, Li J, Casaccia-Bonnefil P. 2005. Histone modifications affect timing of oligodendrocyte progenitor differentiation in the developing rat brain. *J Cell Biol* 169:577-89.

Shen Y, Liu XB, Pleasure DE, Deng W. 2012. Axon-glia synapses are highly vulnerable to white matter injury in the developing brain. *J Neurosci Res* 90:105-21.

Silverstein FS, Naik B, Simpson J. 1991. Hypoxia-ischemia stimulates hippocampal glutamate efflux in perinatal rat brain: an in vivo microdialysis study. *Pediatr Res* 30:587-90.

Simard M, Nedergaard M. 2004. The neurobiology of glia in the context of water and ion homeostasis. *Neuroscience* 129:877-96.

Sivakumar V, Ling EA, Lu J, Kaur C. 2010. Role of glutamate and its receptors and insulin-like growth factors in hypoxia induced periventricular white matter injury. *Glia* 58:507-23.

Skoff RP, Bessert DA, Barks JDE, Song DK, Cerghet M, Silverstein FS. 2001. Hypoxic-ischemic injury results in acute disruption of myelin gene expression and death of oligodendroglial precursors in neonatal mice. *International Journal of Developmental Neuroscience* 19:197-208.

Smith GM, Miller RH, Silver J. 1986. Changing role of forebrain astrocytes during development, regenerative failure, and induced regeneration upon transplantation. *J Comp Neurol* 251:23-43.

Sridhar K, Kumar P, Katariya S, Narang A. 2001. Postasphyxial encephalopathy in preterm neonates. *Indian J Pediatr* 68:1121-5.

Sriram K, Benkovic SA, Hebert MA, Miller DB, O'Callaghan JP. 2004. Induction of gp130-related cytokines and activation of JAK2/STAT3 pathway in astrocytes precedes up-regulation of glial fibrillary acidic protein in the 1-methyl-4-phenyl-1,2,3,6-tetrahydropyridine model of neurodegeneration: key signaling pathway for astrogliosis in vivo? *J Biol Chem* 279:19936-47.

Steinhauser C, Gallo V. 1996. News on glutamate receptors in glial cells. *Trends Neurosci* 19:339-45.

Stolt CC, Rehberg S, Ader M, Lommes P, Riethmacher D, Schachner M, Bartsch U, Wegner M. 2002. Terminal differentiation of myelin-forming oligodendrocytes depends on the transcription factor Sox10. *Genes Dev* 16:165-70.

Stys PK. 1998. Anoxic and ischemic injury of myelinated axons in CNS white matter: from mechanistic concepts to therapeutics. *J Cereb Blood Flow Metab* 18:2-25.

Sullivan SM, Bjorkman ST, Miller SM, Colditz PB, Pow DV. 2010. Morphological changes in white matter astrocytes in response to hypoxia/ischemia in the neonatal pig. *Brain Res* 1319:164-74.

Sunnemark D, Eltayeb S, Wallstrom E, Appelsved L, Malmberg A, Lassmann H, Ericsson-Dahlstrand A, Piehl F, Olsson T. 2003. Differential expression of the chemokine receptors CX3CR1 and CCR1 by microglia and macrophages in myelin-oligodendrocyte-glycoprotein-induced experimental autoimmune encephalomyelitis. *Brain Pathol* 13:617-29.

Takahashi JL, Giuliani F, Power C, Imai Y, Yong VW. 2003. Interleukin-1beta promotes oligodendrocyte death through glutamate excitotoxicity. *Ann Neurol* 53:588-95.

Takashima S, Tanaka K. 1978. Microangiography and vascular permeability of the subependymal matrix in the premature infant. *Can J Neurol Sci* 5:45-50.

Theriault E, Frankenstein UN, Hertzberg EL, Nagy JI. 1997. Connexin43 and astrocytic gap junctions in the rat spinal cord after acute compression injury. *J Comp Neurol* 382:199-214.

Thomas JL, Spassky N, Perez Villegas EM, Olivier C, Cobos I, Goujet-Zalc C, Martinez S, Zalc B. 2000. Spatiotemporal development of oligodendrocytes in the embryonic brain. *J Neurosci Res* 59:471-6.

Thrane AS, Rappold PM, Fujita T, Torres A, Bekar LK, Takano T, Peng W, Wang F, Thrane VR, Enger R and others. 2011. Critical role of aquaporin-4 (AQP4) in astrocytic Ca2+ signaling events elicited by cerebral edema. *Proc Natl Acad Sci U S A* 108:846-51.

Tzarouchi LC, Astrakas LG, Zikou A, Xydis V, Kosta P, Andronikou S, Argyropoulou MI. 2009. Periventricular leukomalacia in preterm children: assessment of grey and white matter and cerebrospinal fluid changes by MRI. *Pediatr Radiol* 39:1327-32.

Vaddi K, Keller M, Newton RC. 1997. The chemokine factsbook. San Diego: Academic Press.

van der Goes A, Brouwer J, Hoekstra K, Roos D, van den Berg TK, Dijkstra CD. 1998. Reactive oxygen species are required for the phagocytosis of myelin by macrophages. *J Neuroimmunol* 92:67-75.

van Neerven S, Nemes A, Imholz P, Regen T, Denecke B, Johann S, Beyer C, Hanisch UK, Mey J. 2010. Inflammatory cytokine release of astrocytes in vitro is reduced by all-trans retinoic acid. *J Neuroimmunol* 229:169-79.

Vannucci RC, Vannucci SJ. 2005. Perinatal hypoxic-ischemic brain damage: evolution of an animal model. *Dev Neurosci* 27:81-6.

Vela JM, Molina-Holgado E, Arevalo-Martin A, Almazan G, Guaza C. 2002. Interleukin-1 regulates proliferation and differentiation of oligodendrocyte progenitor cells. *Mol Cell Neurosci* 20:489-502.

Vincent VA, Tilders FJ, Van Dam AM. 1998. Production, regulation and role of nitric oxide in glial cells. *Mediators Inflamm* 7:239-55.

Volpe JJ. 2000. Overview: normal and abnormal human brain development. *Ment Retard Dev Disabil Res Rev* 6:1-5.

Volpe JJ. 2001. Neurobiology of periventricular leukomalacia in the premature infant. *Pediatr Res* 50:553-62.

Volpe JJ. 2003. Cerebral white matter injury of the premature infant - More common than you think. *Pediatrics* 112:176-180.

Volpe JJ. 2009. Brain injury in premature infants: a complex amalgam of destructive and developmental disturbances. *Lancet Neurol* 8:110-24.

Wallin C, Puka-Sundvall M, Hagberg H, Weber SG, Sandberg M. 2000. Alterations in glutathione and amino acid concentrations after hypoxia-ischemia in the immature rat brain. *Brain Res Dev Brain Res* 125:51-60.

Wang KK, Nath R, Raser KJ, Hajimohammadreza I. 1996. Maitotoxin induces calpain activation in SH-SY5Y neuroblastoma cells and cerebrocortical cultures. *Arch Biochem Biophys* 331:208-14.

Wang X, Li C, Chen Y, Hao Y, Zhou W, Chen C, Yu Z. 2008. Hypoxia enhances CXCR4 expression favoring microglia migration via HIF-1alpha activation. *Biochem Biophys Res Commun* 371:283-8.

Welin AK, Sandberg M, Lindblom A, Arvidsson P, Nilsson UA, Kjellmer I, Mallard C. 2005. White matter injury following prolonged free radical formation in the 0.65 gestation fetal sheep brain. *Pediatr Res* 58:100-5.

Werner P, Pitt D, Raine CS. 2001. Multiple sclerosis: altered glutamate homeostasis in lesions correlates with oligodendrocyte and axonal damage. *Ann Neurol* 50:169-80.

Wilson-Costello D, Friedman H, Minich N, Fanaroff AA, Hack M. 2005. Improved survival rates with increased neurodevelopmental disability for extremely low birth weight infants in the 1990s. *Pediatrics* 115:997-1003.

World Health Organization; March of Dimes; The Partnership for Maternal NCHStC. 2012. World Health Organization; March of Dimes; The Partnership for Maternal, Newborn and Child Health; Save the Children. World Health Organization technical report series.

Wu CY, Kaur C, Sivakumar V, Lu J, Ling EA. 2009. Kv1.1 expression in microglia regulates production and release of proinflammatory cytokines, endothelins and nitric oxide. *Neuroscience* 158:1500-8.

Yan YP, Sailor KA, Lang BT, Park SW, Vemuganti R, Dempsey RJ. 2007. Monocyte chemoattractant protein-1 plays a critical role in neuroblast migration after focal cerebral ischemia. *J Cereb Blood Flow Metab* 27:1213-24.

Yoon BH, Romero R, Kim CJ, Koo JN, Choe G, Syn HC, Chi JG. 1997. High expression of tumor necrosis factor-alpha and interleukin-6 in periventricular leukomalacia. *Am J Obstet Gynecol* 177:406-11.

Yoshioka A, Bacskai B, Pleasure D. 1996. Pathophysiology of oligodendroglial excitotoxicity. *J Neurosci Res* 46:427-37.

Yoshioka A, Hardy M, Younkin DP, Grinspan JB, Stern JL, Pleasure D. 1995. Alpha-amino-3-hydroxy-5-methyl-4-isoxazolepropionate (AMPA) receptors mediate excitotoxicity in the oligodendroglial lineage. *J Neurochem* 64:2442-8.

You Y, Kaur C. 2000. Expression of induced nitric oxide synthase in amoeboid microglia in postnatal rats following an exposure to hypoxia. *Neurosci Lett* 279:101-4.

Zawadzka M, Kaminska B. 2003. Immunosuppressant FK506 affects multiple signaling pathways and modulates gene expression in astrocytes. *Mol Cell Neurosci* 22:202-9.

Zekry D, Epperson TK, Krause KH. 2003. A role for NOX NADPH oxidases in Alzheimer's disease and other types of dementia? *IUBMB Life* 55:307-13.

Zhou Q, Anderson DJ. 2002. The bHLH transcription factors OLIG2 and OLIG1 couple neuronal and glial subtype specification. *Cell* 109:61-73.

Zhu L, Ramboz S, Hewitt D, Boring L, Grass DS, Purchio AF. 2004. Non-invasive imaging of GFAP expression after neuronal damage in mice. *Neurosci Lett* 367:210-2.

In: Glial Cells
Editors: Charanjit Kaur and Eng-Ang Ling
ISBN: 978-1-62618-448-0
© 2013 Nova Science Publishers, Inc.

Chapter 3

ROLE OF MICROGLIA AND ASTROCYTES IN THE PROCESS OF NEUROINFLAMMATION

Anna K. Bal-Price [*] ***and Agnieszka Kinsner-Ovaskainen***
Institute for Health and Consumer Protection,
European Commission Joint Research Centre,
Ispra, VA, Italy

ABSTRACT

Microglial activation represents an increasingly important concept in the pathogenesis of neurodegenerative disorders such as Alzheimer and Parkinson disease, as well as in stroke, traumatic brain injury, demyelinating conditions and pathology associated with CNS infections. At the same time the CNS appears to show marked resistance to inflammation in response to a number of stimuli as compared with peripheral tissues.

These differences reflect the tight regulatory environment of the brain and a balance between inflammation-induced tissue repair and tissue damage. The major resident inflammatory cells in the CNS are microglia. These cells are especially important to guard the integrity and homeostasis of the brain.

In normal conditions they are quiescent cells, but become activated by injury or infection and have been suggested to represent the first line of defence for the CNS. One of the most remarkable properties of microglia is their ability to react to a stress signal from the inside (e.g. stressed or damaged cells, cytokines) as well as from outside (e.g. pathogens) and to direct their reaction for the purpose of tissue repair and for further induction of protective immune responses.

Therefore, the activation of microglia is an important host defence mechanism. However, when the state of glia activation is becoming chronic then activated microglia release various pro-inflammatory cytokines such as tumour necrosis factor-α (TNF-α), interleukin-1β (IL-1β), interleukin-6 (IL-6) (Thomas 1992; Kreutzberg 1996; El Khoury et al. 1998; Aloisi 2001), chemokines (IL-8, MIP-1α, MIP-1β, MCP-1) (Peterson et al.

[*] Corresponding author: Dr Anna Bal-Price;; Institute for Health and Consumer Protection; European Commission JRC, TP 580; Via Fermi 2749, 21027 Ispra (VA), Italy; Tel.: +39 0332 78 6018; Fax: +39 0332 78 5336; Email:anna.price@jrc.ec.europa.eu.

1997; Ehrlich et al. 1998), proteases (Nakanishi 2003), as well as oxidative and nitrosative free radicals (superoxide, nitric oxide, peroxynitrite) leading to the neuronal cell death.

On the other hand microglia can also produce anti-inflammatory mediators, such as TGF-β, PGE_2 and IL-1 receptor antagonist (IL-1ra) (Benveniste et al. 2001) and due to their ability of phagocytosis they can also play the role of scavengers for macromolecules and apoptotic or damaged brain cells as well as pathogens.

In addition to microglia, also the role of astrocytes has to be considered in the context of brain inflammation. Astrocytes are not commonly associated with immunological reactions, and it is well accepted that their role in CNS immunity is largely regulatory.

In this chapter the role or microglia and astrocytes in neuroinflammation involved in the various CNS pathologies will be discussed including the characterization of the inflammatory mediators and the mechanisms of inflammatory-induced neuronal cell death.

1. Characterization of Inflammation in the Central Nervous System (CNS)

The CNS has evolved both anatomically and physiologically to protect its vital functions from damaging immune-mediated inflammation and traditionally has been regarded as immunologically privileged. Nevertheless, increasing evidence indicates that inflammation is involved in the pathogenesis of several neurodegenerative diseases such as Alzheimer's disease, Parkinson's disease, stroke, traumatic brain injury, demyelinating disorders, as well as brain damage associated with CNS infections.

1.1. Specific Aspects of CNS Inflammation

Inflammation in the CNS has several distinct features and the response to pathogenic insults in the brain differs from classical inflammatory response seen in other tissues. An important element in the maintenance of physiological and immunological homeostasis is the blood-brain barrier that restricts the entry of pathogens, plasma proteins and immune cells into the brain parenchyma. Moreover, the types of cells mediating inflammation are quite distinct in the brain tissue as compared to the periphery. During brain inflammation there is little neutrophil recruitment and the major resident inflammatory cells are microglia, which represent the brain macrophages, and astrocytes, shown to release many pro-inflammatory mediators (cytokines, nitric oxide and reactive oxygen species).

The CNS was shown to be markedly resistant to damage in response to a number of pro-inflammatory stimuli. As an example, the acute response of brain parenchyma to a classical pro-inflammatory agent, bacterial lipopolysaccharide (LPS) differs from peripheral tissues (Montero-Menei et al. 1994). Experimental studies in rodents demonstrate that LPS induces a rapid and massive invasion of neutrophils in the skin, but a limited and delayed response in the brain with little signs of vascular reaction and no neutrophil recruitment at any time (Perry and Andersson 1992). The main cells that become activated and dominate the cellular response in the CNS upon LPS treatment are microglia.

Other mechanisms that were proposed to contribute to CNS immune privilege are the local production of anti-inflammatory mediators, e.g., transforming growth factor beta (TGF-β) (Dhandapani and Brann 2003), α-melanocyte-stimulating hormone (α-MSH) (Ter Laak et al. 2003) and vasoactive intestinal peptide (VIP) (Gozes et al. 2003), and the constitutive expression of Fas ligand (FasL) which is responsible for Fas-mediated apoptosis of CNS infiltrating immune cells (Flugel et al. 2000).

Although all the features described above may limit immune-mediated events within the CNS parenchyma, it is now accepted that the brain responds to peripheral inflammatory stimuli, integrates many aspects of the acute phase response and exhibits local inflammatory responses which are crucial for the elimination of pathogens, removal of dead cells and tissue repair. Therefore, a proper balance between pro- and anti-inflammatory processes is important, and an extensive, prolonged neuroinflammation can contribute to both acute and chronic CNS diseases.

1.2. Immunocompetent Cells in the CNS

The CNS is constantly surveyed by a well-developed network of innate immune cells that control all portals of entry of blood-derived pathogens into the brain parenchyma. Macrophages and dendritic cells have been identified in the meninges and choroid plexus, in strategic locations that guard the ventricular/subarachnoid compartment (McMenamin 1999). Perivascular macrophages, which surround small and medium size cerebral vessels, ensure protection of the CNS at the level of the blood-brain barrier displaying phagocytic and immune regulatory functions (Williams et al. 2001). However, if the inflammatory stimulus (e.g. a pathogen or its components) crosses the blood-brain barrier, the CNS parenchyma itself contains other cells – the glial cells – that are capable of reacting to immunological stimuli or neuronal injury, and play an active role in the development of neuroinflammation.

Glial cells are generally classified into two groups: 1) macroglia, which include astrocytes and oligodendrocytes, of ectodermal origin, and 2) microglia, of mesodermal origin, that migrate into the CNS during embryonic development at the time of vascularization (Raine 1999). Glial cells differ morphologically and functionally from the neurons. They do not form synaptic contacts (and therefore cannot transmit transmits information by electrical and chemical signalling) and retain the ability to divide throughout life. The main roles of glial cells include 1) maintaining the ionic milieu of nerve cells, 2) modulating the rate of nerve signal propagation, 3) modulating synaptic action by controlling the uptake of neurotransmitters, 4) providing a scaffold for neural development, and 5) aiding in (or preventing, in some instances) the recovery from neural injury (Raine 1999).

Oligodendrocytes are restricted to the CNS; these cells produce a laminated, lipid-rich wrapping called myelin around some neuronal axons; myelin plays an important role in the conduction of action potential in neurons (increases the speed of potential propagation). Due to the particular role in neuroinflammation, only astrocytes and microglia will be discussed more in detail in the following sections.

1.2.1. Microglia

The major resident inflammatory cells in the CNS are microglia. These are macrophage-like cells, derived from monocytes that populate the brain and spinal cord early during the development, and remain within the CNS as the resident macrophage population. Microglia comprise up to 20% of the total non-neuronal cell population (Davis et al. 1994). These cells are especially important to guard the integrity and homeostasis of the brain. In normal conditions they are quiescent, but become activated by injury or infection and have been suggested to represent the first line of defence for the CNS, which normally lacks professional antigen presenting cells (APCs) and intraparenchymal leukocytes, until they are recruited by pro-inflammatory stimuli (Kreutzberg 1996).

Microglia have several morphological forms depending on their functional and developmental state (Figure 1). During embryonic development monocytes migrate to the CNS and convert into an intermediate form, amoeboid cells, with flat morphology and pseudopodia. It is a transient population present during the late prenatal to early postnatal period. Microglia present in adult brain are called ramified microglia. These cells have a small (5-10 μm) oval cell body with large nucleus and only a little amount of cytoplasm, as well as numerous long, branched processes. Ramified microglia have been characterised as down-regulated (or inactive) macrophages, as they lack most of the characteristic markers and activities of this group (lack of phagocytic and endocytic activity, low expression of leukocyte common antigen (CD45), low levels of membrane ligands and receptors that are essential for mediating or inducing typical macrophage functions) (Davis et al. 1994).

One of the most remarkable properties of microglia is to react to stress signals from the inside (e.g. stressed or damaged cells, cytokines), as well as from outside (e.g. pathogens), to direct their reaction for the purpose of tissue repair and induce protective immune responses. Following the stimulus (e.g. neuronal injury) microglia migrate to the damaged sites of the CNS where they proliferate and become activated. During this process microglia undergo maturation, leading to the acquisition of macrophage differentiation markers and effector properties. They can assume two distinct forms – activated and reactive microglia (Davis et al. 1994). Activated microglia appear like swollen ramified cells and are characterised by a larger cell body with shorter processes. They are practically active macrophages, as they express CR3 complement receptors and class I major histocompatibility complex (MHC) antigens. Reactive microglia are typically small, spherical cells and lack ramified processes. They are fully active macrophages with increased CR3 receptor and class I MHC, as well as expression of class II MHC, thus the ability to present antigens to T-cells. The different forms of brain microglia are schematically presented in Figure 1.

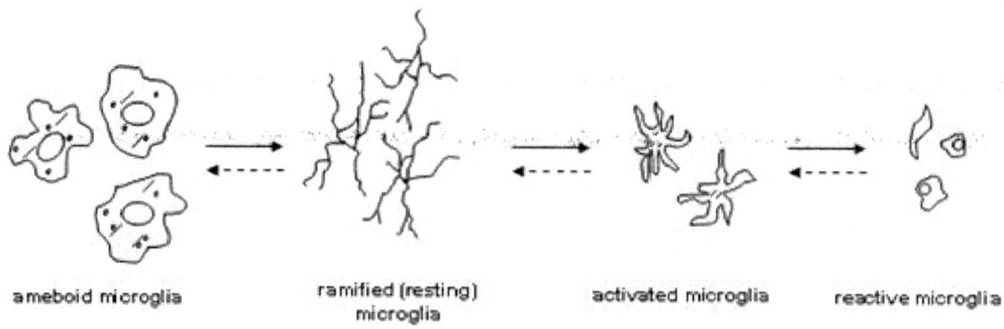

Figure 1. Different cell morphology of brain microglia (resting, activated, reactive).

The activation of microglia is an important host defence mechanism. Activated microglia release various pro-inflammatory cytokines such as tumour necrosis factor-α (TNF-α), interleukin-1β (IL-1β), interleukin-6 (IL-6) (Kreutzberg 1996; Aloisi 2001), chemokines (IL-8, MIP-1α, MIP-1β, MCP-1) (Ehrlich et al. 1998), proteases (Nakanishi 2003), as well as oxidative and nitrosative free radicals (superoxide, nitric oxide, peroxynitrite). Due to their ability of phagocytosis microglia play also the role of scavengers for macromolecules and apoptotic or damaged brain cells as well as pathogens.

Upon activation microglia acquire several innate immune functions, including the induction and regulation of T-cell responses. They are able to act as antigen presenting cells (APCs) and to influence the intracerebral balance of T-helper Th_1 and Th_2 cell-mediated immune responses (Aloisi 2001). In the normal CNS parenchyma the expression of major histocompatibility complex (MHC) antigens is generally very low (Hayes et al. 1987) and resting microglia behave as poor APC, but in virtually all inflammatory and neurodegenerative conditions they become activated and express MHC class II (Kreutzberg 1996).

A constitutive and inducible expression of a variety of other surface receptors is indispensable for microglia to exhibit a proper response to a number of infectious and inflammatory stimuli. The receptors include: 1) pattern recognition receptors (Toll-like receptors, CD14) implicated in the recognition of pathogen associated molecules (such as Gram-positive and Gram-negative bacterial components, viral RNA and proteins, pathogen DNA etc.); 2) complement receptors (called also opsonic receptors), which mediate or enhance phagocytosis; 3) cytokine and chemokine receptors (for both pro- and anti-inflammatory cytokines); these receptors regulate immune functions of microglia (Aloisi 2001).

Although microglia represent the first line of defence in the brain, the activation of these cells can also have negative effects. The inflammatory mediators released from activated microglia can contribute to CNS damage as neurotoxins (Aloisi 2001), and enhance the onset and progression of CNS diseases. Zhang and Fedoroff (1996) showed that in co-culture with neurons, microglial cells at a low degree of activation supported the neuronal survival, but when these microglia were pre-treated with LPS, a known strong activator of immune cells, intensive neurotoxicity was found. The harmful effects of microglia activated with bacterial cell wall components (LPS; lipoteichoic acid, LTA) on neurons cultured *in vitro* were also shown by other authors (Bal-Price and Brown 2001; Kinsner et al., 2005). Therefore, microglial activation can influence the extent of brain injury following an inflammatory stimulus and it is important to control the degree and duration of inflammation in the CNS. Excessive or chronic microglial activation has been implicated in a number of neurodegenerative diseases, such as Alzheimer's disease, Parkinson's disease (McGeer and McGeer 2004; Blasko et al. 2004), as well as trauma, ischemia, brain tumours and infectious diseases (Neumann 2003). Microglia are also involved in several other immune response processes including rejection of transplanted tissue, autoimmune CNS diseases (e.g. multiple sclerosis) and AIDS-associated dementia complex.

1.2.2. Astrocytes

One of the important functions of activated astrocytes is the involvement in the immune functions in the CNS. Several studies performed both *in vivo* (where the expression of a particular molecule or its mRNA was co-localized to reactive astrocytes) as well as *in vitro* (using primary cultures of astrocytes), have demonstrated that activated astrocytes produce a large variety of molecules, which are involved in the initiation and regulation of the inflammatory response. These include several pro- and anti-inflammatory cytokines (IL-1, TNF-α, IL-6, TGF-α, TGF-β), chemokines (IL-8) and eicosanoids (leukotriens B_4 and C_4, prostaglandin E, thromboxanes A_2 and B_2) (Xu et al. 2003; Mrak and Griffin 2005). Activation of astrocytes leads also to the expression of inducible nitric oxide synthase (iNOS) (Brown and Bal-Price 2003). Activated astrocytes express molecules involved in immune responses such as major histocompatibility complex antigens (MHC) (Hoftberger et al. 2004) and are able to present antigens to T lymphocytes. Moreover, they up-regulate the expression of several adhesion molecules (selectins, integrins, adherins), which play a role in the migration of leukocytes through the blood-brain barrier into the CNS parenchyma (Prat et al. 2001; Dietrich 2002).

Apart from being involved in CNS inflammation astrocytes rapidly react to other neurological insults. A series of changes that occur in astrocytes upon activation has a common name of astrocytosis. The main feature of astrocytosis is the increase in the number and size of glial fibrillary acidic protein (GFAP)-expressing cells. GFAP is an intermediate filament cytoskeletal protein considered to be the marker of astrocytes (Raine 1999). The precise function of GFAP molecule is still not clear, as well as it has not yet been established whether the increase in GFAP levels is a result of enhanced production of this protein by the cells or an increase in the number of astrocytes either due to proliferation or migration. Studies using double labelling with GFAP antibodies and bromodeoxyuridine failed to show, at least in acute lesions, mitotic divisions of GFAP-expressing cells (Norton et al. 1992). Furthermore there is no convincing evidence that GFAP-positive cells of adult brain are able to migrate. Therefore it is likely that the appearance of GFAP-positive astrocytes in regions of acute neuronal injury is primarily due to a change in phenotype. Astroglial proliferation, however, cannot be excluded in chronic astrocytosis. Reactive astrocytes form a glial scar in areas of tissue necrosis, excluding the non-neuronal cells from parenchyma and filling in the space which results from neuronal loss (McGraw et al. 2001). They also produce proteases and protease inhibitors (e.g. matrix metalloproteinases), which allow them to remodel the extracellular matrix at sites of neuronal injury and to clear the debris of degenerating cells (Gardner and Ghorpade 2003; Wu et al. 2004). Prominent reactive astrocytosis was found in AIDS dementia complex, a variety of viral infections, prion-associated spongiform encephalopaties, inflammatory demyelinating diseases, acute traumatic brain injury, ischemia (Swanson et al. 2004) and neurodegenerative diseases (e.g. Alzheimer's disease) (Mrak and Griffin 2005).

The primary function of astrocytes is to provide structural, metabolic and trophic support to other cells (Raine 1999). Astrocytes act as a bridge to supply nutrients from blood capillaries to neurons and provide the major site of glycogen storage in the brain. Moreover, they are also able to synthesise and secrete a variety of neurotrophic and growth factors such as nerve growth factor (NGF), brain-derived neurotrophic factor (BDNF), ciliary neurotrophic factor (CNTF) and insulin-like growth factor-1 (IGF-1), which may be beneficial for neuronal survival (Moretto et al. 1994; Rudge et al. 1994).

Astrocytes are responsible for maintaining a homeostatic environment in the brain by: 1) "buffering" or clearance of K^+ released from electrically active neurons (Walz 2000); 2) detoxification of synaptically released glutamate by uptake and metabolic mechanisms (Bezzi et al. 1999); 3) regulation of extracellular ionic gradients and pH (Lascola and Kraig 1997); 4) clearance and metabolism of arachidonic acid (Staub et al. 1995). Astrocytes may also provide glutathione precursors to neurons as they protect neurons against the oxidative stress in a co-culture system (Dringen et al. 2000).

Astrocytes not only support neuronal survival, they may also modulate neuronal signalling (Chvatal and Sykova 2000). Studies of Murphy et al. (1993) and Nedergaard (1994) showed that there is a direct communication between astrocytes and neurons in cultures of brain cells, probably through gap-junction channels (Froes et al. 1999). Moreover, there is growing evidence that astrocytes play an active role in synaptic transmission, not directly forming synaptic contacts, but contributing to the physiological functioning of neurons by the integration of neuronal inputs, exhibition of calcium excitability and modulation of neighbouring neuronal responses (Araque et al. 1999; Araque et al. 2001).

Astrocytes are also essential for the morphological and physiological formation of a functional blood brain barrier in the CNS. The concept of a blood-brain barrier (BBB), which separates the brain from the rest of the body, was developed by Paul Ehlrich in 1906, when he has experimentally shown that some dyes administered intravenously to rats stain all the organs except the brain (Sukriti 2003). The BBB is a physical barrier between blood vessels in the CNS and the brain tissue that plays an important role in the protection of the CNS. It is formed by non-fenestrated endothelial cells that develop tight junctions among adjacent cells providing an increased resistance to passage of solutes between cells. *In vitro* studies have demonstrated that endothelial cells alone, without the presence of astrocytes, cannot provide a tight barrier (Risau et al. 1998). Several studies suggest that astrocytes secrete soluble factors essential for the development of specific BBB properties (Sobue et al. 1999). The presence of a continuous sheet of astrocyte end feet around the capillaries results in a tight interaction between cerebral astrocytes and endothelial cells. This interaction results in a change in morphology and function of the cerebrovascular endothelium, and is especially important for the maturation and differentiation of tight junctions between endothelial cells (Prat et al. 2001; Abbott 2002), induction of specific metabolic properties of the endothelial cells, such as the expression of alkaline phosphatase and γ-glutamyltransferase (Roux et al. 1994).

The nature of the BBB can vary depending on the location. Certain areas of the brain, associated with ventricular organs and areas of endocrine regulation, commonly known as circumventricular system, have an extensive vasculature and lack of a normal lack the BBB. The integrity of the BBB can be also altered in some pathological conditions such as infection (bacterial, viral, parasitic), inflammation, brain injury, tumours and hypertensive encephalopathy, as well as by some drugs and hyperosmotic agents (e.g. mannitol). In these conditions, the increase in BBB permeability may allow access of leukocytes into the brain parenchyma where they can release neurotoxins, activate endogenous inflammatory processes or, in the case of macrophages, phagocytose cell debris.

2. Mediators of Inflammation in the CNS

Most of the key mediators of inflammation identified in the peripheral tissues are also expressed in the inflamed brain. The primary mediators of inflammation include cytokines, chemokines, eicosanoids, platelet activating factor (PAF), reactive oxygen species (ROS) and nitric oxide (NO). All these factors have been reported to be expressed and/or released by glial cells in the response to insult to the CNS *in vivo* and *in vitro*.

2.1. Cytokines

Cytokines are signalling molecules (secreted, cell-membrane associated or stored in the extracellular matrix) that transmit signals from the extracellular environment to the nucleus through specific receptors and intracellular signal transduction or second messenger molecular pathways. They are key regulators of innate and adaptive immune responses. A number of cytokines are induced in the brain in response to cerebral ischemia, injury, infectious and autoimmune diseases; they include the pro-inflammatory IL-1α, IL-1β, IL-2, IL-6, IL-8 and TNF-α, as well as some anti-inflammatory cytokines such as TGF-β, IL-10 (Aloisi 2001). The sources of cytokines in the CNS are mainly microglia and astrocytes, but also tissue infiltrating immune cells and CNS-associated macrophages (Raivich and Banati 2004). Receptors for most cytokines have been described in the CNS, some of them at very low level, although rapid up-regulation can occur after injury (Szelenyi 2001).

2.1.1. Pro-inflammatory cytokines

The two main pro-inflammatory cytokines with pleiotropic and largely overlapping functions are TNF-α and IL-1β. Intracerebrally produced TNF-α can be involved in initiating CNS tissue destruction and inflammation (Akassoglou et al. 1998). TNF-α induced neurotoxicity was observed *in vivo*, as mice overexpressing TNF-α developed neuropathological symptoms (Probert et al. 1995). *In vitro*, TNF-α has been shown to stimulate secretion of glutamate from glial cells (Piani and Fontana 1994) and to potentiate glutamate neurotoxicity in human foetal brain cells (Chao and Hu 1994).

Two different TNF-α receptors have been characterised: TNF-RI (or p55), mediating most actions of soluble TNF-α and known to induce apoptosis, and TNF-RII (p75), more sensitive to transmembranous TNF-α and shown to have anti-apoptotic effects (Pan et al. 1997). Moreover, members of the TNF-receptor family activate several transcription factors, including NF-κB, which themselves induce the transcription of mediators of inflammation (Koedel et al. 2000).

IL-1β induces inflammatory effects similar to TNF-α. In many CNS diseases IL-1β concentrations have been shown to correlate significantly with TNF-α concentrations and with neurological complications (van Deuren 1994; Jain et al. 2000). Convincing evidence suggests a prominent role of IL-1β in acute neuronal injury. Increased expression of IL-1β is seen in the CNS after a variety of brain insults and administration of exogenous IL-1β to animals undergoing ischemic or excitotoxic challenges leads to a dramatic increase in cell death. On the other hand, the administration of a selective IL-1 receptor antagonist (IL-1ra) markedly reduces the extent of cell death induced by ischemic or excitotoxic injury in rats (Hailer et al. 2005). Similarly, inhibition of caspase-1 (which is required for the release of active IL-1β) and the administration of anti-IL-1β antibodies, have been also shown to decrease neuronal injury (Rothwell and Luheshi 2000; Touzani et al. 2002). Recent studies have employed transgenic animals with specific modifications of selected genes to investigate the contribution of inflammation to neurodegeneration. Mice deficient in pro-inflammatory cytokines (Ohtaki et al. 2003) show a reduction in cell death in response to different insults when compared to their wild-type counterparts, whereas in mice deficient in anti-inflammatory cytokines neuronal injury is increased (Grilli et al. 2000).

TNF-α and IL-1β are known to cause blood-brain barrier breakdown, mainly through their ability to induce in cerebrovascular endothelial cells and astrocytes the expression of adhesion molecules and of chemokines, which facilitate leukocyte extravasation and recruitment into the CNS (Sedgwick et al. 2000). Intrathecal injection of TNF-α or IL-1β leads to blood-brain barrier injury, influx of leukocytes and serum proteins across the BBB into the CSF, brain oedema, increase in intracranial pressure and CSF lactate levels, reduction in cerebral oxygen uptake and in cerebral blood flow, and neuronal apoptosis (Allan 2000; Allan and Rothwell 2001). Both cytokines also up-regulate endothelial derived adhesion molecules (P-selectin, E-selecin) in cerebral vasculature, which promotes the recruitment of granulocytes to the site of inflammation (Tang et al. 1996). TNF-α and IL-1β have been shown to induce the expression of iNOS and trigger the release of NO from glial cells, as well as vascular endothelium (Bonmann et al. 1997). TNF-α and IL-1β are also known to induce glial reactions and to promote astrogliosis and microgliosis (Herx and Yong 2001; Basu et al. 2002).

Another cytokine produced in the CNS by microglia and astrocytes is interleukin-6 (IL-6), a multifunctional mediator, which plays an important role in cell-cell signalling under normal and pathophysiological conditions (Gruol and Nelson 1997). IL-6 can exert both pro- and anti-inflammatory effects (Gadient and Otten 1997). The levels of IL-6, which are low in the normal brain, are strongly up-regulated following brain injury or inflammation *in vivo* (Clark et al. 1999), and in response to LPS or TNF-α treatment *in vitro* (Gruol and Nelson 1997). In the brain, IL-6 has mainly a neurotrophic and neuroprotective role (Chao et al. 1995). Both *in vitro* and *in vivo* studies demonstrated that IL-6 promotes survival of neurons against several neurotoxic agents (glutamate, MPP+, NMDA), presumably through inhibition of apoptosis (Hirota et al. 1996; Umegaki et al. 1996). Apart from its protective effects on neurons, IL-6 can also mediate glial activation and has mitogenic effects on astrocytes cultured *in vitro* (Selmaj et al. 1990). Severe astrogliosis and increased microglial reactions were observed in mice overexpressing IL-6.

In the CNS glial cells are considered the major sources of cytokines that stimulate the humoral and cell-mediated immune responses, such as IL-12 (Aloisi et al. 1997), and IL-18 (Prinz and Hanisch 1999). These cytokines are produced during infections and autoimmune diseases and are critically involved in the development of Experimental Allergic Encephalomyelitis (EAE), an animal model of multiple sclerosis (Segal et al. 1998; Shevach et al. 1999).

2.1.2. Anti-Inflammatory Cytokines

Although most studies concentrate on glia-derived pro-inflammatory cytokines, attention has been devoted also to the role of CNS cells in the processes that down-modulate inflammation and immunity. Microglia were shown to produce anti-inflammatory cytokines, such as TGF-β, IL-10, and IL-1 receptor antagonist (IL-1ra), whereas astrocytes secrete TGF-β and IL-10 (Kiefer et al. 1998; Liu et al. 1998; De Groot et al. 1999; Aloisi et al. 1999). IL-1ra has a major role in counteracting the biological effects of IL-1, thanks to its ability to bind to IL-1 receptor I (IL-1RI) without initiating signal transduction, and thus blocking the IL-1 receptor. IL-10 was found in large amounts in the CSF during bacterial meningitis (van Furth et al. 1995). It inhibits the production of IL-1β, IL-6, IL-8 and TNF-α by monocytes and the release of reactive oxygen species (ROS) by macrophages (Bogdan et al. 1991; Cunha et al. 1992). TGF-β is also an anti-inflammatory cytokine that can deactivate microglia by suppressing the release of hydrogen peroxide (Tsunawaki et al. 1988) and nitric oxide (Matsuno et al. 2001). It also inhibits endothelial granulocyte adhesion and the production of several cytokines including IL-1, TNF-α, IL-6 and IFN-γ. In addition, TGF-β protects neurons from N-methyl-D-aspartate (NMDA) induced calcium overload and from excitotoxic death (Hailer et al. 2001), as well as from β-amyloid induced neurotoxicity (Chao et al. 1994). TGF-β, IL-4 and IL-10 are known to inhibit microglia activation, down-regulate the expression of molecules associated with antigen presentation on these cells, and inhibit the production of pro-inflammatory cytokines, chemokines, nitrogen and oxygen radicals (Aloisi et al. 1999; O'Keefe et al. 1999).

2.2. Chemokines

Chemokines are a group of cytokines that play a major role in the recruitment of leukocytes from the blood into the CNS and the migration of some cells, including microglia.

Chemokines are a superfamily of small peptides, which based on the cysteine motif are divided into four families (CXC, CC, C, and CX3C). They interact with receptors that have seven G protein coupled transmembrane domains expressed on a wide variety of immune and non-immune cells (Zlotnik and Yoshie 2000).

The potential sources of chemokines produced intracerebrally during CNS inflammation are endothelial cells, astrocytes and microglia (Hesselgesser and Horuk 1999). Chemokines of the CXC family (IL-8, IP-10) and of the CC family (MIP-1α, MIP-1β, MCP-1 and RANTES) are produced by adult microglia and may contribute to the recruitment of T-cells, macrophages and dendritic cells to the CNS parenchyma (De Groot and Woodroofe 2001). Also human embryonic microglia release MIP-1α, MIP-1β, and MCP-1 upon LPS stimulation (Lee et al. 2002).

The panel of chemokines released by astrocytes is slightly different (Hua and Lee 2000). Astrocytes were shown to release IP-10, IL-8, MCP-1 and RANTES, but not MIP-1 and MIP-2, upon stimulation with LPS, viruses, pro-inflammatory cytokines (IL-1β and TNF-α) (Hua and Lee 2000) and complement derived anaphylatoxins (Jauneau et al. 2003). Intracisternal injection of MIP-1 and MIP-2 causes an increase in CSF protein levels and the appearance of leukocytes, indicating an important role of these chemokines in bacterial meningitis (Zwijnenburg et al. 2003).

Increasing evidence suggests that chemokines could also stimulate the migration of microglia to injured or inflammatory sites (Rappert et al. 2004; Marella and Chabry 2004). Expression of chemokine receptors on microglia has been demonstrated *in vitro* as well as *in vivo* in the course of infectious and autoimmune diseases (McManus et al. 2000).

2.3. Eicosanoids and Leukotriens

Activation of phospholipase A_2 induces the hydrolysis of cell membrane phospholipids and the release of arachidonic acid and platelet-activating factor (PAF). Prostaglandins (PG) and thromboxanes, collectively called eicosanoids, are synthesized from arachidonic acid through cyclooxygenase (COX) pathway and are important regulators of inflammation and immune responses. The activation of lipooxygenase leads to the release of leukotriens.

Increased levels of eicosanoids and inducible COX-2 isoforms have been demonstrated in several CNS inflammatory pathologies and evidence has been provided that microglia and astrocytes produce large amounts of PGE_2 *in vitro* (Ajmone-Cat et al. 2003; Teather et al. 2003). Cultured microglia produce also PGD_2 and thromboxane B_2 (Giulian et al. 1996; Mohri et al. 2003).

PGE_2 is thought to have a protective role in inflammation due to its ability to inhibit macrophage pro-inflammatory functions and to down-regulate Th_1 responses (Goodwin and Ceuppens 1983). It also inhibits production of pro-inflammatory cytokines and nitric oxide as well as expression of MHC class II molecules in microglia (Zhang and Rivest 2001). These findings suggest that PGE_2 is a factor that locally down-regulates the immune and inflammatory responses in CNS.

Platelet-activating factor is a potent inflammatory mediator derived from endothelial cells, macrophages and platelets. PAF plays an important role in normal CNS functions but also in brain damage and cerebral inflammation. In the rat brain PAF is intensely expressed by microglia. It is interesting that both pneumococcal call wall components and PAF share a common phosphocholine unit.

Pneumococci can bind to the PAF receptor and via this "gate" invade the CNS (Ring et al. 1998). Inhibition of signalling from the PAF receptor attenuates inflammation, particularly leukocytosis, during pneumococcal meningitis.

2.4. Metalloproteinases

Metalloproteinases (MMPs) are zinc-dependent endoproteases that can degrade components of the extracellular matrix. They play a physiological role in embryonic development and tissue morphogenesis.

Over the past few years clinical and experimental studies provided evidence for a role of matrix MMPs in neuroinflammation and brain damage involving blood brain barrier breakdown, neuroinflammation, glial reactivity, neuronal death (Kieseier et al. 2001; Rosenberg 2002).

In particular, MMPs have been implicated in the pathogenesis of gliomas (tumours of glial origin), viral infections, multiple sclerosis, Alzheimer's disease, brain trauma and ischemia (Kaczmarek et al. 2002). MMPs can be produced by glial cells, both astrocytes and microglia (Toft-Hansen et al. 2004). In normal conditions their expression in the brain is low (Kaczmarek et al. 2002), but is up-regulated in diseased tissue, e.g. within CNS lesions in animal models of multiple sclerosis (MS) and in tissue from patients with this disease.

The expression of MMPs contributes to tissue destruction and inflammation in MS (Leppert et al. 2001). In bacterial meningitis MMPs contribute to blood-brain barrier breakdown and facilitate leukocyte extravasation (Paul et al. 1998).

The two main MMPs involved in meningitis are MMP-8 and MMP-9. The increase of MMP-9 was found to be a specific feature of bacterial meningitis and CSF levels of MMP-9 in bacterial meningitis are 10 - 1000 folds higher than in viral meningitis (Kolb et al. 1998). Inhibition of MMPs is one of the potential therapeutic alternatives in meningitis.

Indeed, treatment with a broad-spectrum inhibitor of MMPs decreases MMP-9 and TNF-α concentrations in CSF and reduces the neocortical neuronal damage (Leib et al. 2001).

3. Mechanisms of Inflammatory Induced Neuronal Cell Death

3.1. Oxidative and Nitrosative Stress

Oxidative stress occurs when oxygen and nitrogen free radicals are generated in excess and the endogenous antioxidant systems are no more capable to remove the radicals overload. The biologically relevant free radicals are superoxide anion ($O_2^{\cdot-}$), perhydroxyl radical (protonated superoxide anion ($HO_2^{\cdot-}$), the hydroxyl radical ($HO^{\cdot}$) and free radical nitric oxide ($NO^{\cdot}$). The production of ROS occurs at the site of inflammation and contributes to tissue damage. The brain has several features that render it particularly sensitive to oxidative stress. It has the highest oxygen metabolic rate of any organ in the body, consuming approximately 20% of the total amount of oxygen yet representing only 2 - 5% of the total body weight (Dringen et al. 2000). This increases the probability that excessive levels of reactive oxygen species will be produced. Neurons are very vulnerable to ROS because of the high local oxygen tension, high levels of polyunsaturated fatty acids that can be oxidized by ROS, and high concentration of iron, which has been associated with free radical injury (Dringen et al. 2000). Also, local levels of endogenous antioxidants in the CNS are relatively low (Bolanos 1995). Oxidative stress was shown to mediate neuronal damage in wide range of neurological disorders including cerebral ischemia, cerebral trauma, primary neurodegenerative disorders, Alzheimer's and Parkinson's disease, and infectious diseases (e.g. meningitis) (Brown and Bal-Price 2003).

3.1.1. Reactive Oxygen Species (ROS)

Superoxide anion ($O_2^{\cdot-}$) is the most commonly occurring oxygen free radical. Tissue toxicity from extracellular superoxide is based on its direct reaction with biological targets, such as lipids, catecholamines, DNA, RNA, steroids, as well as is a result of the secondary formation of other oxygen radicals (Cuzzocrea et al. 2001). Nature has evolved a class of superoxide dismutase enzymes (SOD) to remove the deleterious free radical by-product of oxygen metabolism. These enzymes react rapidly with superoxide and dismutate the radical to non-radical products, H_2O_2 and oxygen, faster than superoxide can react with potential biological targets. Dismutation leads to the production of H_2O_2, which can concomitantly reduce ferric ion to ferrous ion. Reduction of ferric iron in the presence of hydrogen peroxide (also described as Haber-Weiss reaction) leads to the formation of the most active free oxygen radical - the hydroxyl radical ($HO^{\cdot}$) that may cleave covalent bonds in proteins and carbohydrates, cause lipid peroxidation, and destroy cell membranes.

Alteration in the equilibrium between the production of ROS and the antioxidative processes in favour of the formation of ROS results in oxidative stress, and can cause the destruction of both neurons and vascular cells. The production of ROS can lead to neuronal injury through: 1) destruction of cellular membrane lipids by their peroxidation (Cuzzocrea et al. 2001); 2) cleavage of DNA during the hydroxylation of guanine and methylation of cytosine (Hemnani and Parihar 1998; Vincent and Maiese 1999); 3) oxidation of proteins that yield protein carbonyl derivatives and nitrotyrosine (Cuzzocrea et al. 2001).

ROS are able to activate or suppress the activities of protein tyrosine kinases, serine/threonine kinases and phosphatases (Wang et al. 2003), and to induce the activation of several transcription factors including activator protein-1 (AP-1), nuclear factor κB (NF-κB), and p53, thereby modulating cellular responses (Kamata and Hirata 1999). However, the possibility that mild ROS generation may also initiate protective mechanisms through activation of pro-survival factors cannot be ruled out. In addition to the detrimental effects on cellular integrity, reactive oxygen species can inhibit complex enzymes in the electron transport chain of the mitochondria resulting in blockage of mitochondrial respiration (Yamamoto et al. 2002; Huang and Manton 2004).

3.1.2. Reactive Nitrogen Species

Nitric oxide (NO) influences many physiological and/or pathophysiological pathways in the CNS, resulting in either beneficial or detrimental effects to the nervous tissue. NO is produced from oxidation of L-arginine to L-citrulline via an enzymatically catalyzed process (Bredt 1999). The enzymes that produce NO have been divided into two classes depending on their special features: constitutive and inducible NO synthases (Wang and Marsden 1995). The brain expresses all three identified nitric oxide synthases (NOS) isoforms. Moreover NOS activity in the brain is higher than in any other tissue of the body (Duncan and Heales 2005).

The constitutively expressed isoforms of nitric oxide synthase (cNOS) include neuronal NOS (nNOS or type 1) and endothelial NOS (eNOS or type 3). Their function is dependent on the changes in intracellular Ca^{2+} levels and binding to calmoduline (Moncada et al. 1995). These enzymes can produce relatively small amounts of NO, mainly under physiological conditions. Nitric oxide has several physiological functions in the CNS. It can act as a neurotransmitter, as well as co-transmitter. A subset of neurons termed as "nitrergic nerves" were shown to release NO (Moncada et al. 1995) and a large body of evidence suggests that these neurons play a role in the control of neuroendocrine secretion in the hypothalamus, behavioural changes, as well as in learning and memory (Holscher 1997). NO's role as a neurotransmitter in the hippocampus appears to be important in the phenomenon of "long term potentiation", which is a form of synaptic plasticity associated with learning and memory (Arancio et al. 1996). NO produced by eNOS also functions as a vasodilator in the brain, acting on smooth muscle cells of the arteries and arterioles. It regulates the local blood flow and is believed to help to preserve the cerebral blood flow in cases of brain ischemia (Alderton et al. 2001). The role in maintaining uninterrupted circulation is vital, since the brain (and especially neurons) have high metabolic demand and do not tolerate reduced blood flow.

In contrary to the constitutive nNOS and eNOS, the expression of the inducible form of the enzyme (iNOS or type 2) is evoked only by appropriate stimuli such as bacterial lipopolysaccharide (LPS), and/or pro-inflammatory cytokines (IFN-γ, IL-1β, TNF-α, IL-6) (MacMicking et al. 1997). iNOS, first identified in macrophages, is expressed in many brain cells, but not under normal, physiological conditions. Astrocytes *in vitro* can be stimulated to express iNOS and generate up to 1 μM NO in the extracellular medium within few hours (Brown 1995). Human microglial cells have also been shown to express iNOS both *in vivo* and *in vitro* (Kitamura et al. 1998). Some neurons can express iNOS and release NO at least under *in vitro* conditions (Moro et al. 1998).

Unlike the constitutive forms of nitric oxide synthases, iNOS can produce high amounts of NO for relatively long periods. Induction of iNOS may have either toxic or protective effects, depending on the type of the insult, the tissue type, the level and duration of iNOS expression. In high local concentration NO can be cytostatic and cytotoxic for fungal, bacterial and protozoal organisms, as well as for tumour cells (Ascenzi et al. 2003; Xu et al. 2002). On the other hand, prolonged exposure to high concentration of NO may be also cytotoxic for the host cells (Abramson et al. 2001; Wink et al. 2001).

The iNOS is regulated at the expression level by transcriptional and post-transcriptional mechanisms (Kleinert et al. 2003). The main regulator of iNOS expression at transcriptional level seems to be nuclear factor-κB (NF-κB). Pharmacological inhibition of NF-κB significantly attenuates iNOS mRNA expression and NO production in cytokine stimulated cells (Taylorand Geller 2000). The important role for NF-κB binding sites in the induction of iNOS has been shown in murine (Blanchette et al. 2003), rat (Eberhardt et al. 1998) and human cells (Chu et al. 1998; Marks-Konczalik et al. 1998). Several other transcription factors were demonstrated to have an important function in the regulation of iNOS at the promoter level, among which are the octamer factor (Oct), interferon regulatory factor-1 (IRF-1), signal transducer and activator of transcription-1α (STAT-1 α), cAMP-induced transcription factors CREB and C/EBP, activating protein-1 (AP-1), peroxisome proliferator-activated receptors (PPAR) (extensively reviewed by Kleinert et al. 2003). Along with the transcriptional control, post-transcriptional mechanisms play an important role in regulation of iNOS expression. Several RNA binding proteins seem to destabilize iNOS mRNA and inhibit translational efficiency (reviewed by Taylor and Geller 2000). Also transforming growth factor β1 (TGF-β1) was shown to destabilise iNOS mRNA, retard the synthesis of iNOS protein and accelerate its degradation (Vodovotz et al. 1996).

Once produced, NO has a short half-life, and it decomposes rapidly to nitrite (NO_2^-) and nitrate (NO_3^-) (Singh and Evans 1997). These two NO-metabolites can be detected using a colorimetric assay – Griess reaction (Green et al. 1982). However, NO can also combine rapidly with the superoxide anion (O_2^-) and form peroxynitrite ($OONO^-$), which can damage DNA and proteins, cause lipid peroxidation as well as inhibition of cellular respiration. Peroxynitrite can diffuse much faster through the cell membrane and exerts more toxic effects than hydroxyl radicals. Many of the toxic effects previously attributed to superoxide and nitric oxide alone may be in fact due to peroxynitrite. Peroxynitrite was described to cause cell death and tissue damage in a number of neurodegenerative diseases such as Parkinson's disease, Alzheimer's disease, amyotrophic lateral sclerosis (ALS) and brain ischemia (Ebadi and Sharma 2003), as well as in toxic shock, arthritis, acute reperfusion injury (Boveris et al. 2002; Wang et al. 2003).

There are *in vitro* observations showing that NO and peroxynitrite can trigger DNA damage as a result of nitrosylation and deamination of nucleic acids leading to single strand and double strand breaks in DNA. In addition, damage to DNA can cause activation of the poly-(ADP-ribose) polymerase (PARP). PARP is an enzyme that is activated during DNA damage and is suggested to regulate gene expression and gene amplification, cellular differentiation, cellular division and malignant transformation as well as apoptotic cell death. Upon binding to DNA PARP becomes activated and cleaves NAD^+ in an ATP dependent manner. Therefore, excessive activation of PARP leads to the depletion of cellular NAD^+ and

ATP pools, and contributes to cellular energy depletion (Cosi and Marien 1999). It was shown that ROS and RNS activate PARP not only via DNA damage but also directly (Hasko et al. 2002). Evidence shows that PARP activation resulting from oxidative/nitrosative stress is involved in the pathogenesis of neurodegenerative diseases (Virag and Szabo 2002).

Another mechanism leading to neuronal damage induced by NO and peroxynitrite is the inhibition of mitochondrial respiration compromising cellular energy metabolism. RNS are known to interact and inhibit irreversibly components of the electron transport chain in mitochondria and in particular complex I, complex II and complex IV (Duncan and Heales 2005).

There are differences in the susceptibility of brain cells to NO. Upon *in vitro* exposure to NO astrocytes appear more resistant to the effects of RNS, when compared to neurons. This may be explained by the astrocytes' ability to up-regulate glycolysis, as following NO-mediated inhibition of respiration these cells rapidly increase the activity of key regulatory enzymes of glycolysis. Another factor influencing the difference in susceptibility to RNS between astrocytes and neurons appears to be related to the cellular availability of anti-oxidative reduced glutathione (GSH). In astrocytic cultures the levels of GSH are approximately double than in neuronal cultures (Bolanos et al. 1995). Moreover astrocytes were shown to up-regulate quickly the biosynthesis of GSH upon exposure to NO (Heales et al. 2004).

Although astrocytes may have a neuroprotective role, increasing the GSH availability for neuronal cells, prolonged co-culture of neurons with NO generating astrocytes leads to mitochondrial dysfunction and to neuronal cell death (Stewart et al. 2003) probably due to the formation of more potent oxidizing species such as peroxynitrite.

3.1.3. Anti-Oxidative Mechanisms

Reactive oxygen species are generated in high amounts during normal oxidative metabolism in the brain. Neuronal cells are highly susceptible to oxidative and nitrosative stress, therefore in the brain there are several antioxidative mechanisms, which protect neurons by inactivating the excess of ROS and RNS. Antioxidants may be classified according to their chemical nature and mode of function into: 1) enzymes that act on specific radicals after they are formed and degrade them to less harmful products (e.g. superoxide dismutase, catalase); 2) preventive antioxidants that act by binding to and sequestering oxidation promoters and transition metal ions (iron, copper), which strongly accelerate free radical formation; 3) scavenging antioxidants (with different mechanisms of action).

Reduced glutathione (GSH) is a tripeptide (Glu-Cys-Gly) considered to act as a major defence mechanism against ROS/RNS toxicity in the brain (Dringen et al. 2000). GSH oxidation occurs in the presence of GSH peroxidases, which catalyse the conversion of H_2O_2 to H_2O and O_2 in the cytoplasm, forming GSH disulphide (GSSG). The oxidation product can subsequently be regenerated to GSH by the NADPH dependent enzyme GSH reductase (Dringen et al. 2000). GSH directly reacts with RNS and ROS. Intact reduced glutathione pools are of extreme importance for the cells as they provide protection from oxidant induced injury.

Another important mechanism that protects brain cells against excessive ROS production is dysmutation of O_2- by superoxide dismutase (SOD). There are three forms of SOD: mitochondrial (Mn, SOD2), cytosolic (Cu/Zn, SOD1), and linked with extracellular surfaces (SOD3). SODs catalyze the formation of oxygen and H_2O_2 from two O_2^-. Hydrogen peroxide that is formed in this reaction is subsequently transformed by another enzyme - catalase - into oxygen and water. Under normal conditions SOD keeps under control the formation of superoxide; however in acute and chronic inflammation the formation of O_2^- overwhelms the capacity of SOD to remove it.

The brain contains also some antioxidant proteins, which bind metal ions that are co-factors in reactions of ROS formation (lactoferrin, transferrin – bind ferric ions; ceruloplasmin binds copper). Other antioxidant substances that are important for the CNS are scavengers of ROS/RNS such as α-tocoferol (vitamin E), ascorbic acid (vitamin C), carotene (pro-vitamin A) and coenzyme Q. Also melatonin, an endogenous substance produced in the pineal gland, is a powerful antioxidant of particular interest for the CNS (Gupta et al. 2003).

In the brain astrocytes are considered to play an important role in the defence against oxidative stress and have a higher capacity to detoxify ROS than other CNS cells (Dringen et al. 2000). They maintain high intracellular concentrations of certain antioxidants, which makes them more resistant to oxidative stress compared to oligodendrocytes and neurons (Wilson 1997). Astrocytes are the main source of reduced glutathione and contain the highest quantities of GSH from all CNS cells. Neurons have significantly lower GSH content, which is considered to be one of the reasons for higher susceptibility of this cell type to oxidative stress (Dringen et al. 2000). Following reactive gliosis, the neuroprotective role of astrocytes may be accentuated because of increases in a number of activities: 1) expression of antioxidant enzymes; 2) transport and metabolism of glucose that yields reducing equivalents for antioxidant regeneration and lactate for neuronal metabolism; 3) synthesis of glutathione; 4) recycling of vitamin C (Wilson 1997).

Attempts for new therapies in many inflammatory CNS diseases are based on the control of oxidative stress. There are three strategies to protect the tissues from locally produces oxygen radicals: 1) deliver SOD or SOD mimetics; 2) deliver catalase or related peroxynitrite scavenger; 3) chelate and thereby inactivate the trace iron that catalyses the reaction. Until now, pharmacological interventions to reduce ROS generation in shock, inflammation and ischemia/reperfusion include: 1) vitamin E-like antioxidants; 2) N-acetylcysteine; 3) SOD mimetics (e.g. MnTBAP) (Szabo 1996); 4) peroxynitrite decomposition catalysts (e.g. FeTPPS) (Crow 2000); and 5) iNOS inhibitors (Southan and Szabo 1996).

3.2. Excitotoxicity

Excitotoxicity is a process, in which excessive amounts of excitatory amino acids, in particular glutamate, induce neuronal toxicity. Under normal conditions glutamate is cleared from the neuronal synapses by astrocytes via glutamate transporters and is converted into glutamine, which is released and in turn taken up by neurons (Simard and Nedergaard, 2004). This prevents that glutamate reaches excitotoxic levels in the extracellular space. Astrocytes can also themselves release glutamate that modulates the activity of both excitatory and inhibitory synapses.

However, when released in excess, glutamate induces neurotoxicity interfering with the NMDA and/or AMPA receptors, which results in the overload of neurons with Ca^{2+} and Na^+. Increased levels of Ca^{2+} can stimulate the production of ROS and nitric oxide (via activation of nNOS) and cause mitochondrial dysfunction, which leads to the opening of the mitochondrial permeability transition pore (MPTP), release of apoptosis inducing factor

(AIF) and cytochrome *c* to the cytoplasm, and finally to apoptotic death. On the other hand, nitric oxide itself can be a trigger of excitotoxicity. Recently it has been shown that NO, at concentrations that inhibit respiration, cause release of glutamate from neurons (McNaught and Brown 1998), microglia (Barger and Basile 2001) and astrocytes (Bal-Price et al. 2002). Excitotoxicity contributes to the pathogenesis of several neurodegenerative diseases such as Alzheimer's disease, Parkinson's disease, amyotrophic lateral sclerosis, ischemia and brain injury (Arundine and Tymianski 2004; Hynd et al. 2004).

3.3. Mitochondrial Dysfunction

Mitochondria are vital organelles that maintain the cellular energy reserves by production of ATP in the respiratory electron transfer chain. Besides, they are known to be a significant source of superoxide radicals and other ROS that are associated with oxidative stress (Nohl et al. 2005). Impairment of the electron transfer chain at the flavin mononucleotide group of complex I (NADPH ubiquinone oxidoreductase) or at the ubiquinone site of complex III (ubiquinone-cytochrome *c* reductase) results in active generation of ROS. Once generated ROS further impair mitochondrial electron transport and enhance ROS production (Nohl et al. 2005).

It has been widely shown that mitochondrial dysfunction resulting from oxidative stress is the cause of neuronal cell death (Kirkland et al. 2002). The permeability of the mitochondrial membrane is dependent upon the mitochondrial permeability transition pore (MPTP) located at the contact sites between the inner and outer mitochondrial membrane (Crompton 1999; Bernardi et al. 2001). Additionally, it has been demonstrated that nitric oxide generated following anoxia (Mander et al. 2005) or released from glial cells activated with pro-inflammatory stimuli (e.g. LPS) (Bal-Price and Brown 1999; Bal-Price and Brown 2001) causes depolarization of mitochondrial membrane, subsequent release of cytochrome *c* and activation of caspases.

4. Neuroinflammation and Neurodegenerative Diseases

The role of neuroinflammation in a number of CNS diseases has been recognised only recently. The concept of "neuroinflammation" implies that specific innate immune responses in the brain are mediated mainly by activated microglia and astrocytes, which precedes and causes neuronal degeneration. Before neuroinflammation became a commonly used term, neuroscientists recognised "reactive gliosis" as the endogenous CNS tissue response to acute brain injury.

Acute pathological conditions such as cerebral ischemia and traumatic brain injury are characterised by rapid and usually severe insults to the brain, which lead to substantial loss of nerve cells and subsequent functional deficits. Several processes have been implicated in the neuronal damage including increased glutamate release (excitotoxicity), oxidative stress and disturbances in ionic homeostasis (Morimoto et al. 2002; Chavarria and Alcocer-Varela 2004). There are also data suggesting the active role of inflammatory processes in these diseases - the activation of inflammatory cells (microglia, astrocytes) and increased expression of inflammatory mediators (cytokines, complement) (McGeer and McGeer 2001).

Although such specific responses in acute brain injury might be included in the term "neuroinflammation", it is more commonly applied to chronic CNS diseases. Any chronic inflammatory process can damage healthy tissue and the brain may be particularly vulnerable, since neurons are post-mitotic cells and once lost cannot be replaced. There is vast evidence indicating that chronic inflammation in the brain may play an important role in the progressive neuronal cell death in many chronic CNS diseases such as Alzheimer's disease (AD), Parkinson's disease (PD), amyotrophic lateral sclerosis (ALS) or multiple sclerosis (MS).

The greatest evidence of the role of inflammation in chronic CNS disorders comes from studies on Alzheimer's disease which is the most common neurodegenerative disease - approximately 10% of all people over the age of 65 and as many as 50% of those over the age of 85 are diagnosed with the condition. It is an irreversible, progressive disorder characterised by a loss of neurons predominantly in the cerebral cortex and hippocampus (Poulin and Zakzanis 2002). Evidence for the importance of inflammation in AD comes from two directions. Firstly, extensive immunohistochemical and molecular biology studies of brain tissues collected from patients who suffered from AD revealed the presence of many hallmarks of inflammation, including microglial activation, expression of cytokines, activation of the complement system, invasion of immune cells (McGeer and McGeer 2001). Secondly, there is an ongoing a debate on the value of non-steroidal anti-inflammatory drugs (NSAIDs, e.g. aspirin, ibuprofen) in AD treatment. Epidemiological studies suggest that patients on long term anti-inflammatory treatment (mainly because of arthritis) have a significantly reduced risk of developing AD (Szekely et al. 2004).

As in the case of many neurodegenerative diseases, the aetiology of AD is not clear, however, evidences suggest that accumulation of β-amyloid in neuritic plaques and remnants of a cytoskeletal protein tau (neurofibrillary tangles) act as irritants, causing activation of complement system, the initiation of reactive changes in microglia, the release cytokines (IL-1β, IL-6, IL-8) (McGeer and McGeer 1998) and potentially neurotoxic products such as reactive oxygen species, nitric oxide, excessive extracellular glutamate (Klegeris et al. 1997). All these toxic inflammatory products contribute to neuronal cell death, which further activates the immune reactions and leads to a chronic and progressive neurodegeneration.

Similar processes are observed in Parkinson's disease, a chronic, progressive neurodegenerative disorder characterised by degeneration of the nigrostriatal dopamine (DA) neurons in the substantia nigra. According to a common hypothesis, neurodegeneration in PD lays in abnormal accumulation of the protein α-synuclein in neurons, that similarly to β-amyloid in AD, aggregates and triggers activation of glial cells and the progression of inflammation. Indeed, activated microglia, and to a lesser extent reactive astrocytes, are found in the area associated with neuronal cell loss (Teismann and Schulz 2004), possibly contributing to the inflammatory process by the release of pro-inflammatory cytokines such as TNF-α, IL-1β and IL-6 (Nagatsu and Sawada 2005), prostaglandins (PGE_2, PGD_2), reactive oxygen and nitrosative species (NO). The anti-inflammatory treatment with NSAID or dexamethasone has demonstrated to have a beneficial role also in PD, although it is much less evident than in the case of AD (Minghetti 2004; Kurkowska-Jastrzebska et al. 2004).

Multiple sclerosis is another example of a disease involving inflammation of the brain and associated neurological impairment. The key feature of MS is demyelination of axons in peripheral nerves and brain areas that leads to their subsequent degeneration and formation of plaques (Bitsch et al. 2000). The aetiology of MS is still not fully understood. Considerable evidence suggests the main role of autoimmune reactions to an unknown antigen and the activation of T lymphocytes (or deactivation of suppressor T cells) that, together with macrophages, invade the CNS. There are suggestions that an initial infection – viral or bacterial – can trigger inflammation and activation of T cells cross-reacting with autoantigens present in the CNS. Many studies demonstrate that the cytokines TNF-α and IFN-γ mediate some aspects of the disease (Bettelli and Nicholson 2000). They are both toxic to oligodendrocytes and can stimulate local inflammatory cytokines production (Benveniste and Benos 1995). Also clinical studies report the increased expression of cytokines in the brain parenchyma and CSF (Olsson et al. 1990; Rieckmann et al. 1995), but the therapeutic strategies targeted to block TNF-α and IFN-γ have not yet been successful. The current treatments of MS use immunosuppressive drugs, anti-inflammatory approaches and the treatment with interferon-β. The mechanism of action of IFN-β is not fully known, but in *in vitro* studies it was shown to suppress many actions of IFN-γ, inhibit the expression and release of IL-1 and TNF-α, and induce the release of IL-1ra (Jungo et al. 2001).

5. Neuroinflammation and Infectious Diseases of the CNS

Infections of the CNS are rare but life-threatening complications of systemic infections caused by diverse microorganisms. Due to its anatomy, the CNS represents a special milieu for bacterial, fungal, viral and parasitic infections. The brain and spinal cord are protected by bone and meningeal coverings that compartmentalise infection; they are separated from the systemic circulation by the blood-brain barrier, which largely prevents macromolecules from entering the brain parenchyma. The CNS lacks an intrinsic immune system, therefore immunoglobulins and immune competent cells are scarce, except at foci of inflammation. Moreover, the brain and the spinal cord have a unique compact structure and space between cells in the parenchyma is too small to permit passage even of a virus (some viruses travel through the CNS by axoplasmic flow).

The infections in the CNS comprise several forms. The most common one is meningitis - an inflammation of the pia-arachnoid meninges, caused by a variety of different agents (bacteria, fungi, or parasites) growing within the subarachnoidal space. The most common, but also quite benign, is viral meningitis, primarily caused by echoviruses, coxackie viruses, mumps. Bacteria are the second cause of meningitis, however the clinical symptoms and the complications of this disease are much more severe.

Another form of CNS infection is the brain abscess - a focus of purulent infection of the brain parenchyma, usually caused by bacteria. Brain abscesses develop from either a contiguous focus of infection (such as the ears, the sinuses or the teeth) or hematogenous spread from a distant focus (such as the lungs or heart, particularly with chronic purulent pulmonary disease, sub-acute bacterial endocarditis or cyanotic congenital heart disease). Many brain abscesses have a mixed flora of aerobic and anaerobic bacteria. Approximately 60 to 70% contain streptococci; *Staphylococcus aureus,* enterobacteria and *Bacteroides* are frequently present. Fungi cause fewer than 10% of brain abscesses. Generally, the brain abscess is a condition very difficult to cure, requiring multiple antibiotic treatment and sometimes surgical interventions.

Unlike an abscess, which is a localized area of bacterial or fungal growth, encephalitis (often defined as inflammation of the brain) is usually due to viruses that produce more widespread intracellular infections. Many viruses, including enteroviruses, mumps and lymphocytic choriomeningitis viruses, cause mild forms of encephalitis. Life-threatening viral encephalitis is due primarily to herpes simplex viruses (HSV-1 and HSV-2) and arboviruses (mainly togaviruses, flaviviruses, and bunyaviruses).

Some infections in the CNS can develop into a chronic form. Today, the most important example of a chronic brain infection is HIV encephalitis, in which the HIV virus enters and persists in the CNS (in monocytes, perivascular cells and microglia) (Garden 2002). HIV infection is uniquely different from all other CNS infections in that the virus targets and disables these cells that are key players in neuroinflammation – the microglia in the brain and T lymphocytes in the periphery. Chronic infection can occur also in the course of syphilis (caused by the bacteria *Treponema pallidum*), which persist over many years with the unpredictable appearance of varied neurological complications. Chronic brain inflammation has been implicated also in the pathogenesis of prion infectious diseases, including transmissible spongiform encephalopathies in animals (e.g. scrapie, bovine spongiform encephalopathy - BSE) and humans (Creutzfeld-Jakob disease - CJD).

Although meningitis is an inflammatory disease of the meninges, usually it is not restricted to these membranes, but brain cells are also implicated, both as effectors and as objects of inflammatory injury. Therefore, neurological injury in bacterial meningitis is not only due to meningeal inflammation but also to cerebral vasculitis, cerebral oedema, cerebral necrosis, intracranial haemorrhage (Nau and Bruck 2002). The induction of symptoms requires initiation of the inflammatory response, which is triggered by bacterial components such as the cell wall (e.g. lipopolysaccharide in Gram-negative bacteria, lipoteichoic acid and peptidoglycan in Gram-positive bacteria). Within the CSF bacteria multiply, lyse spontaneously and release pro-inflammatory and toxic compounds by autolysis or secretion. The bacterial products can traffic easily from the CSF to the brain parenchyma via the CNS paravascular fluid circulation.

Bacterial components can directly induce some neuronal toxicity (e.g. the *S. pneumoniae* toxin pneumolysin has been shown to directly damage neurons but most evidence suggests that they stimulate glial cells (astrocytes and microglia) and resident macrophages to release several host-derived inflammatory mediators (cytokines, nitric oxide, ROS), which play a dominant role in neuronal damage (Bal-Price and Brown 2001; Bal-Price et al. 2002; Kinsner et al. 2005; Kinsner et al. 2006). A rapid increase of pro-inflammatory cytokines (TNF-α, IL-1β, IL-6) and chemokines (IL-8, MIP-1, MIP-2) is observed in the CSF in response to bacterial cell wall components, and their levels correlate with bacterial counts, severity of disease and occurrence of complications.

Neuronal injury in meningitis is not a single event and several mechanisms are interacting with each other ultimately leading to the death of neurons. As previously discussed, cells functionally involved during meningitis include glial cells (astrocytes and microglia), meningeal macrophages, endothelial cells of the intracerebral vessels, and later also immunocompetent cells (monocytes, lymphocytes) recruited from the systemic circulation. The main factors triggering inflammation are the bacterial components released into the CSF, that are recognised by glial cells and involve innate immune functions stimulating Toll-like receptors (TLRs) and inducing translocation of nuclear factor κB (NF-κB), the activation of mitogen activated protein kinases (MAPK) and the transcription of genes encoding inflammatory mediators (Akira and Hemmi 2003). This initial inflammatory response from the brain parenchyma - and in particular astrocytes and microglia - seems to be an important factor contributing to neuronal damage. As demonstrated in some *in vitro* studies, heat-inactivated pneumococci injure both neurons co-cultured with glial cells (Kim and Tauber 1996) and neurons in organotypic hippocampal cultures (Schmidt et al. 2001). Neuronal damage can be induced by pneumococcal lipoteichoic acid (Kinsner et al. 2006), peptidoglycan and bacterial DNA (Schmidt et al. 2001; Kim and Tauber 1996).

The mechanisms of ischemic or hypoxic lesions in meningitis are 1) vasculitis, vasospasm and obstruction of cerebral arteries, 2) generalised cerebral oedema, 3) impairment of cerebral autoregulation, leading to hypoxic lesions during hypotension. The pro-inflammatory mediators released by activated glial cells are largely responsible for these events.

Conclusion

Neuroinflammation has been implicated in the pathology of many neurodegenerative disorders for decades. Still it is not fully understood when and how inflammation arises in the course of these diseases and whether inflammation is an underling cause or a resulting condition in those pathologies. Based on the results discussed in this review microglial activation followed by astrocytes reactivity contributes to neuronal damage in many neurodegenerative diseases. Astrocytes and microglia, undergo activation in response to stimuli such as injury, illness, or infection. The glial response can mediate a variety of deleterious events related to the production of pro-inflammatory cytokines, chemokines or reactive oxygen and nitrogen species. However, glial cells produce also anti-inflammatory cytokines and may be the source of trophic factors and can protect against oxidative stress and glutamate release. The extent and the mechanisms by which in vivo inflammatory-activated microglia and astrocytes damage neurons (or protect) requires further research.

References

Abbott N. J. (2002) Astrocyte-endothelial interactions and blood-brain barrier permeability. *J Anat* 200, 629-638.

Abramson S. B., Amin A. R., Clancy R. M., and Attur M. (2001) The role of nitric oxide in tissue destruction. *Best Pract Res Clin Rheumatol* 15, 831-845.

Ajmone-Cat M. A., Nicolini A., and Minghetti L. (2003) Prolonged exposure of microglia to lipopolysaccharide modifies the intracellular signalling pathways and selectively promotes prostaglandin E2 synthesis. *J Neurochem* 87, 1193-1203.

Akassoglou K., Bauer J., Kassiotis G., Pasparakis M., Lassmann H., Kollias G., and Probert L. (1998) Oligodendrocyte apoptosis and primary demyelination induced by local TNF/p55TNF receptor signalling in the central nervous system of transgenic mice:

models for multiple sclerosis with primary oligodendrogliopathy. *Am J Pathol* 153, 801-813.

Akira S. and Hemmi H. (2003) Recognition of pathogen-associated molecular patterns by TLR family. *Immunol Lett* 85, 85-95.

Alderton W. K., Cooper C. E., and Knowles R. G. (2001) Nitric oxide synthases: structure, function and inhibition. *Biochem J* 357,593-615.

Allan S. M. (2000) The role of pro- and antiinflammatory cytokines in neurodegeneration. *Ann N Y Acad Sci* 917, 84-93.

Allan S. M. and Rothwell N. J. (2001) Cytokines and acute neurodegeneration. *Nat Rev Neurosci* 2, 734-744.

Aloisi F. (2001) Immune function of microglia. *Glia* 36, 165-179.

Aloisi F., De Simone R., Columba-Cabezas S., and Levi G. (1999) Opposite effects of interferon-gamma and prostaglandin E2 on tumor necrosis factor and interleukin-10 production in microglia: a regulatory loop controlling microglia pro- and anti-inflammatory activities. *J Neurosci Res* 56, 571-580.

Aloisi F., Penna G., Cerase J., Menendez I. B., and Adorini L. (1997) IL-12 production by central nervous system microglia is inhibited by astrocytes. *J Immunol* 159, 1604-1612.

Arancio O., Kiebler M., Lee C. J., Lev-Ram V., Tsien R. Y., Kandel E. R., and Hawkins R. D. (1996) Nitric oxide acts directly in the presynaptic neuron to produce long-term potentiation in cultured hippocampal neurons. *Cell* 87, 1025-1035.

Araque A., Carmignoto G., and Haydon P. G. (2001) Dynamic signalling between astrocytes and neurons. *Annu Rev Physiol* 63, 795-813.

Araque A., Sanzgiri R. P., Parpura V., and Haydon P.G. (1999) Astrocyte-induced modulation of synaptic transmission. *Can J Physiol Pharmacol* 77, 699-706.

Arundine M. and Tymianski M. (2004) Molecular mechanisms of glutamate-dependent neurodegeneration in ischemia and traumatic brain injury. *Cell Mol Life Sci* 61, 657-668.

Ascenzi P., Bocedi A., and Gradoni L. (2003) The anti-parasitic effects of nitric oxide. *IUBMB Life* 55, 573-578.

Bal-Price A., Borutaite V., and Brown G. C. (1999) Mitochondria mediate nitric oxide-induced cell death. *Ann N Y Acad Sci* 893, 376-378.

Bal-Price A. and Brown G. C. (2001) Inflammatory neurodegeneration mediated by nitric oxide from activated glia-inhibiting neuronal respiration, causing glutamate release and excitotoxicity. *J Neurosci* 21, 6480-6491.

Bal-Price A., Moneer Z., and Brown G. C. (2002) Nitric oxide induces rapid, calcium-dependent release of vesicular glutamate and ATP from cultured rat astrocytes. *Glia* 40, 312-323.

Barger S. W. and Basile A. S. (2001) Activation of microglia by secreted amyloid precursor protein evokes release of glutamate by cystine exchange and attenuates synaptic function. *J Neurochem* 76, 846-854.

Basu A., Krady J. K., O'Malley M., Styren S. D., DeKosky S. T., and Levison S. W. (2002) The type 1 interleukin-1 receptor is essential for the efficient activation of microglia and the induction of multiple proinflammatory mediators in response to brain injury. *J Neurosci* 22, 6071-6082.

Benveniste E. N., and Benos D. J. (1995) TNF-alpha- and IFN-gamma-mediated signal transduction pathways: effects on glial cell gene expression and function. *FASEB J* 9, 1577-1584.

Bernardi P., Petronilli V., Di Lisa F., and Forte M. (2001) A mitochondrial perspective on cell death. *Trends Biochem Sci* 26, 112-117.

Bettelli E. and Nicholson L. B. (2000) The role of cytokines in experimental autoimmune encephalomyelitis. *Arch Immunol Ther Exp* 48, 389-398.

Bezzi P., Vesce S., Panzarasa P., and Volterra A. (1999) Astrocytes as active participants of glutamatergic function and regulators of its homeostasis. *Adv Exp Med Biol* 468, 69-80.

Bitsch A., Schuchardt J., Bunkowski S., Kuhlmann T., and Bruck W. (2000) Acute axonal injury in multiple sclerosis. Correlation with demyelination and inflammation. *Brain* 123 (Pt 6), 1174-1183.

Blanchette J., Jaramillo M., and Olivier M. (2003) Signalling events involved in interferon-gamma-inducible macrophage nitric oxide generation. *Immunology* 108, 513-522.

Blasko I., Stampfer-Kountchev M., Robatscher P., Veerhuis R., Eikelenboom P., and Grubeck-Loebenstein B. (2004) How chronic inflammation can affect the brain and support the development of Alzheimer's disease in old age: the role of microglia and astrocytes. *Aging Cell* 3, 169-176.

Bogdan C., Vodovotz Y., and Nathan C. (1991) Macrophage deactivation by interleukin 10. *J Exp Med* 174, 1549-1555.

Bolanos J. P., Heales S. J., Land J. M., and Clark J. B. (1995) Effect of peroxynitrite on the mitochondrial respiratory chain: differential susceptibility of neurones and astrocytes in primary culture. *J Neurochem* 64, 1965-1972.

Bonmann E., Suschek C., Spranger M., and Kolb-Bachofen V. (1997) The dominant role of exogenous or endogenous interleukin-1 beta on expression and activity of inducible nitric oxide synthase in rat microvascular brain endothelial cells. *Neurosci Lett* 230, 109-112.

Boveris A., Alvarez S., and Navarro A. (2002) The role of mitochondrial nitric oxide synthase in inflammation and septic shock. *Free Radic Biol Med* 33, 1186-1193.

Bredt D. S. (1999) Endogenous nitric oxide synthesis: biological functions and pathophysiology. *Free Radic Res* 31, 577-596.

Brown G.C. (1995) Nitric oxide regulates mitochondrial respiration and cell function by inhibiting cytochrome oxidase. *FEBS Lett* 369, 136-139.

Brown G. C. and Bal-Price A. (2003) Inflammatory neurodegeneration mediated by nitric oxide, glutamate, and mitochondria. *Mol Neurobiol* 27, 325-355.

Chao C. C. and Hu S. (1994) Tumor necrosis factor-alpha potentiates glutamate neurotoxicity in human fetal brain cell cultures. *Dev Neurosci* 16, 172-179.

Chao C. C., Hu S., and Peterson P. K. (1995) Glia, cytokines, and neurotoxicity. *Crit Rev Neurobiol* 9, 189-205.

Chavarria A. and Alcocer-Varela J. (2004) Is damage in central nervous system due to inflammation? *Autoimmun Rev* 3, 251-260.

Chu S. C., Marks-Konczalik J., Wu H. P., Banks T. C., and Moss J. (1998) Analysis of the cytokine-stimulated human inducible nitric oxide synthase (iNOS) gene: characterisation of differences between human and mouse iNOS promoters. *Biochem Biophys Res Commun* 248, 871-878.

Chvatal A. and Sykova E. (2000) Glial influence on neuronal signalling. *Prog Brain Res* 125, 199-216.

Clark W. M., Rinker L. G., Lessov N. S., Hazel K., and Eckenstein F. (1999) Time course of IL-6 expression in experimental CNS ischemia. *Neurol Res* 21, 287-292.

Cosi C. and Marien M. (1999) Implication of poly (ADP-ribose) polymerase (PARP) in neurodegeneration and brain energy metabolism. Decreases in mouse brain NAD+ and ATP caused by MPTP are prevented by the PARP inhibitor benzamide. *Ann N Y Acad Sci* 890, 227-239.

Crompton M. (1999) The mitochondrial permeability transition pore and its role in cell death. *Biochem J* 341, 233-249.

Crow J.P. (2000) Peroxynitrite scavenging by metalloporphyrins and thiolates. *Free Radic Biol Med* 28, 1487-1494.

Cunha F. Q., Moncada S., and Liew F. Y. (1992) Interleukin-10 (IL-10) inhibits the induction of nitric oxide synthase by interferon-gamma in murine macrophages. *Biochem Biophys Res Commun* 182, 1155-1159.

Cuzzocrea S., Riley D. P., Caputi A. P., and Salvemini D. (2001) Antioxidant therapy: a new pharmacological approach in shock, inflammation, and ischemia/reperfusion injury. *Pharmacol Rev* 53, 135-159.

Davis E. J., Foster T. D., and Thomas W. E. (1994) Cellular forms and functions of brain microglia. *Brain Res Bull* 34, 73-78.

De Groot C. J., Montagne L., Barten A. D., Sminia P., and Van D., V (1999) Expression of transforming growth factor (TGF)-beta1, -beta2, and -beta3 isoforms and TGF-beta type I and type II receptors in multiple sclerosis lesions and human adult astrocyte cultures. *J Neuropathol Exp Neurol* 58, 174-187.

Dhandapani K. M. and Brann D. W. (2003) Transforming growth factor-beta: a neuroprotective factor in cerebral ischemia. *Cell Biochem Biophys* 39, 13-22.

Dietrich J. B. (2002) The adhesion molecule ICAM-1 and its regulation in relation with the blood-brain barrier. *J Neuroimmunol* 128, 58-68.

Dringen R., Gutterer J. M., and Hirrlinger J. (2000) Glutathione metabolism in brain metabolic interaction between astrocytes and neurons in the defense against reactive oxygen species. *Eur J Biochem* 267, 4912-4916.

Duncan A.J. and Heales S.J. (2005) Nitric oxide and neurological diseases. *Mol Asp Med* 26, 67-96.

Ebadi M. and Sharma S. K. (2003) Peroxynitrite and mitochondrial dysfunction in the pathogenesis of Parkinson's disease. *Antioxid Redox Signal* 5, 319-335.

Eberhardt W., Pluss C., Hummel R., and Pfeilschifter J. (1998) Molecular mechanisms of inducible nitric oxide synthase gene expression by IL-1beta and cAMP in rat mesangial cells. *J Immunol* 160, 4961-4969.

Ehrlich L. C., Hu S., Sheng W. S., Sutton R. L., Rockswold G. L., Peterson P. K., and Chao C. C. (1998) Cytokine regulation of human microglial cell IL-8 production. *J Immunol* 160, 1944-1948.

Flugel A., Schwaiger F. W., Neumann H., Medana I., Willem M., Wekerle H., Kreutzberg G. W., and Graeber M. B. (2000) Neuronal FasL induces cell death of encephalitogenic T lymphocytes. *Brain Pathol* 10, 353-364.

Froes M. M., Correia A. H., Garcia-Abreu J., Spray D. C., Campos de Carvalho A. C., and Neto M. V. (1999) Gap-junctional coupling between neurons and astrocytes in primary central nervous system cultures. *Proc Natl Acad Sci U S A* 96, 7541-7546.

Gadient R. A. and Otten U. H. (1997) Interleukin-6 (IL-6) - a molecule with both beneficial and destructive potentials. *Prog Neurobiol* 52, 379-390.

Garden G. (2002) Microglia in human immunodeficiency virus-associated neurodegeneration. *Glia* 40, 240-251.

Gardner J. and Ghorpade A. (2003) Tissue inhibitor of metalloproteinase (TIMP)-1: the TIMPed balance of matrix metalloproteinases in the central nervous system. *J Neurosci Res* 74, 801-806.

Giulian D., Corpuz M., Richmond B., Wendt E., and Hall E. R. (1996) Activated microglia are the principal glial source of thromboxane in the central nervous system. *Neurochem Int* 29, 65-76.

Goodwin J. S. and Ceuppens J. (1983) Regulation of the immune response by prostaglandins. *J Clin Immunol* 3, 295-315.

Gozes I., Divinsky I., Pilzer I., Fridkin M., Brenneman D. E., and Spier A. D. (2003) From vasoactive intestinal peptide (VIP) through activity-dependent neuroprotective protein (ADNP) to NAP: a view of neuroprotection and cell division. *J Mol Neurosci* 20, 315-322.

Green L. C., Wagner D. A., Glogowski J., Skipper P. L., Wishnok J. S., and Tannenbaum S. R. (1982) Analysis of nitrate, nitrite, and [15N]nitrate in biological fluids. *Anal Biochem* 126, 131-138.

Grilli M., Barbieri I., Basudev H., Brusa R., Casati C., Lozza G., and Ongini E. (2000) Interleukin-10 modulates neuronal threshold of vulnerability to ischaemic damage. *Eur J Neurosci* 12, 2265-2272.

Gruol D. L. and Nelson T. E. (1997) Physiological and pathological roles of interleukin-6 in the central nervous system. *Mol Neurobiol* 15, 307-339.

Gupta Y. K., Gupta M., and Kohli K. (2003) Neuroprotective role of melatonin in oxidative stress vulnerable brain. *Indian J Physiol Pharmacol* 47, 373-86.

Hailer N. P., Vogt C., Korf H. W., and Dehghani F. (2005) Interleukin-1beta exacerbates and interleukin-1 receptor antagonist attenuates neuronal injury and microglial activation after excitotoxic damage in organotypic hippocampal slice cultures. *Eur J Neurosci* 21, 2347-2360.

Hasko G., Mabley J. G., Nemeth Z. H., Pacher P., Deitch E. A., and Szabo C. (2002) Poly(ADP-ribose) polymerase is a regulator of chemokines production: relevance for the pathogenesis of shock and inflammation. *Mol Med* 8, 189-283.

Hayes G. M., Woodroofe M. N., and Cuzner M. L. (1987) Microglia are the major cell type expressing MHC class II in human white matter. *J Neurol Sci* 80, 25-37.

Heales S. J., Lam A. A., Duncan A. J., and Land J. M. (2004) Neurodegeneration or neuroprotection: the pivotal role of astrocytes. *Neurochem Res* 29, 513-519.

Hemnani T. and Parihar M. S. (1998) Reactive oxygen species and oxidative DNA damage. *Indian J Physiol Pharmacol* 42, 440-452.

Herx L. M. and Yong V. W. (2001) Interleukin-1 beta is required for the early evolution of reactive astrogliosis following CNS lesion. *J Neuropathol Exp Neurol* 60, 961-971.

Hesselgesser J. and Horuk R. (1999) Chemokine and chemokine receptor expression in the central nervous system. *J Neurovirol* 5, 13-26.

Hirota H., Kiyama H., Kishimoto T., and Taga T. (1996) Accelerated Nerve Regeneration in Mice by upregulated expression of interleukin (IL) 6 and IL-6 receptor after trauma. *J Exp Med* 183, 2627-2634.

Hoftberger R., Aboul-Enein F., Brueck W., Lucchinetti C., Rodriguez M., Schmidbauer M., Jellinger K., and Lassmann H. (2004) Expression of major histocompatibility complex class I molecules on the different cell types in multiple sclerosis lesions. *Brain Pathol* 14, 43-50.

Holscher C. (1997) Nitric oxide, the enigmatic neuronal messenger: its role in synaptic plasticity. *Trends Neurosci* 20, 298-303.

Hua L. L. and Lee S. C. (2000) Distinct patterns of stimulus-inducible chemokine mRNA accumulation in human fetal astrocytes and microglia. *Glia* 30, 74-81.

Huang H. and Manton K. G. (2004) The role of oxidative damage in mitochondria during aging: a review. *Front Biosci* 9, 1100-1117.

Hynd M. R., Scott H. L., and Dodd P. R. (2004) Glutamate-mediated excitotoxicity and neurodegeneration in Alzheimer's disease. *Neurochem Int* 45, 583-595.

Jain M., Aneja S., Mehta G., Ray G. N., Batra S., and Randhava V. S. (2000) CSF interleukin-1 beta, tumor necrosis factor-alpha and free radicals production in relation to clinical outcome in acute bacterial meningitis. *Indian Pediatr* 37, 608-614.

Jauneau A. C., Ischenko A., Chan P., and Fontaine M. (2003) Complement component anaphylatoxins upregulate chemokine expression by human astrocytes. *FEBS Lett.* 27, 17-22.

Jungo F., Dayer J. M., Modoux C., Hyka N., and Burger D. (2001) IFN-beta inhibits the ability of T lymphocytes to induce TNF-alpha and IL-1beta production in monocytes upon direct cell-cell contact. *Cytokine* 14, 272-282.

Kaczmarek L., Lapinska-Dzwonek J., and Szymczak S. (2002) Matrix metalloproteinases in the adult brain physiology: a link between c-Fos, AP-1 and remodeling of neuronal connections? *EMBO J* 21, 6643-6648.

Kamata H. and Hirata H. (1999) Redox regulation of cellular signalling. *Cell Signal* 11, 1-14.

Kiefer R., Schweitzer T., Jung S., Toyka K. V., and Hartung H. P. (1998) Sequential expression of transforming growth factor-beta1 by T-cells, macrophages, and microglia in rat spinal cord during autoimmune inflammation. *J Neuropathol Exp Neurol* 57, 385-395.

Kieseier B. C., Schneider C., Clements J. M., Gearing A. J., Gold R., Toyka K. V., and Hartung H. P. (2001) Expression of specific matrix metalloproteinases in inflammatory myopathies. *Brain* 124, 341-351.

Kim Y. S. and Tauber M. G. (1996) Neurotoxicity of glia activated by gram-positive bacterial products depends on nitric oxide production. *Infect Immun* 64, 3148-3153.

Kinsner A., Pilotto V., Deininger S., Brown G. C., Coecke S., Hartung T., and Bal-Price A. (2005) Inflammatory neurodegeneration induced by lipoteichoic acid from *Staphylococcus aureus* is mediated by glia activation, nitrosative and oxidative stress, and caspase activation. *Journal of Neurochemistry*; 95, 1132-43.

Kinsner A., Boveri M. , Hareng L., Brown G. C., Coecke S., Hartung T., and Bal-Price A. (2006) Highly purified lipoteichoic acid induced pro-inflammatory signalling in primary culture of rat microglia through Toll-like receptor 2: selective potentiation of nitric oxide production by muramyl dipeptide. *Journal of Neurochemistry,* 99,596-607

Kirkland R. A., Windelborn J. A., Kasprzak J. M., and Franklin J. L. (2002) A Bax-induced pro-oxidant state is critical for cytochrome c release during programmed neuronal death. *J Neurosci* 22, 6480-6490.

Kitamura Y., Matsuoka Y., Nomura Y., Taniguchi T. (1998) Induction of inducible nitric oxide synthase and heme oxygenase-1 in rat glial cells. *Life Sci* 62, 1717-1721.

Klegeris A., Walker D. G., and McGeer P. L. (1997) Regulation of glutamate in cultures of human monocytic THP-1 and astrocytoma U-373 MG cells. *J Neuroimmunol* 78, 152-161.

Kleinert H., Schwarz P. M., and Forstermann U. (2003) Regulation of the expression of inducible nitric oxide synthase. *Biol Chem* 384, 1343-1364.

Koedel U., Bayerlein I., Paul R., Sporer B., and Pfister H. W. (2000) Pharmacologic interference with NF kappaB activation attenuates central nervous system complications in experimental Pneumococcal meningitis. *J Infect Dis* 182, 1437-1445.

Kolb S. A., Lahrtz F., Paul R., Leppert D., Nadal D., Pfister H. W., and Fontana A. (1998) Matrix metalloproteinases and tissue inhibitors of metalloproteinases in viral meningitis: upregulation of MMP-9 and TIMP-1 in cerebrospinal fluid. *J Neuroimmunol* 84, 143-150.

Kreutzberg G. W. (1996) Microglia: a sensor for pathological events in the CNS. *Trends Neurosci* 19, 312-318.

Kurkowska-Jastrzebska I., Litwin T., Joniec I., Ciesielska A., Przybylkowski A., Czlonkowski A., and Czlonkowska A. (2004) Dexamethasone protects against dopaminergic neurons damage in a mouse model of Parkinson's disease. *Int Immunopharmacol* 4, 1307-1318.

Lascola C. and Kraig R. P. (1997) Astroglial acid-base dynamics in hyperglycemic and normoglycemic global ischemia. *Neurosci Biobehav Rev* 21, 143-150.

Lee S. J. and Lee S. (2002) Toll-like receptors and inflammation in the CNS. *Curr Drug Targets Inflamm Allergy* 1, 181-191.

Leib S. L., Clements J. M., Lindberg R. L., Heimgartner C., Loeffler J. M., Pfister L. A., Tauber M. G., and Leppert D. (2001) Inhibition of matrix metalloproteinases and tumour necrosis factor alpha converting enzyme as adjuvant therapy in pneumococcal meningitis. *Brain* 124, 1734-1742.

Leppert D., Lindberg R. L., Kappos L., and Leib S. L. (2001) Matrix metalloproteinases: multifunctional effectors of inflammation in multiple sclerosis and bacterial meningitis. *Brain Res Brain Res Rev* 36, 249-257.

Liu J. S., Amaral T. D., Brosnan C. F., and Lee S. C. (1998) IFNs are critical regulators of IL-1 receptor antagonist and IL-1 expression in human microglia. *J Immunol* 161, 1989-1996.

MacMicking J., Xie Q. W., and Nathan C. (1997) Nitric oxide and macrophage function. *Annu Rev Immunol* 15, 323-350.

Mander P., Borutaite V., Moncada S., and Brown G. C. (2005) Nitric oxide from inflammatory-activated glia synergises with hypoxia to induce neuronal death. *J Neurosci Res* 79, 208-215.

Marella M. and Chabry J. (2004) Neurons and astrocytes respond to prion infection by inducing microglia recruitment. *J Neurosci* 24, 620-627.

Marks-Konczalik J., Chu S. C., and Moss J. (1998) Cytokine-mediated transcriptional induction of the human inducible nitric oxide synthase gene requires both activator protein 1 and nuclear factor kappaB-binding sites. *J Biol Chem* 273, 22201-22208.

Matsuno R., Aramaki Y., and Tsuchiya S. (2001) Involvement of TGF-beta in inhibitory effects of negatively charged liposomes on nitric oxide production by macrophages stimulated with lps. *Biochem Biophys Res Commun* 281, 614-620.

McGeer P. L. and McGeer E. G. (1998) Mechanisms of cell death in Alzheimer disease - immunopathology. *J Neural Transm Suppl* 54, 159-166.

McGeer P. L. and McGeer E. G. (2001) Inflammation, autotoxicity and Alzheimer disease. *Neurobiol Aging* 22, 799-809.

McGeer P. L. and McGeer E. G. (2004) Inflammation and neurodegeneration in Parkinson's disease. *Parkinsonism Relat Disord* 10, 3-7.

McGraw J., Hiebert G. W., and Steeves J. D. (2001) Modulating astrogliosis after neurotrauma. *J Neurosci Res* 63, 109-115.

McManus C. M., Weidenheim K., Woodman S. E., Nunez J., Hesselgesser J., Nath A., and Berman J. W. (2000) Chemokine and chemokine-receptor expression in human glial elements: induction by the HIV protein, Tat, and chemokine autoregulation. *Am J Pathol* 156, 1441-1453.

McMenamin P. G. (1999) Distribution and phenotype of dendritic cells and resident tissue macrophages in the dura mater, leptomeninges, and choroid plexus of the rat brain as demonstrated in wholemount preparations. *J Comp Neurol* 405, 553-562.

McNaught K. S. and Brown G. C. (1998) Nitric oxide causes glutamate release from brain synaptosomes. *J Neurochem* 70, 1541-1546.

Minghetti L. (2004) Cyclooxygenase-2 (COX-2) in inflammatory and degenerative brain diseases. *J Neuropathol Exp Neurol* 63, 901-910.

Mohri I., Eguchi N., Suzuki K., Urade Y., and Taniike M. (2003) Hematopoietic prostaglandin D synthase is expressed in microglia in the developing postnatal mouse brain. *Glia* 42, 263-274.

Moncada S, Higgs EA. (1995) Molecular mechanisms and therapeutic strategies related to nitric oxide. *FASEB J* 9, 1319-1330

Montero-Menei C. N., Sindji L., Pouplard-Barthelaix A., Jehan F., Denechaud L., and Darcy F. (1994) Lipopolysaccharide intracerebral administration induces minimal inflammatory reaction in rat brain. *Brain Res* 653, 101-111.

Moretto G., Xu R. Y., Walker D. G., and Kim S. U. (1994) Co-expression of mRNA for neurotrophic factors in human neurons and glial cells in culture. *J Neuropathol Exp Neurol* 53, 78-85.

Morimoto K., Murasugi T., and Oda T. (2002) Acute neuroinflammation exacerbates excitotoxicity in rat hippocampus in vivo. *Exp Neurol* 177, 95-104.

Moro M. A., De Alba J., Leza J. C., Lorenzo P., Fernandez A. P., Bentura M. L., Bosca L., Rodrigo J., and Lizasoain I. (1998) Neuronal expression of inducible nitric oxide synthase after oxygen and glucose deprivation in rat forebrain slices. *Eur J Neurosci.* 10, 445-456.

Mrak R. E. and Griffin W. S. (2005) Glia and their cytokines in progression of neurodegeneration. *Neurobiol Aging* 26, 349-354.

Murphy T. H., Blatter L. A., Wier W. G., and Baraban J. M. (1993) Rapid communication between neurons and astrocytes in primary cortical cultures. *J Neurosci* 13, 2672-2679.

Nagatsu T. and Sawada M. (2005) Inflammatory process in Parkinson's disease: role for cytokines. *Curr Pharm Des* 11, 999-1016.

Nakanishi H. (2003) Microglial functions and proteases. *Mol Neurobiol* 27, 163-176.

Namura S., Nagata I., Takami S., Masayasu H., and Kikuchi H. (2001) Ebselen reduces cytochrome c release from mitochondria and subsequent DNA fragmentation after transient focal cerebral ischemia in mice. *Stroke* 32, 1906-1911.

Nau R. and Bruck W. (2002) Neuronal injury in bacterial meningitis: mechanisms and implications for therapy. *Trends Neurosci* 25, 38-45.

Nedergaard M. (1994) Direct signalling from astrocytes to neurons in cultures of mammalian brain cells. *Science* 263, 1768-1771.

Neumann H. (2003) Molecular mechanisms of axonal damage in inflammatory central nervous system diseases. *Curr Opin Neurol* 16, 267-273.

Nohl H., Gille L., Staniek K. (2005) Intracellular generation of reactive oxygen species by mitochondria. *Biochem Pharmacol.* 69, 719-723.

Norton W. T., Aquino D. A., Hozumi I., Chiu F. C., and Brosnan C. F. (1992) Quantitative aspects of reactive gliosis: a review. *Neurochem Res* 17, 877-885.

O'Keefe G. M., Nguyen V. T., and Benveniste E. N. (1999) Class II transactivator and class II MHC gene expression in microglia: modulation by the cytokines TGF-beta, IL-4, IL-13 and IL-10. *Eur J Immunol* 29, 1275-1285.

Ohtaki H., Funahashi H., Dohi K., Oguro T., Horai R., Asano M., Iwakura Y., Yin L., Matsunaga M., Goto N., and Shioda S. (2003) Suppression of oxidative neuronal damage after transient middle cerebral artery occlusion in mice lacking interleukin-1. *Neurosci Res* 45, 313-324.

Olsson T., Zhi W. W., Hojeberg B., Kostulas V., Jiang Y. P., Anderson G., Ekre H. P., and Link H. (1990) Autoreactive T lymphocytes in multiple sclerosis determined by antigen-induced secretion of interferon-gamma. *J Clin Invest* 86, 981-985.

Pan G., O'Rourke K., Chinnaiyan A. M., Gentz R., Ebner R., Ni J., and Dixit V. M. (1997) The receptor for the cytotoxic ligand TRAIL. *Science* 276, 111-113.

Paul R., Lorenzl S., Koedel U., Sporer B., Vogel U., Frosch M., and Pfister H. W. (1998) Matrix metalloproteinases contribute to the blood-brain barrier disruption during bacterial meningitis. *Ann Neurol* 44, 592-600.

Perry V. H. and Andersson P. B. (1992) The inflammatory response in the CNS. *Neuropathol Appl Neurobiol* 18, 454-459.

Piani D. and Fontana A. (1994) Involvement of the cystine transport system xc- in the macrophage-induced glutamate-dependent cytotoxicity to neurons. *J Immunol* 152, 3578-3585.

Poulin P. and Zakzanis K. K. (2002) In vivo neuroanatomy of Alzheimer's disease: evidence from structural and functional brain imaging. *Brain Cogn* 49, 220-225.

Prat A., Biernacki K., Wosik K., and Antel J. P. (2001) Glial cell influence on the human blood-brain barrier. *Glia* 36, 145-155.

Prinz M. and Hanisch U. K. (1999) Murine microglial cells produce and respond to interleukin-18. *J Neurochem* 72, 2215-2218.

Probert L., Akassoglou K., Pasparakis M., Kontogeorgos G., and Kollias G. (1995) Spontaneous inflammatory demyelinating disease in transgenic mice showing central nervous system-specific expression of tumor necrosis factor alpha. *Proc Natl Acad Sci U S A* 92, 11294-11298.

Raine C. S. (1999) Neurocellular anatomy. In *Basic Neurochemistry: molecular, cellular and medical aspects.* (Siegel G. J., Agranoff B.W., Albers R.W., Fisher S.K., and Uhler M.D., eds), pp. 3-30, Lippincott Williams and Wilkins, Philadelphia, U.S.

Raivich G. and Banati R. (2004) Brain microglia and blood-derived macrophages: molecular profiles and functional roles in multiple sclerosis and animal models of autoimmune demyelinating disease. *Brain Research Reviews* 46, 261-281.

Rappert A., Bechmann I., Pivneva T., Mahlo J., Biber K., Nolte C., Kovac A. D., Gerard C., Boddeke H. W., Nitsch R., and Kettenmann H. (2004) CXCR3-dependent microglial recruitment is essential for dendrite loss after brain lesion. *J Neurosci* 24, 8500-8509.

Rieckmann P., Albrecht M., Ehrenreich H., Weber T., and Michel U. (1995) Semi-quantitative analysis of cytokine gene expression in blood and cerebrospinal fluid cells by reverse transcriptase polymerase chain reaction. *Res Exp Med (Berl)* 195, 17-29.

Ring A., Weiser J. N., and Tuomanen E. I. (1998) Pneumococcal trafficking across the blood-brain barrier. Molecular analysis of a novel bidirectional pathway. *J Clin Invest* 102, 347-360.

Risau W., Esser S., and Engelhardt B. (1998) Differentiation of blood-brain barrier endothelial cells. *Pathol Biol (Paris)* 46, 171-175.

Rosenberg G. A. (2002) Matrix metalloproteinases in neuroinflammation. *Glia* 39, 279-291.

Rothwell N. J. and Luheshi G. N. (2000) Interleukin-1 in the brain: biology, pathology and therapeutic target. *Trends Neurosci* 23, 618-625.

Roux F., Durieu-Trautmann O., Chaverot N., Claire M., Mailly P., Bourre J. M., Strosberg A. D., and Couraud P. O. (1994) Regulation of gamma-glutamyl transpeptidase and alkaline phosphatase activities in immortalized rat brain microvessel endothelial cells. *J Cell Physiol* 159, 101-113.

Rudge J. S., Morrissey D., Lindsay R. M., and Pasnikowski E. M. (1994) Regulation of ciliary neurotrophic factor in cultured rat hippocampal astrocytes. *Eur J Neurosci* 6, 218-229.

Schmidt H., Tlustochowska A., Stuertz K., Djukic M., Gerber J., Schutz E., Kuhnt U., and Nau R. (2001) Organotypic hippocampal cultures. A model of brain tissue damage in Streptococcus pneumoniae meningitis. *J Neuroimmunol* 113, 30-39.

Sedgwick J. D., Riminton D. S., Cyster J. G., and Korner H. (2000) Tumor necrosis factor: a master-regulator of leukocyte movement. *Immunol Today* 21, 110-113.

Segal B. M., Dwyer B. K., and Shevach E. M. (1998) An interleukin (IL)-10/IL-12 immunoregulatory circuit controls susceptibility to autoimmune disease. *J Exp Med* 187, 537-546.

Selmaj K. W., Farooq M., Norton W. T., Raine C. S., and Brosnan C. F. (1990) Proliferation of astrocytes in vitro in response to cytokines. A primary role for tumor necrosis factor. *J Immunol* 144, 129-135.

Shevach E. M., Chang J. T., and Segal B. M. (1999) The critical role of IL-12 and the IL-12R beta 2 subunit in the generation of pathogenic autoreactive Th1 cells. *Springer Semin Immunopathol* 21, 249-262.

Simard M. and Nedergaard M. (2004) The neurobiology of glia in the context of water and ion homeostasis. *Neuroscience* 129; 877-896.

Singh S. and Evans T. W. (1997) Nitric oxide, the biological mediator of the decade: fact or fiction? *Eur Respir J* 10, 699-707.

Sobue K., Yamamoto N., Yoneda K., Hodgson M. E., Yamashiro K., Tsuruoka N., Tsuda T., Katsuya H., Miura Y., Asai K., and Kato T. (1999) Induction of blood-brain barrier properties in immortalized bovine brain endothelial cells by astrocytic factors. *Neurosci Res* 35, 155-164.

Southan G.J. and Szabo C. (1996) Selective pharmacological inhibition of distinct nitric oxide synthase isoforms. *Biochem Pharmacol* 51, 383-394.

Sukriti N. (2003) Pathophysiology of Blood–Brain Barrier Breakdown *Met Mol Med* 89, 97-120.

Staub F., Winkler A., Peters J., Goerke U., Kempski O., and Baethmann A. (1995) Clearance and metabolism of arachidonic acid by C6 glioma cells and astrocytes. *Neurochem Res* 20, 1449-1456.

Stewart V. C. and Heales S. J. (2003) Nitric oxide-induced mitochondrial dysfunction: implications for neurodegeneration. *Free Radic Biol Med* 34, 287-303.

Swanson R. A., Ying W., and Kauppinen T. M. (2004) Astrocyte influences on ischemic neuronal death. *Curr Mol Med* 4, 193-205.

Szabo C., Day B.J., and Salzman A.L. (1996) Evaluation of the relative contribution of nitric oxide and peroxynitrite to the suppression of mitochondrial respiration in immunostimulated macrophages using a manganese mesoporphyrin superoxide dismutase mimetic and peroxynitrite scavenger. *FEBS Lett* 381, 82-86.

Szekely C. A., Thorne J. E., Zandi P. P., Ek M., Messias E., Breitner J. C., and Goodman S. N. (2004) Nonsteroidal anti-inflammatory drugs for the prevention of Alzheimer's disease: a systematic review. *Neuroepidemiology* 23, 159-169.

Szelenyi J. (2001) Cytokines and the central nervous system. *Brain Res Bull* 54, 329-338.

Tang T., Frenette P. S., Hynes R. O., Wagner D. D., and Mayadas T. N. (1996) Cytokine-induced meningitis is dramatically attenuated in mice deficient in endothelial selectins. *J Clin Invest* 97, 2485-2490.

Taylor B. S. and Geller D. A. (2000) Molecular regulation of the human inducible nitric oxide synthase (iNOS) gene. *Shock* 13, 413-424.

Teather L. A. and Wurtman R. J. (2003) Cyclooxygenase-2 mediates platelet-activating factor-induced prostaglandin E2 release from rat primary astrocytes. *Neurosci Lett* 340, 177-180.

Ter Laak M. P., Brakkee J. H., Adan R. A., Hamers F. P., and Gispen W. H. (2003) The potent melanocortin receptor agonist melanotan-II promotes peripheral nerve regeneration and has neuroprotective properties in the rat. *Eur J Pharmacol* 462, 179-183.

Toft-Hansen H., Nuttall R.K., Edwards D.R., and Owens T. (2004) Key metalloproteinases are expressed by specific cell types in experimental autoimmune encephalomyelitis. *J Immunol* 173, 5209-5218.

Touzani O., Boutin H., LeFeuvre R., Parker L., Miller A., Luheshi G., and Rothwell N. (2002) Interleukin-1 influences ischemic brain damage in the mouse independently of the interleukin-1 type I receptor. *J Neurosci* 22, 38-43.

Tsunawaki S., Sporn M., Ding A., and Nathan C. (1988) Deactivation of macrophages by transforming growth factor-beta. *Nature* 334, 260-262.

Umegaki H., Yamada K., Naito M., Kameyama T., Iguchi A., and Nabeshima T. (1996) Protective effect of interleukin-6 against the death of PC12 cells caused by serum deprivation or by the addition of a calcium ionophore. *Biochem Pharmacol* 52, 911-916.

Van Deuren M. (1994) Kinetics of tumour necrosis factor-alpha, soluble tumour necrosis factor receptors, interleukin 1-beta and its receptor antagonist during serious infections. *Eur J Clin Microbiol Infect Dis* 13, 12-16.

Van Furth A.M., Seijmonsbergen E.M., Langermans J.A., Groeneveld P.H., de Bel C.E. and van Furth R (1995) High levels of interleukin 10 and tumor necrosis factor alpha in cerebrospinal fluid during the onset of bacterial meningitis. *Clin Infect Dis* 21, 220-222

Vincent A. M. and Maiese K. (1999) Nitric oxide induction of neuronal endonuclease activity in programmed cell death. *Exp Cell Res* 246, 290-300.

Virag L and Szabo C. (2002) The therapeutic potential of poly-(ADP-ribose) polymerase inhibitors. *Pharmacol Rev* 54, 375-429.

Vodovotz Y., Geiser A. G., Chesler L., Letterio J. J., Campbell A., Lucia M. S., Sporn M. B., and Roberts A. B. (1996) Spontaneously increased production of nitric oxide and aberrant expression of the inducible nitric oxide synthase in vivo in the transforming growth factor beta 1 null mouse. *J Exp Med* 183, 2337-2342.

Walz W. (2000) Role of astrocytes in the clearance of excess extracellular potassium. *Neurochem Int* 36, 291-300.

Wang J. Y., Shum A. Y., Ho Y. J., and Wang J. Y. (2003) Oxidative neurotoxicity in rat cerebral cortex neurons: synergistic effects of H2O2 and NO on apoptosis involving activation of p38 mitogen-activated protein kinase and caspase-3. *J Neurosci Res* 72, 508-519.

Wang Y. and Marsden P. A. (1995) Nitric oxide synthases: gene structure and regulation. *Adv Pharmacol* 34, 71-90.

Williams K., Alvarez X., and Lackner A. A. (2001) Central nervous system perivascular cells are immunoregulatory cells that connect the CNS with the peripheral immune system. *Glia* 36, 156-164.

Wilson J. X. (1997) Antioxidant defense of the brain: a role for astrocytes. *Can J Physiol Pharmacol* 75, 1149-1163.

Wink D. A., Miranda K. M., and Espey M. G. (2001) Cytotoxicity related to oxidative and nitrosative stress by nitric oxide. *Exp Biol Med (Maywood)* 226, 621-623.

Wu C. Y., Hsieh H. L., Jou M. J., and Yang C. M. (2004) Involvement of p42/p44 MAPK, p38 MAPK, JNK and nuclear factor-kappa B in interleukin-1beta-induced matrix metalloproteinase-9 expression in rat brain astrocytes. *J Neurochem* 90, 1477-1488.

Xu J., Chalimoniuk M., Shu Y., Simonyi A., Sun A. Y., Gonzalez F. A., Weisman G. A., Wood W. G., and Sun G. Y. (2003) Prostaglandin E2 production in astrocytes: regulation by cytokines, extracellular ATP, and oxidative agents. *Prostaglandins Leukot Essent Fatty Acids* 69, 437-448.

Xu W., Liu L. Z., Loizidou M., Ahmed M., and Charles I. G. (2002) The role of nitric oxide in cancer. *Cell Res* 12, 311-320.

Yamamoto T., Maruyama W., Kato Y., Yi H., Shamoto-Nagai M., Tanaka M., Sato Y., and Naoi M. (2002) Selective nitration of mitochondrial complex I by peroxynitrite: involvement in mitochondria dysfunction and cell death of dopaminergic SH-SY5Y cells. *J Neural Transm* 109, 1-13.

Zhang J. and Rivest S. (2001) Anti-inflammatory effects of prostaglandin E2 in the central nervous system in response to brain injury and circulating lipopolysaccharide. *J Neurochem* 76, 855-864.

Zhang S. C. and Fedoroff S. (1996) Neuron-microglia interactions in vitro. *Acta Neuropathol (Berl)* 91, 385-395.

Zlotnik A. and Yoshie O. (2000) Chemokines: a new classification system and their role in immunity. *Immunity* 12, 121-127.

Zwijnenburg P. J., Polfliet M. M., Florquin S., van den Berg T. K., Dijkstra C. D., van Deventer S. J., Roord J. J., van der P. T., and van Furth A. M. (2003) CXC-chemokines

KC and macrophage inflammatory protein-2 (MIP-2) synergistically induce leukocyte recruitment to the central nervous system in rats. *Immunol Lett* 85, 1-4.

Reviewed by: Helena Hogberg, PhD, Johns Hopkins Center for Alternatives to Animal Testing (CAAT), Johns Hopkins University Bloomberg School of Public Health, 615 N. Wolfe St., W7032, Baltimore, MD, 21205; Phone: +1 410 614 4980; Fax: +1 410 614 2871 (hhogberg@jhsph.edu).

In: Glial Cells
Editors: Charanjit Kaur and Eng-Ang Ling
ISBN: 978-1-62618-448-0
© 2013 Nova Science Publishers, Inc.

Chapter 4

GLIA AND THE PATHOLOGY OF VARIANT CREUTZFELDT-JAKOB DISEASE (VCJD)

Richard A. Armstrong*
Vision Sciences, Aston University, Birmingham, UK

ABSTRACT

Glia may be implicated in the pathology of variant Creutzfeldt-Jakob disease (vCJD) in several ways: (1) glial cells could be involved in the formation of prion protein (PrP^{sc}) deposits, (2) PrP^{sc} deposits could stimulate the production of astrocytes and microglia, (3) PrP^{sc} deposits could damage adjacent glial cells, and (4) glial cells could remove aggregates of PrP^{sc} from the brain. To clarify the significance of glial cells in vCJD, the relationship between PrP^{sc} deposits and their associated glia, together with neurons and blood vessels, was studied in six cases of vCJD. Multicentric PrP^{sc} deposits were the largest and least frequent type of deposit observed and were more commonly associated with glial cells, neuronal perikarya, and blood vessels than the more common diffuse and florid PrP^{sc} deposits. Diffuse PrP^{sc} deposits were more frequently associated with glial cells and neurons than the florid deposits. The ratio of astrocytes to oligodendrocytes adjacent to PrP^{sc} deposits was similar to normal brain but the ratio of astrocytes or oligodendrocytes to microglia was less than in normal brain. The intensity of immunolabelling of multicentric PrP^{sc} deposits was positively correlated with the presence of associated vacuoles and negatively correlated with the frequency of microglia. The patterns of correlation between deposit morphology and associated glial cells and neurons were similar for the diffuse and florid type PrP^{sc} deposits. Deposit size was most consistently correlated with the number of associated neurons and vacuoles. The data suggest in vCJD: (1) there was no evidence that glia were necessary for the formation of PrP^{sc} deposits, (2) there is an increase in microglia which may be an attempt to remove PrP^{sc} from the bain, and (3) PrP^{sc} deposits could affect adjacent astrocytes and damage the blood brain barrier (BBB).

* Corresponding Author: Dr. R.A. Armstrong, Vision Sciences, Aston University, Birmingham, B4 7ET, UK. Tel 0121-359-3611, Fax 0121-333-4220, EMail: R.A.Armstrong@aston.ac.uk.

Keywords: Variant Creutzfeldt-Jakob disease (vCJD), astrocytes, oligodendrocytes, microglia, neurons, blood vessels

INTRODUCTION

A number of diseases have been described in animals and humans caused by proteinaceous infectious particles called prions (Prusiner, 1995) and referred to as the 'transmissible spongiform encephalopathies' (TSE). Prions are composed mainly of protein and differ significantly in behaviour from bacteria and viruses. Prion diseases include 'scrapie' in sheep, 'bovine spongiform encephalopathy' (BSE) in cattle, and Creutzfeldt-Jakob disease (CJD) in humans. These diseases are important because they can be transmitted between members of the same species and may also cross the species barrier and adapt to new hosts. Of particular concern is whether a subtype of CJD in humans, largely found in the United Kingdom (UK) and termed variant CJD (vCJD), can be acquired from cattle with BSE (Will et al., 1996; Ironside, 2000).

Prion Diseases

There are four human TSE caused by prions. In addition to CJD itself, three other human prion diseases have been identified. First, 'kuru' occurred in the past in the 'Fore highlanders', natives of Papua and New Guinea, and was probably transmitted as a consequence of ritual cannibalism. Second, 'fatal familial insomnia' (FFI) is a recently described genetic disorder that is characterized initially by sleep disturbance, insomnia, and agitation and later, by the development of hallucinations, stupor, and coma (Collins et al., 2001). Third, Gerstman-Straussler-Scheinker (GSS) disease is a rare genetic disorder first described in 1936 and characterized by ataxia, dementia, limb weakness, and speech problems (Collins et al., 2001).

Prions and Prion Disease

The first description of CJD was published independently by Creutzfeldt (Creutzfeldt, 1921) and Jakob (Jakob, 1921), and is the most important human form of TSE. Patients develop dementia, which may be preceded by ataxia and loss of coordination, with death resulting in about 3-12 months after the onset of symptoms. The characteristic pathological signs of prion disease are observed in the gray matter of the brain including vacuolation ('spongiform change'), neuronal loss, the proliferation of astrocytes, and the deposition of prion protein (PrP) in the form of discreet deposits or plaques. PrP exists in two forms, viz., normal cellular PrP (PrP^{c}), which does not cause disease and a disease specific form of PrP (PrP^{sc}), the presence of which can induce prion disease (DeArmond and Prusiner, 1995). Within a species, these two forms of PrP are identical in amino acid composition but differ in molecular conformation and in the composition of the attached chains of carbohydrates. Normal PrP^{c} comprises four α–helices with virtually no β–sheets whereas PrP^{sc} displays an identical primary structure to PrP^{c} but differs in secondary and tertiary structure (Caughey,

2001). Hence, PrP^{sc} displays a four-stranded β–sheet configuration covered on one face by two α-helices. Prusiner (1995) found that transgenic mice reared without the gene for PrP^{c} could not be infected with scrapie suggesting that PrP^{c} was required for the disease to develop. Normal PrP^{c} is converted into pathogenic PrP^{sc} in the presence of PrP^{c}, the process being auto-catalytic and proceeding at a rapid rate within the brain. Conversion of PrP^{c} to PrP^{sc} may be mediated via several chaperone molecules (Stockel and Hartl, 2001) and a conserved sequence of PrP (residues 90-121) may also be critical for PrP^{sc} generation (Stockel and Hartl, 2001). PrP^{sc}, because of its β–sheet structure, has a greater tendency than PrP^{c} to form insoluble aggregates or deposits in brain tissue. Hence, the deposition of PrP^{sc} in the form of deposits may result in the death of neurons and the development of vacuolation. Within the nervous system, PrP^{sc} appears to target specific nerve cell populations and may spread through the brain via cerebral spinal fluid or cell to cell by anatomical connections (Prusiner and DeArmond, 1994; Armstrong et al., 2000). No significant immune response has been detected in prion disease but complement proteins (C1q, C3b) have been found associated with PrP^{sc} deposits and the membrane attack complex (MAC) with neurons (Kovacs et al., 2004).

Subtypes of CJD

There are three major subtypes of CJD: (1) cases associated with genetic factors (familial or fCJD), (2) cases resulting from the transmission of PrP^{sc} (iatrogenic or iCJD), and (3) cases that occur sporadically within the population (sporadic or sCJD). About 10-15% of cases of CJD are genetic and this condition is inherited as an autosomal dominant gene. Point mutations of the coding region of the *PrP* gene on chromosome 20 have been identified in a number of these cases (Goldfarb et al., 1994). A small number of CJD cases can be traced to a transmissible cause. Possible sources of transmission include corneal transplant (Hogan and Cavanagh, 1995), the use of electrodes implanted in the brain, neurosurgery, dura mater grafts, and the use of growth hormone. Disease acquired as a result of the use of growth hormone extracted from human pituitary glands has largely been eliminated as a result of the use of genetically engineered growth hormone. About 85% of recorded cases of CJD are sporadic. The mean age of onset of sCJD is 60 years of age and its incidence is approximately 1/1,000,000. Two theories have been proposed to explain the sporadic cases. First, a mutation of the *PrP* gene could result in the formation of PrP^{sc} rather that PrP^{c} or second, PrP^{c} could be converted spontaneously to PrP^{sc}.

Variant CJD

The appearance of a new subtype of CJD, viz., vCJD, which may be related to BSE, has caused considerable concern especially in the UK. The first cases of vCJD were recorded in 1995 and by 2012, the total number of deaths ascribed to the disease was 176 (National CJD Surveillance Unit data). The new variant of CJD differs significantly from other subtypes in having an earlier age of onset (mean 28 years) and a prolonged duration of illness (up to 2 years) (Will et al., 1996; Ironside, 2000). Presentation of the disease is largely psychiatric with patients exhibiting anxiety, depression, and behavioural changes. After a period of weeks or months, a cerebellar syndrome develops and the patient experiences problems in walking and with movement. Memory problems develop late in the clinical course and the patient ultimately becomes mute and unable to move. Myoclonus occurs at some stage in the disease in the majority of patients. In addition, the pathology of vCJD differs from other forms of the disease in the presence of widespread and concentrated deposits of PrP^{sc} throughout the brain in the form of 'florid deposits' (Grigoriev et al., 1999; Ironside, 2000; Ironside et al., 1996; Armstrong et al., 2003a). In addition, the PrP^{sc} of vCJD has a uniform glycotype (PrP^{sc}, Type 4) and is distinct from that observed in sCJD (Hill et al., 1999, Ironside et al., 2000).

Types of PrP^{sc} deposit

Different types of PrP^{sc} deposits have been identified in the various TSE (Watanabe and Duchen, 1993). These PrP^{sc} deposits differ in morphology and contain varying amounts of loosely interwoven amyloid fibrils (Fournier et al., 2000).

They have been classified into different morphological subtypes including multicentric, unicentric, 'kuru', neuritic, diffuse, synaptic, and perivascular types of deposit (Watanabe and Duchen, 1993). In addition, the different types of deposit appear to be associated with specific prion diseases. Hence the 'kuru-type' deposit with its solid core, radiating fibrils, and lack of dystrophic neurites and reactive cells is particularly associated with the disease 'kuru' while 'synaptic-type' deposits appear to be particularly characteristic of sCJD (Armstrong et al., 2001). Different morphological forms of PrP^{sc} deposit have also been identified in the brains of patients with vCJD. One of the commonest types of deposit in vCJD is the 'florid deposit', composed of a central core and a rim of peripheral vacuoles.

These deposits more closely resemble the 'classic' β-amyloid (Aβ) deposits observed in Alzheimer's disease (AD) (Armstrong, 1998) than the 'kuru-type' deposits found in kuru (Liberski et al., 2000). In addition to the florid deposits, various other types of PrP^{sc} deposit are often present (Grigoriev et al., 1999) including diffuse and multicentric-type deposits.

A unique distribution of PrP^{sc} deposits is also present in vCJD affecting all of the cerebral cortex, cerebellum, basal ganglia, thalamus, and brain stem. Whether the diffuse deposits evolve into florid deposits as the disease progresses or whether they represent unique morphological forms of PrP^{sc} remains to be resolved (Armstrong et al., 2003a).

Glial Cells and PrP^{sc} Deposits

Glial cells are non-neural cells which have a variety of functions in the central nervous system (CNS). The ratio of glia to neurons is 1:1 in the brain as a whole but 2:1 in the cerebral gray matter. Glia have four main functions in the CNS: (1) to surround neurons and hold them in place, (2) to supply nutrients and oxygen to neurons, (3) to insulate one neuron from another, and (4) to modulate neurotransmission. Hence, in the hippocampus and cerebellum, glia may be involved in synaptic transmission, in regulating the clearance of neurotransmitters from the synaptic cleft, and in the release of transmitters such as ATP. Of the different types of glia, astrocytes are crucial in the clearance of neurotransmitters from the synaptic cleft and in the prevention of the accumulation of glutamate. In addition, astrocytes can enlarge and proliferate and can release inhibitory compounds that prevent the regrowth of damaged axons. Astrocytes also have numerous projections which anchor neurons to their blood supply and are important in the establishment of the blood brain barrier (BBB). Consequently, damage to glia could have widespread effects in the CNS including an affect on the BBB and the release of blood proteins (Armstrong et al., 2003b). By contrast, oligodendrocytes coat axons in the CNS resulting in the formation of myelin sheaths while microglia are specialised macrophages involved in phagocytosis and in the protection of neurons. Microglia are mobile and often proliferate in response to damage or neurodegeneration and might therefore, along with astrocytes, be expected to increase in the brain in vCJD.

OBJECTIVES

Glia may potentially interact with PrP^{sc} deposits in vCJD in a variety of ways. First, glial cells could be involved in the formation and subsequent growth of PrP^{sc} deposits and in the possible evolution of the diffuse-type to florid-type deposits (Armstrong et al., 2003a). Second, PrP^{sc} deposits could stimulate the production of glial cells, especially microglia. Third, PrP^{sc} deposits may damage adjacent glial cells as well as neurons thus influencing CNS function. Fourth, glial cells could be involved in attempts to remove PrP^{sc} deposits from the brain. Hence, the objective of this chapter was to investigate the association between diffuse, florid, and multicentric PrP^{sc} deposits with astrocytes, oligodendrocytes, and microglia, together with neurons and cerebral microvessels, to determine the significance of glia in vCJD.

MATERIALS AND METHODS

Cases

Table 1. Demographic details and gross brain pathology of variant Creutzfeldt-Jakob disease cases studied

Case	Sex	Age at onset (yrs)	Duration (yrs)	Brain weight (gm)	Atrophy
A	F	39	2	586 (L)	None
B	F	28	1	1375	None
C	F	28	1	NA	NA
D	M	19	1	NA	NA
E	M	30	1	699 (R)	None
F	M	48	2	1470	None

Abbreviations: M = Male, F = Female, R = Right hemisphere, L = Left hemisphere, NA = data not available.

Six cases of vCJD (3 male, 3 female) (details in Table 1) were studied at the Brain Bank, Department of Neuropathology, Institute of Psychiatry, King's College London, UK. Brain material was obtained from the National CJD Surveillance Unit, Western General Hospital, Edinburgh, UK and included two cases (A,B) which were among the first published description of vCJD (Will et al., 1996). All cases fulfilled the neuropathological diagnostic criteria for vCJD (Ironside, 2000). None of the cases had any of the known mutations of the PrP gene or family history of prion disease, and there was no evidence of the known types of iatrogenic aetiology. The pattern of PrP^{sc} deposition characteristic of vCJD was observed with florid deposits in the cerebral cortex, cerebellum, basal ganglia, thalamus, and brain stem. All vCJD cases studied were homozygous for methionine at codon 129 of the PrP gene (Cervenakova et al., 1998).

Histological Methods

Blocks of the frontal cortex (B8) at the level of the genu of the corpus callosum, parietal cortex (B7) at the level of the splenium of the corpus callosum, occipital cortex including the calcarine sulcus and parahippocampal gyrus (B28) were studied. Tissue was fixed in 10% phosphate buffered formal-saline and embedded in paraffin wax.

Coronal 7μm sections were immunolabelled against PrP using the monoclonal antibody 12F10 (dilution 1:250) which binds to a region of human PrP downstream of the neurotoxic domain adjacent to helix region 2: residues 142-160 (Krasemann et al., 1996) and kindly provided by Prof. G. Hunsmann, The German Primate Centre, Gottingen, Germany).

Immunoreactivity was enhanced by formic acid (98% for 5 minutes) and autoclaving (121°C for 10 minutes) pretreatment. Sections were treated with Dako Biotinylated Rabbit anti-Mouse (RAM) (dilution 1:100) and Dako ABComplex HRP kit for 45 minutes (Amersham, UK). Diaminobenzidine tetrahydrochloride was used as the chromogen. Immunolabelled sections were counterstained with haematoxylin for 1 minute to stain glial cell nuclei and the nissl substance of neurons.

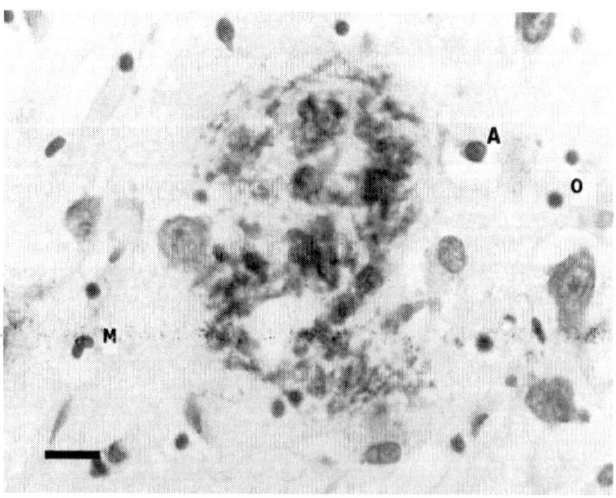

Figure 1. Glial cells (A = Astrocyte nucleus, O = Oligodendrocyte nucleus, M = Microglia nucleus) associated with a diffuse prion protein (PrP^{sc}) deposit a case of variant Creutzfeldt-Jakob disease (vCJD). (PrP immunostaining, Haematoxylin; Bar = 10μm).

In such preparations, surviving neurons were identified as cells containing at least some stained cytoplasm in combination with larger shape and non-spherical outline (Armstrong, 1996). Small spherical or asymmetrical nuclei without cytoplasm, but with the presence of a thicker nuclear membrane and more heterogeneous chromatin, were identified as glial cells. the nuclei of non-neural cells (Figure 1) were considered to fall into three groups: (1) larger more lightly stained glial nuclei (astrocytes), (2) smaller more darkly stained nuclei (oligodendrocytes), and (3) darkly stained angular-shaped nuclei (microglia) (Nauta and Feirtag, 1986). Tissue sections were also immunolabelled with GFAP and CD68 to confirm these morphological interpretations for astrocytes and microglia respectively. In addition, neurons were divided into two groups: (1) larger neurons, maximum diameter of cell body >25 μm and (2) smaller neurons, diameter <25 μm. Blood vessel profiles were also present in the sections lined with the crescent-shaped nuclei of endothelial cells.

Morphometric Methods

In each cortical gyrus studied, guidelines were marked at random on the slide extending from the pia mater to the white matter. All PrP^{sc} deposits touching a guideline were then included in the measured sample. Guidelines were drawn until a total of at least 50 PrP^{sc} deposits were sampled within each region.

The following data were collected from each PrP^{sc} deposit: (1) whether the deposit occurred within a sulcus or the crest of a gyrus, (2) the distance of the deposit below the pia mater, (3) the greatest diameter of the deposit, (4) the shape of the deposit measured as the ratio of the smallest to the largest diameter, (5) the depth of immunolabelling of the deposit measured on a five point scale from 1 (light stain) to 5 (heavy stain), (6) the length of any blood vessel profile actually touching the deposit, (7) the number of neuronal perikarya contained within or touching the deposit divided into larger (>25 mm) and smaller (<25 mm) neurons (Armstrong, 1995), (9) the number of astrocytic, oligodendrocytic, and microglia cell nuclei contained within or directly touching the deposit, and (10) the number of vacuoles touching or contained within the deposit.

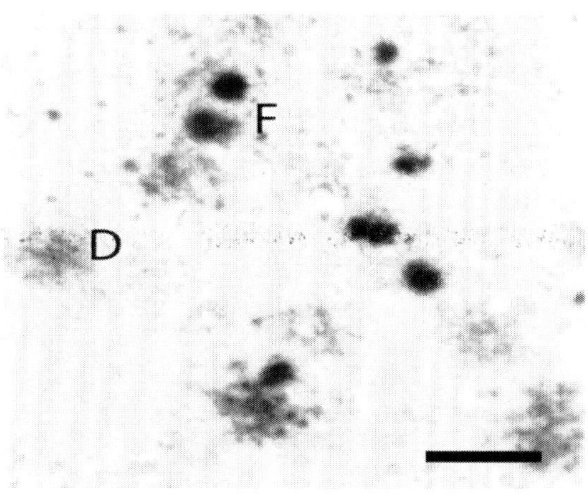

Figure 2. Diffuse (D) and florid (F) prion protein (PrP^{sc}) deposits in the cerebral cortex of a case of variant Creutzfeldt-Jakob disease (vCJD). (PrP immunostaining, Haematoxylin; Bar = 40μm).

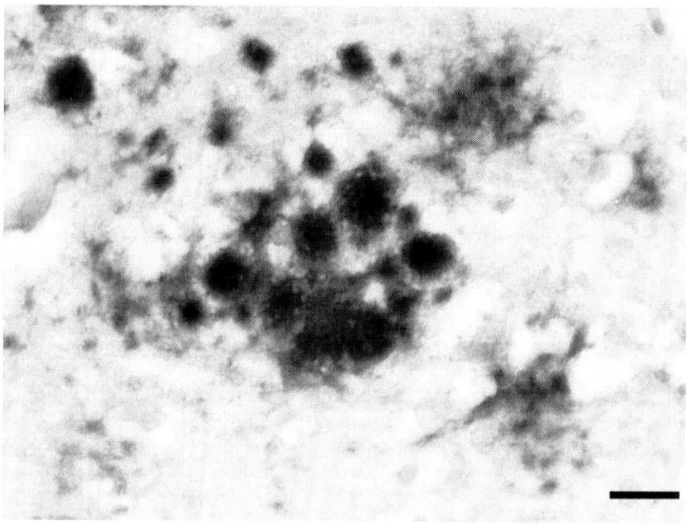

Figure 3. A multicentric prion protein (PrP^{sc}) deposits in the cerebral cortex of a case of variant Creutzfeldt-Jakob disease (vCJD). (PrP immunostaining, Haematoxylin; Bar = 30μm).

In addition, each PrP^{sc} deposit was classified into the three subtypes: diffuse, florid, and multicentric using previously published criteria (Armstrong et al., 2003a).

Hence, florid deposits were unicentric and consisted of a dense core of PrP^{sc} (Figure 2), diffuse deposits were unicentric and always lacked a solid core (Figure 2), and multicentric deposits (Figure 3) consisted of a cluster of several small solid deposits (Watanabe and Duchen, 1993).

Data Analysis

Two statistical analyses were carried out (STATISTICA software, Statsoft Inc., 2300 East 14th St, Tulsa, Ok, 74104, USA). First, to determine whether there were differences in the morphology of the diffuse and florid PrP^{sc} deposits between patients and brain regions, the data were averaged for each brain region for each patient. These data were analysed by a two-factor, split-plot analysis of variance (ANOVA) to determine whether each morphological attribute or associated structure varied between patients, deposit type, or brain region. Second, correlations (Pearson's 'r') were calculated between the morphological characteristics of the diffuse or florid PrP^{sc} deposits (diameter, shape, degree of immunolabelling) and each associated cell type (neurons, glial cell nuclei, blood vessels, vacuoles). Multicentric deposits were significantly rarer than the diffuse and florid types, were pooled from all brain regions and patients, and then analysed as a separate group.

RESULTS

The major quantitative characteristics of the three subtypes of PrP^{sc} deposit in vCJD, viz., diffuse, florid, and multicentric deposits are summarised in Table 2. The diffuse and florid

PrP^{sc} deposits were evenly represented in the sample while multicentric deposits were rare and contributed only 3.3% to the total sample. In addition, there were some PrP^{sc} deposits which could not be identified with confidence to any of the three deposit types but these accounted for less than 4% of the sample. On average, multicentric deposits had the largest diameters and were the most frequently associated with blood vessel profiles, neuronal cell bodies, glial cell nuclei, and vacuoles. Diffuse PrP^{sc} deposits were larger, less symmetrical in shape, and were more lightly stained than the florid PrP^{sc} and more frequently associated with neurons, glial cell nuclei, and vacuoles compared with the florid PrP^{sc} deposits.

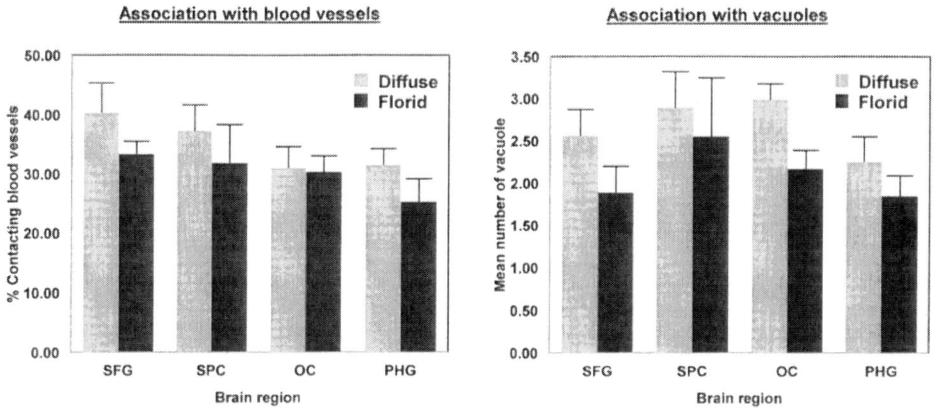

Figure 4. Degree of association of the diffuse and florid prion protein (PrP^{sc}) deposits with blood vessel profiles and vacuoles in cases of variant Creutzfeldt-Jakob disease (vCJD). ANOVA: Blood vessels Brain region $F = 1.92$ ($P > 0.05$), Deposit type $F = 7.24$ ($P < 0.05$), Interaction $F = 0.63$ ($P > 0.05$), Patients $F = 4.34$ ($P > 0.05$); Vacuoles Brain region $F = 1.28$ ($P > 0.05$), Deposit type $F = 9.04$ ($P < 0.01$), Interaction $F = 0.37$ ($P > 0.05$), Patient $F = 2.54$ ($P < 0.05$).

Table 2. Summary of the morphological characteristics and associated glia and neurons of the prion protein (PrP^{sc}) deposits in cases of variant Creutzfeldt-Jakob disease (vCJD). Data for glia and neurons are mean numbers per deposit

	PrPsc deposit type		
Feature	Diffuse	Florid	Multicentric
Number of deposits	561	549	40
% deposits touching blood vessel	47	46	3.3
Largest diameter (μm)	35.0	30.2	65
Shape	0.78	0.94	0.80
Immunolabelling	2.6	4.8	4.7
Number of large neurons	1.54	0.13	1.92
Number of small neurons	0.63	0.15	0.73
Number of astrocytes	0.09	0.05	0.05
Number of oligodendrocytes	0.49	0.17	0.40
Number of microglia	0.38	0.15	0.43
Number of vacuoles	2.68	2.12	6.08

Table 3. Aspects of the morphology of diffuse and florid prion protein (PrP^{sc}) deposits (mean, SE in parentheses) in different brain regions (FC = Frontal cortex, PC = parietal cortex, OC = Occipital cortex, PHG = Parahippocampal gyrus) in cases of variant Creutzfeldt-Jakob disease (vCJD)

		Region			
Morphology	Subtype	FC	PC	OC	PHG
Diameter	Diffuse	39 (1.57)	39.7 (1.85)	42.55 (1.35)	32.9 (1.68)
	Florid	11 (1.58)	13.38 (1.03)	14.8 (0.75)	12.45 (0.58)
Shape	Diffuse	0.76 (0.02)	0.79 (0.01)	0.76 (0.02)	0.80 (0.01)
	Florid	0.95 (0.02)	0.94 (0.02)	0.92 (0.02)	0.94 (0.01)
Immunolabel	Diffuse	2.6 (0.11)	2.72 (0.24)	2.61 (0.09)	2.61 (0.13)
	Florid	4.9 (0.06)	4.86 (0.06)	4.94 (0.03)	4.64 (0.09)

Analysis of variance (ANOVA): Deposit size: Brain region F = 23.12 ($P < 0.001$), Deposit type F = 1070.61 ($P < 0.001$), Interaction F = 5.03 ($P < 0.01$), Patients F = 15.15 ($P < 0.01$); Shape: Brain region F = 2.23 ($P > 0.05$), Deposit type F = 252.80 ($P < 0.001$), Interaction F = 0.87 ($P > 0.05$), Patient F = 3.73 ($P < 0.05$); Immunolabelling: Brain region F =0.67 ($P > 0.05$), Deposit type F = 968.06 ($P < 0.001$), Interaction F = 0.93 ($P > 0.05$), Patient F = 1.24 ($P > 0.05$).

Variations in the morphology of the PrP^{sc} deposits in four cortical areas are shown in Table 3. The diffuse PrP^{sc} deposits were consistently larger, more symmetrical in shape, and more lightly stained than the florid PrP^{sc} deposits in all brain regions studied. There was less difference in size between the diffuse and florid deposits in the PHG compared with other cortical areas. The mean number of vacuoles associated with the deposit and the frequency of blood vessels touching the deposits are shown in Figure 4. The diffuse PrP^{sc} deposits were consistently associated with more vacuoles and blood vessels than the florid PrP^{sc} deposits and this difference was present in all regions. The mean number of cells associated with PrP^{sc} deposits is shown in Figure 5.

The diffuse PrP^{sc} deposits were associated with more neuronal cell bodies, and all three types of glial cell nuclei than the florid deposits. This difference was present in all regions with the exception of the occipital cortex, where the diffuse PrP^{sc} deposits were associated with a greater number of neurons.

A summary of the correlations between the morphology of the diffuse and florid PrP^{sc} deposits and associated cells is shown in Table 4. There were few positive correlations between deposit size, shape, and immunolabelling and the frequency of associated blood vessels, small neurons, astrocytes, oligodendrocytes, or microglia. The most consistent correlations were a positive correlation between deposit size and the number of associated large neurons and with the number of vacuoles. There was no essential difference in the pattern of correlation between the different cell types and the diffuse and florid PrP^{sc} deposits. The correlation matrix for the sample of multicentric deposits is shown in Table 5. There were no significant correlations between deposit size or shape and the frequency of associated cells. However, intensity of immunolabelling was positively correlated with the frequency of associated vacuoles ($r = 0.45$, $P < 0.01$) and negatively correlated with the frequency of microglial nuclei ($r = -0.38$, $P < 0.05$).

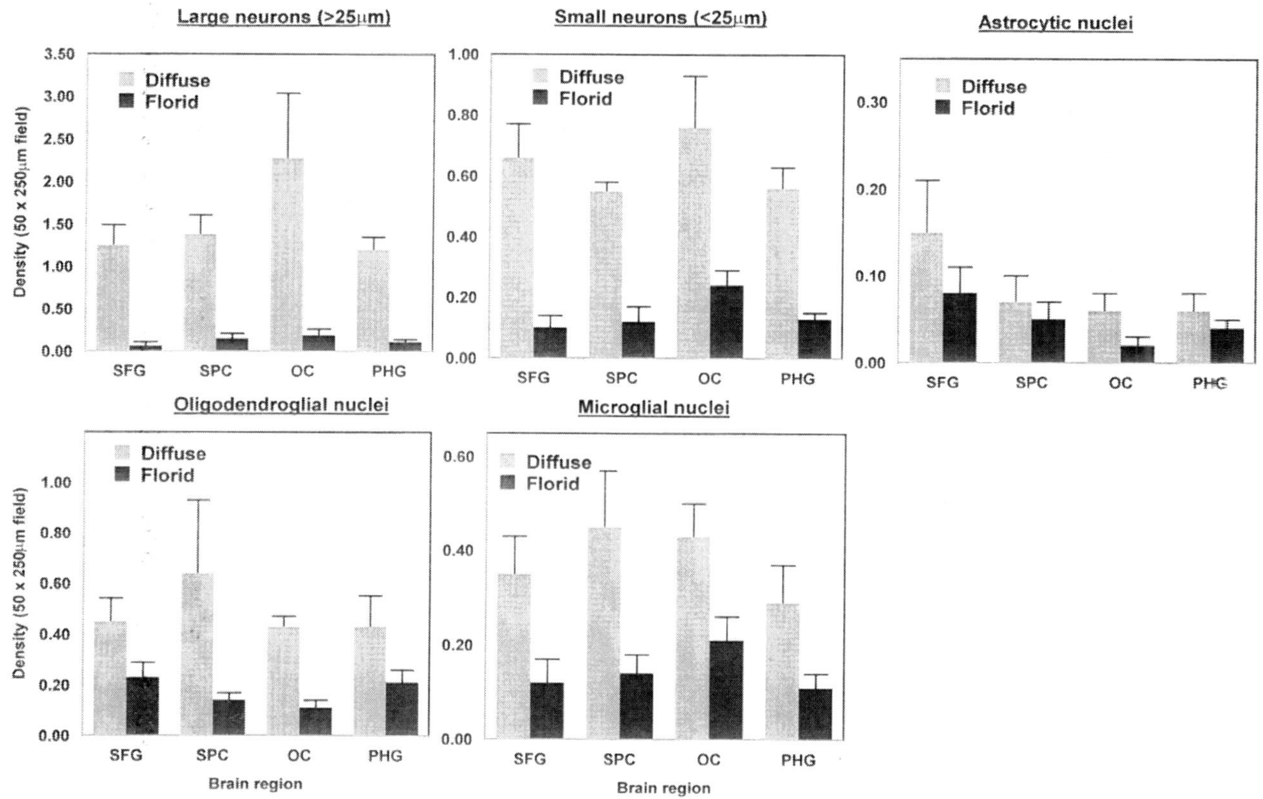

Figure 5. Degree of association of the diffuse and florid prion protein (PrP^{sc}) deposits with neuronal cell bodies and glial cell nuclei in cases of variant Creutzfeldt-Jakob disease (vCJD). ANOVA: Large neurons Brain region $F = 12.24$ ($P < 0.001$), Deposit type $F = 223.52$ ($P < 0.001$), Interaction $F = 6.23$ ($P<0.01$), Patients $F = 2.72$ ($P > 0.05$); Small neurons Brain region $F = 1.84$ ($P > 0.05$), Deposit type $F = 59.91$ ($P < 0.001$), Interaction $F = 0.32$ ($P > 0.05$), Patient $F = 0.44$ ($P < 0.05$); Astrocytes, Brain region $F = 1.02$ ($P > 0.05$), Deposit type $F = 1.73$ ($P > 0.05$), Interaction $F = 0.60$ ($P > 0.05$), Patients $F = 3.59$ ($P < 0.05$); Oligodendrocytes, Brain region $F = 0.50$ ($P > 0.05$), Deposit type $F = 15.30$ ($P < 0.001$), Interaction $F = 0.67$ ($P > 0.05$), Patient $F = 3.45$ ($P < 0.05$); Microglia, Brain region $F = 2.56$ ($P > 0.05$), Deposit type $F = 48.94$ ($P < 0.001$), Interaction $F = 0.61$ ($P > 0.05$), Patient $F = 10.09$ ($P < 0.001$).

Table 4. Correlation matrix between the morphological features (BV = blood vessels, SH = Shape of deposit, IL = Intensity of immunolabelling, LN = Large neurons, SN = Small neurons, A = Astrocytes, O = Oligodendrocytes, Mg = Microglia, V = Vacuoles) of the multicentric prion protein (PrP^sc^) deposits

	Variables									
	BV	Size	SH	IM	LN	SN	A	O	Mg	V
BV	-	0.08	-0.02	-0.19	-0.08	0.21	-0.07	-0.10	0.22	-0.12
Size		-	0.18	0.14	0.16	0.10	-0.01	0.07	-0.03	0.22
SH			-	-0.08	0.01	-0.20	0.01	0.10	0.10	-0.18
IM				-	0.23	-0.12	0.13	0.05	-0.38*	0.45**
LN					-	-0.10	0.10	-0.31*	-0.21	0.29
SN						-	-0.05	-0.14	0.12	0.01
A							-	-0.12	-0.14	0.17
O								-	0.38*	-0.17
Mg									-	0.03
V										-

Table 5. Frequency of correlations (Pearson's 'r') between the morphology of the diffuse and florid PrP^sc^ deposits (SH = deposit shape, IL = Intensity of immunolabelling) and associated histological features in vCJD

	Diffuse deposits				Florid deposits		
Feature	'r'	Size	SH	IL	Size	SH	IL
Blood vessels	+	1	2	0	4	0	1
	-	0	2	0	0	2	2
	ns	23	20	24	20	22	19
Large neurons	+	9	0	1	6	0	0
	-	0	0	0	0	5	0
	ns	15	23	22	15	19	22
Small neurons	+	2	2	2	2	0	0
	-	0	0	0	0	3	1
	ns	22	22	21	19	15	21
Astrocytes	+	1	1	0	1	0	0
	-	1	1	1	0	0	1
	ns	12	15	17	16	19	17
Oligodendrocytes	+	3	0	1	4	0	0
	-	0	0	0	0	1	2
	ns	21	24	23	20	23	20
Microglia	+	6	1	0	5	0	0
	-	0	2	0	0	2	1
	ns	18	21	24	16	20	18
Vacuoles	+	14	1	8	15	0	0
	-	0	1	0	0	1	1
	ns	10	22	16	9	23	21

DISCUSSION

The majority (up to 96%) of PrP^{sc} deposits in the vCJD cases could be assigned with confidence to one of three morphological types, viz., diffuse, florid, or multicentric deposits, the latter being considerably rarer than the diffuse and florid types.

The morphological attributes of these PrP^{sc} deposits and their pattern of association with glia, neurons, blood vessels, and vacuoles were similar in different regions of the cerebral cortex. The one exception was the greater association of diffuse and florid PrP^{sc} deposits with larger neuronal cell bodies in the occipital cortex. The visual cortex and especially area V1, however, has a significantly higher density of neurons than other cortical areas (Armstrong et al., 2002) which may explain this correlation.

Are Glia Involved in the Formation of Prp^{sc} Deposits?

Spatial associations between PrP^{sc} deposits and astrocytic nuclei were relatively rare suggesting that astrocytes are unlikely to be involved in the initial formation of the deposits. A number of studies, however, have described associations between PrP^{sc} deposits and microglia (Liberski et al., 2000). In mice infected by the scrapie agent (Williams et al., 1994), for example, there is a marked astrocytic and microglia response related to the appearance of vacuoles and the accumulation of PrP^{sc}. Some authors have claimed that microglia are essential for the formation of PrP^{sc} deposits (Guiroy et al., 1994) with ferritin-immunoreactive microglia observed in association with unicentric, multicentric, and diffuse PrP^{sc} deposits. Nevertheless, only about 30% of PrP^{sc} deposits appear to be associated with microglia (Guiroy et al., 1994) and an even smaller proportion of florid PrP^{sc} deposits are associated with microglia in the present study. In addition, authors have reported that microglia may be associated with the formation of vacuolation rather than PrP^{sc} deposition (Sazaki et al., 1993). Hence, it is unlikely that microglia are necessary for the formation of PrP^{sc} deposits.

Is There an Increase in Glia in vCJD?

The ratio of astrocytes to oligodendrocytes in normal brain is approximately 0.23 (Table 6) very similar to the ratio for glia in association with either the diffuse or florid PrP^{sc} deposits. This suggests that the presence of PrP^{sc} deposits has little effect on the numbers of astrocytes and oligodentrocytes.

Table 6. Ratios of astrocytes (A), oligodendrocytes (O), and microglia (Mg) in association with various types of prion protein (PrP^{sc}) deposit in variant Creutzfeldt-Jakob disease (vCJD) compared with normal brain

Ratio	Normal brain	vCJD		
		Diffuse	Florid	Multicentric
A:O	0.23	0.18	0.29	0.13
A:Mg	2.66	0.23	0.33	0.12
O:Mg	11.63	1.29	1.13	0.93

The ratio of astrocytes to oligodendrocytes adjacent to multicentric deposits, however, was lower than in normal brain, suggesting either an increase in astrocytes or a reduction in oligodendrocytes. There is a highly significant reduction in the ratio of both astrocytes and oligodendrocytes to microglia adjacent to PrP^{sc} deposits consistent with an increase in microglia in vCJD. This increase could be an attempt to remove PrP^{sc} from some deposits resulting in the possible shrinkage or even removal of the deposit (Armstrong, 2007). Diffuse and florid-type PrP^{sc} deposits have a characteristic size frequency distribution in vCJD reflecting the pattern of growth of the deposits (Armstrong, 2007).

Two statistical models have been proposed to explain the frequency distribution of sizes of PrP^{sc} deposits in CJD: (1) a 'power-law model' suggesting that processes of aggregation/disaggregation of PrP^{sc} predominate in the growth of the protein deposits and (2) a 'log-normal' model suggesting that surface diffusion and molecular binding to PrP^{sc} is the critical factor. In a study of eleven patients with vCJD, the size frequency distributions of the florid deposits were fitted by a power-law function in all brain areas studied suggesting processes of aggregation and disaggregation are particularly important in explaining the growth of the florid PrP^{sc} deposits in vCJD. It is likely that glial cells play a major role in removing PrP^{sc} from the brain in vCJD.

Do PrP^{sc} Deposits Damage Glia in vCJD?

All three types of PrP^{sc} deposit demonstrate a similar pattern of correlation with associated glia and neurons. All three deposit types also exhibit a correlation with blood vessel profiles and vacuoles, the multicentric deposits having the greatest degree of association with these structures. These differences are likely to reflect difference in average size of the PrP^{sc} deposits, larger deposits being more likely to contact more cells than smaller deposits. Hence, individually, the larger multicentric PrP^{sc} deposits are likely to damage more glia than the smaller diffuse and florid deposits but are far less numerous. Larger neurons are also more frequently associated with PrP^{sc} deposits than small neurons, and oligodendrocytes and microglia are more frequently associated with PrP^{sc} deposits than astrocytes.

Abnormalities of parvalbumin-immunoreactive neurons, an important group of inhibitory neurons in the cortex, have been shown to be damaged in CJD (Ferrier et al., 1993), affected cells having reduced and short fragmented dendrites and large numbers of dendritic varicosities. In addition, abundant abnormally swollen neurons have been observed Japanese cases of CJD with extensive white matter degeneration (Kato et al., 1992).

Significant correlations have been also reported between PrP^{sc} deposits and the frequency of astrocytes in CJD (MacDonald et al., 1995). In addition, α-B crystallin has been reported in astrocytes, the most intense immunolabelling being in regions with extensive vacuolation (Renkawek et al., 1992) suggesting a stress response in neurons to the developing pathology. Damage to astrocytes in vCJD could affect the BBB (Armstrong et al., 2003b). Florid PrP^{sc} deposits are on average a third of the size of the diffuse PrP^{sc} deposits, but have a frequency of association with blood vessels and vacuoles greater than would be expected by their size. Previous studies have also suggested a positive association between florid deposits and vacuoles (Grigoriev et al., 1999) and with blood vessel profiles (Armstrong et al., 2003b).

A previous study of vCJD cases suggested: (1) florid PrP^{sc} deposits were clustered around the larger diameter blood vessels, the dimension of the clusters varying with brain region and (2) the density of florid deposits declined as a negative exponential function with distance from a larger diameter blood vessel. Hence, diffusion from blood vessels resulting from damage to astrocytes and a compromised BBB could be involved in the pathogenesis of the florid deposits (Armstrong, 2010).

CONCLUSION

In conclusion, three morphological types of prion protein (PrP^{sc}) deposit occur in the cerebral cortex of cases of variant Creutzfeldt-Jakob disease (vCJD), viz., diffuse, florid and multicentric deposits (plaques). Multicentric deposits were, on average, the largest deposits observed and were more frequently associated with glial cells, neuronal perikarya, and blood vessels. Diffuse deposits were larger, less symmetrical in shape and more lightly immunolabelled than the florid deposits and more frequently associated with glial cells and neurons. The patterns of correlation of morphology and associated glial cells and neurons were essentially similar for the diffuse and florid type deposits. The data suggest in vCJD: (1) there is no evidence that glia are directly involved in the formation of PrP^{sc} deposits, (2) there is an increase in microglia which may be an attempt to remove PrP^{sc}, and (3) PrP^{sc} deposits could damage adjacent astrocytes affecting the blood brain barrier (BBB).

ACKNOWLEDGMENTS

The assistance of the National CJD Surveillance Unit, Western General Hospital, Edinburgh and the Brain Bank, Institute of Psychiatry, King's College London in supplying cases for this study and in preparation of tissue sections is gratefully acknowledged.

REFERENCES

Armstrong RA. Factors determining the morphology of β-amyloid (Aβ) deposits in Down's syndrome. *Neurodegeneration* 1995, 4, 179-186.

Armstrong RA. Correlations between the morphology of diffuse and primitive b-amyloid (Ab) deposits and the frequency of associated cells in Down's syndrome. *Neuropathology and Applied Neurobiology,* 1996, 22, 527-530.

Armstrong RA. β-amyloid deposits: stages in life history or independent origin? *Dementia and Geriatric Cognitive Disorders,* 1998, 9, 227-238.

Armstrong RA. Size frequency distributions of abnormal protein deposits in Alzheimer's disease and variant Creutzfeldt-Jakob disease. *Folia Neuropathologica,* 2007, 45, 108-114.

Armstrong RA. Dispersion of prion protein deposits around blood vessels in variant Creutzfeldt-Jakob disease. *Folia Neuropathologica,* 2010, 48, 227-232.

Armstrong RA, Cairns NJ, Lantos PL. The spatial pattern of the vacuolation in patients with sporadic Creutzfeldt-Jakob disease. *Neuroscience Letters,* 2000, 281, 187-190.

Armstrong RA, Cairns NJ, Lantos PL. The spatial patterns of prion protein deposits in Creutzfeldt-Jakob disease: comparison with β-amyloid deposits in Alzheimer's disease. *Neuroscience Letters*, 2001, 298: 53-56.

Armstrong RA, Cairns NJ, Ironside JW, Lantos PL Quantification of vacuolation, ('spongiform change'), surviving neurons and prion protein deposition in eleven cases of variant Creutzfeldt-Jakob disease. *Neuropathology and Applied Neurobiology,* 2002, 28, 129-135.

Armstrong RA, Lantos PL, Ironside JW, Cairns NJ. Differences in the density and spatial distribution of florid and diffuse plaques in variant Creutzfeldt-Jakob disease (vCJD). *Clinical Neuropathology*, 2003a, 22, 209-214.

Armstrong RA, Cairns NJ, Ironside JW, Lantos PL. Florid prion protein (PrP) plaques in patients with variant Creutzfeldt-Jakob disease (vCJD) are spatially related to blood vessels. *Neuroscience Research Communications,* 2003b, 32, 29-36.

Caughey B. Interactions between prion protein isoforms: the kiss of death? *Trends in Biochemical Science*, 2001, 26, 235-242.

Cervenakova L, Goldfarb LG, Garruto R, Lee HS, Gajdusek DC, Brown P. Phenotype-genotype studies in kuru: implications for new variant Creutzfeldt-Jakob disease. *Proceedings of the National Academy of Science, USA*, 1998, 95, 13239-13241.

Collins S, McLean CA, Masters CL. Gerstmann-Straussler-Scheinker syndrome, fatal familial insomnia and kuru: a review of these less common human transmissible spongiform encephalopathies. *Journal of Clinical Neuroscience,* 2001, 8, 387-397.

Creutzfeldt HG. Über eines eigenartige herd-formige Erkrankung des Zentralnervensystems. In: Nissl F, Alzheimer A, eds., *Histologische und Histopathologische Arbeiten uber die Grosshirnrinde*, Jena, Gustav Fisher, 1921, 1-48.

DeArmond SJ, Prusiner SB. Etiology and pathogenesis of prion disease. *American Journal of Pathology,* 1995, 146, 785-804.

Ferrier I, Casas R, Rivera R. Parvalbumin-immunoreactive cortical neurons in Creutzfeldt-Jakob disease. *Annals of Neurology*, 1993, 34, 864-866.

Fournier JG, Kopp N, Streichenberger N, Escaig-Haye F, Langeveldt J, Brown P. Electron microscopy of brain amyloid deposits from a patient with new variant Creutzfeldt-Jakob disease. *Acta Neuropathology*, 2000, 99, 637-642.

Goldfarb LG, Brown P, Cervenakova L, Gajdusek DC. Genetic analysis of Creutzfeldt-Jakob disease and related disorders. *Philosophical Transactions of the Royal Society*, Series B, 1994, 343, 379-384.

Grigoriev V, Escarg-Haye F, Streichenberger N, Kopp N, Langeveld J, Brown P, Fournier JG. Submicroscopic immunodetection of prion protein in the brain of a patient with new variant Creutzfeldt-Jakob disease. *Neuroscience Letters,* 1999, 264, 57-60.

Guiroy DC, Wakayama I, Liberski PP, Gajdusek DC. Relationship of microglia and scrapie amyloid-immunoreactive deposits in kuru, Creutzfeldt-Jakob disease and Gerstmann-Staussler syndrome. *Acta Neuropathologica* 1994, 87, 526-530.

Hill AF, Butterworth RJ, Joiner S, Jackson G, Rossor MN, Thomas DJ, Frosh A, Tolley N, Bell JE, Spencer M, King A, Al-Sarraj S, Ironside JW, Lantos PL, Collinge J. Investigation of variant Creutzfeldt-Jakob disease and other human prion diseases with tonsil biopsy samples. *Lancet,* 1999, 353, 183-189.

Hogan RN, Cavanagh HD. Transplantation of corneal tissue from donors with disease of the central nervous system. *Cornea,* 1995, 14, 533-547.

Ironside JW. Pathology of variant Creutzfeldt-Jakob disease. *Archives of Virology* [Suppl], 2000, 16, 143-151.

Ironside JW, Sutherland K, Bell JE, McCardle L, Barrie C, Estebeiro K, Zeidler M, Will RG. A new variant of Creutzfeldt-Jakob disease: neuropathological and clinical features. *Cold Spring Harbour Symposium of Quantitative Biology*, 1996, LXI, 523-530.

Ironside JW, Head MW, Bell JE, McCardle L, Will RG. Laboratory diagnosis of variant Creutzfeldt-Jakob disease. *Histopathology*, 2000, 37, 1-9.

Jakob A. Uber eigenartige Erkrankungen des Zentralnervensystems mit bemerkenswerten anatomischen Befunden (spastische Pseudosklerose-Encephalomyelopathic mit disseminierten Degenerationsherden). *Dtsch Z Nervenheilk,* 1921, 70, 132-146.

Kato S, Hirano A, Umahara T, Wena JF, Herz F, Ohama E. Ultrastructural and immunohistochemical studies on ballooned cortical neurons in Creutzfeldt-Jakob disease: expression of alpha-B crystalline, ubiquitin and stress response protein-27. *Acta Neuropathologica*, 1992, 84, 443-448.

Kovacs GG, Gasque P, Strobel T, Lindeck-Pozza E, Strohschneider M, Ironside JW, Buddka H, Guentchev M. Complement activation in human prion disease. *Neurobiology of Disease*, 2004, 15, 21-28.

Krasemann S, Groschup MH, Harmeyer L, Hunsmann G, Bodemer W. Generation of monoclonal antibodies against human prion proteins in PrPO/O mice. *Molecular Medicine*, 1996, 2, 725-734.

Liberski PP, Ironside JW, McCardle L, Shering A. Ultrastructure analysis of the florid deposit in variant Creutzfeldt-Jakob disease. *Folia Neuropathologica*, 2000, 38, 167-170.

MacDonald ST, Sutherland K, Ironside JW. Prion protein genotype and pathological phenotype studied in sporadic Creutzfeldt-Jakob disease. *Neuropathology and Applied Neurobiology*, 1996, 22: 285-292.

Nauta WJH, Feirtag M. *Fundamental Neuroanatomy.* WH Freeman and Co., New York, 1986.

Prusiner SB. The prion diseases. *Scientific American*, 1995; 31-37.

Prusiner SB, DeArmond SJ. Prion diseases and neurodegeneration. *Annual Revue of Neuroscience,* 1994, 17, 311-339.

Renkawek K, Dejong WW, Merck KB, Frenken CW, Van Workum FP, Bosman GJ. Alpha-B-crystallin is present in reactive glia in Creutzfeldt-Jakob disease. *Acta Neuropathologica*, 1992, 83, 324-327.

Sasaki A, Hirato J, Nakajato Y. Immunohistochemical study of microglia in the Creutzfeldt-Jakob diseased brain. *Acta Neuropathologica,* 1993, 86, 337-344.

Stockel J, Hartl FU. Chaperonin-mediated *de novo* generation of prion protein aggregates. *Journal of Molecular Biology*, 2001, 313, 861-872.

Will RG, Ironside JW, Zeidler M, Cousins SN, Estebeiro K, Alperovitch A, Poser S, Pocchiari M, Hofman A, Smith PG. A new variant of Creutzfeldt-Jakob disease in the United Kingdom. *Lancet* 1996, 347, 921-925.

Williams AE, Lanson LJ, Perry VH, Fraser H. Characterisation of the microglial response in murine scrapie. *Neuropathology and Applied Neurobiology,* 1994, 20, 47-55.

Watanabe R, Duchen LW. Cerebral amyloid in human prion disease. *Neuropathology and Applied Neurobiology,* 1993, 19, 253-260.

In: Glial Cells
Editors: Charanjit Kaur and Eng-Ang Ling
ISBN: 978-1-62618-448-0
© 2013 Nova Science Publishers, Inc.

Chapter 5

Glial Fibrillary Acidic Protein and S100 Calcium-Binding Protein B in the Cerebrospinal Fluid of Children with Acute Neurological Disorders

Keisuke Nakajima[1], Masaharu Hayashi[*2], Rie Miyata[2], Naoyuki Tanuma[2] and Shuki Mizutani[1]
[1] Department of Pediatrics, Tokyo Medical and Dental University, Tokyo, Japan
[2] Department of Brain Development and Neural Regeneration, Tokyo Metropolitan Institute of Medical Science, Tokyo, Japan

Abstract

In order to investigate the pathogenesis of acute neurological diseases in children, we examined cerebrospinal fluid (CSF) levels of 2 specific markers for astrocytes: glial fibrillary acidic protein (GFAP) and S100 calcium-binding protein B (S100B). We introduce the significance of examination of astrocytic markers in adult and pediatric neurological disorders by reviewing the findings of previous reports with regard to changes in CSF and/or serum levels of GFAP and S100B. We also explain acute encephalopathy with biphasic seizures and late reduced diffusion (AESD) and discuss problems in its pathogenesis. We then summarize our data on ELISA analysis of CSF levels of GFAP and S100B in controls and patients with meningitis, AESD, and status epilepticus (SE). Because the CSF level of GFAP but not S100B showed an age-dependent change in controls, we propose the "Glial index (S100B/GFAP)" in order to deepen our understanding of correlations between GFAP and S100B. CSF levels of both GFAP and S100B were static in patients with viral meningitis in comparison with controls and were significantly elevated in patients with bacterial meningitis, consistent with findings in the previous literature. In contrast, CSF levels of GFAP were decreased in patients with SE and AESD, whereas levels of S100B were increased. Such contrasting

* Corresponding author: E-mail: hayashi-ms@igakuken.or.jp; Tel: +81-3-6834-2334; Fax: +81-3-5316-3150, Department of Brain Development and Neural Regeneration, Tokyo Metropolitan Institute of Medical Science, 2-1-6 Kamikitazawa, Setagayaku, Tokyo 156-8506, Japan.

changes in CSF levels of GFAP and S100B led to an increase in the glial index in SE and AESD patients. Similarly, in the receiver operating characteristic (ROC) analysis comparing AESD patients to the controls, the area under the curve (AUC) in the glial index was high. The glial index may be a reliable marker for early diagnosis of AESD. Considering the frequent comorbidity of human herpesvirus 6 infection in AESD, the data may suggest a possible relationship between astrocytic dysfunction and human herpes virus-6 infection.

INTRODUCTION

Astrocytes participate in all essential functions of the central nervous system (CNS), including blood flow regulation, energy metabolism, ion and water homeostasis, immune reaction, neurotransmission, and adult neurogenesis [1]. Several markers specific for astrocytes have been proposed and examined in the cerebrospinal fluid (CSF). Glial fibrillary acidic protein (GFAP) and S100 calcium-binding protein B (S100B) are the best known of these markers. GFAP is the main intermediate filament protein in mature astrocytes and is expressed exclusively in the CNS [2]. On the other hand, S100B is a member of the S100 calcium-binding protein family and is detected in protoplasmic and fibrillary astrocytes [3,4]. At least 80–90% of the total S100B pool is found in the nervous tissue; the remainder is found in non-neuronal tissues. Increased secretion of GFAP and S100B in cultured astrocytes occurs a few minutes after activation of adenosine or glutamate receptors (Figure 1). In addition, release of GFAP and S100B into the CSF may also occur after damage to astrocytes caused by destructive lesions in the brain tissue.

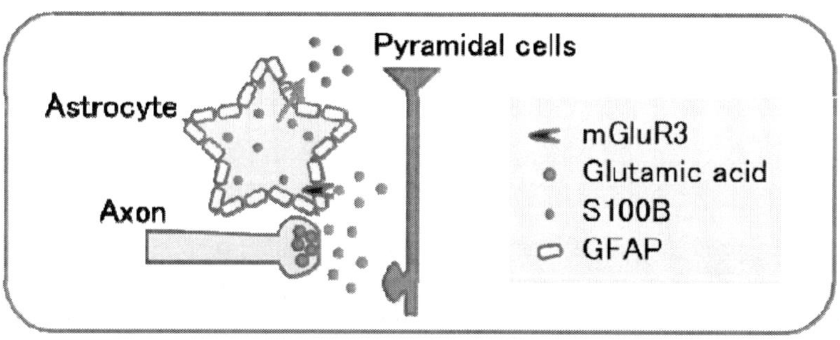

Abbreviations are as follows: mGluR3, metabotropic glutamate receptor 3; GFAP, glial fibrillary acidic protein; S100B, S100 calcium-binding protein B.

Figure 1. Image of secretion of astrocytic markers.

In adults, changes in CSF levels of GFAP and S100B have been reported in various disorders, and the clinical significance of these has been discussed. Increased CSF levels of GFAP and/or S100B have been found in autoimmune disorders such as multiple sclerosis, neuromyelitis optica, and acute disseminated encephalomyelitis [5, 6]. Patients with neurodegenerative disorders, including Alzheimer disease [7], amyotrophic lateral sclerosis [8], and spinocerebellar ataxia [9], also show an increase in the CSF levels of GFAP and/or S100B. A correlation between serum levels of astrocytic markers and clinical severity or the subsequent outcome has been reported in patients with cerebrovascular disorders such as stroke and subarachnoid hemorrhage [10, 11], probably because the increase of GFAP and S100B in the CSF partially reflects the degree of brain tissue damage. In children, CSF levels of GFAP and S100B have been examined in acute neurological disorders such as bacterial meningitis and traumatic brain injury [12-14]. The changes in these levels may occur just after the insult and seem to be correlated with functional outcome [13, 14]. An increase in the CSF levels of astrocytic markers has been reported in other heterogeneous disorders, including perinatal asphyxia in full-term neonates [15], hydrocephalus after shunt operation [16], genetically confirmed Alexander disease [17], and other metabolic white-matter disorders [18]. Children with malignancies such as Langerhans cell histiocytosis [19] and acute lymphoblastic leukemia [20] also show differences between CSF levels of GFAP measured before and after treatment.

Acute Encephalopathy with Biphasic Seizures and Late Reduced Diffusion (AESD)

Acute encephalopathy is the generic term for acute brain dysfunction caused by various agents, such as infection, metabolic disease, hepatic or renal dysfunction, or hypertension. The use of MRI has contributed to the identification of several subcategories of acute encephalopathy. Several forms of encephalopathy in children have been recently identified in Japan [21]. Acute encephalopathy with biphasic seizures and late reduced diffusion (AESD) is one of these new subcategories [22]. It is characterized clinically by biphasic seizures; that is, seizures that are accompanied by fever—usually continuous—with status epilepticus (SE) as the initial neurological symptom [23]. The initial seizures are followed by secondary ones, which occur most often as a cluster of complex partial seizures at days 3 to 5, finally resulting in variable levels of neurologic sequelae. The brain MRI shows no changes within the first 2 days; however, during days 3 to 9, it indicates reduced diffusion in the frontal subcortical white matter with sparing of the perirolandic region [24]. A representative clinical course of AESD patients is shown in Figure 2. The patient developed signal changes in the subcortical white matter on diffusion-weighted MRI images at day 6, and the brain atrophy subsequently increased. Because AESD is associated with biphasic epileptic events, consisting of SE or clusters of seizures, the involvement of excitotoxicity has been speculated on the basis of changes observed with MR spectroscopy [22, 24]. Cytokine storm may also be implicated in AESD, as it is in patients with other encephalitis/encephalopathies associated with influenza virus and human herpesvirus 6 (HHV-6) [25, 26]. However, this hypothesis has not been fully verified. On the other hand, the CSF GFAP level has been reported to increase in patients with nonprogressive and progressive neurological encephalopathies [27] and SE [28]. Screening AESD from SE at the acute disease phase can enable early and comprehensive treatment, and the detailed analysis of CSF markers in AESD patients may contribute to such early detection of AESD. We compared the CSF levels of total tau protein and neuron-specific enolase (NSE)—markers of axonal and neuronal damage—in patients with febrile seizure (FS) and AESD [29]. The CSF levels of total tau protein (but not NSE) in AESD patients were higher than those in FS patients. This indicates that evaluation of the CSF level of total tau protein may be useful for early screening of AESD. Interestingly, an age-dependent change was observed in the CSF level of total tau protein in controls; it is high in infants and drops rapidly with age. In addition, Shiihara et al. also examined the CSF levels of total tau protein and S100B in patients with AESD and FS and evaluated the area under the curve (AUC) using receiver operating characteristic (ROC) analysis [30]. The positive predictive value for AESD using the combination of CSF levels of S100B and total tau protein is approximately 80%. Taking these findings into consideration, we planned a comprehensive analysis of the CSF levels of GFAP and S100B in children with acute neurological disorders, including meningitis, AESD, and SE, in order to clarify their pathogenesis and establish markers for early disease.

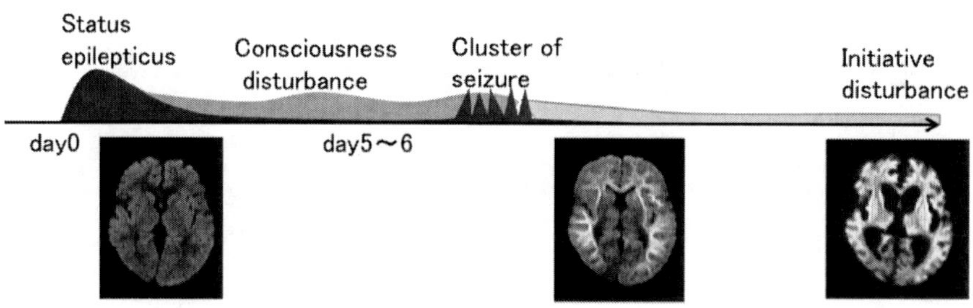

Figure 2. Clinical course of acute encephalopathy with biphasic seizures and late reduced diffusion (AESD).

CSF Astrocytic Markers in Meningitis and AESD

The subjects included 17 controls without any organic changes in the CNS, 20 patients with bacterial meningitis, 7 patients with viral meningitis, 23 patients with AESD, and 21 patients with SE. All patients were younger than 3 years. First, we examined the presence and absence of age dependence in CSF levels of astrocytic markers in controls. Next, we compared the levels of astrocytic markers and the glial index (S100B/GFAP), which we proposed, in patients with bacterial or viral meningitis, SE, and AESD. In addition, we performed an ROC analysis, to determine the AUC for CSF levels of GFAP and S100B and for the glial index. This study was approved by the Medical Ethical Committee of the Tokyo Metropolitan Institute of Medical Science, and patients and/or parents granted permission for lumbar punctures and further analyses of the CSF. Written informed consent was obtained from the parents. CSF samples were obtained from each subject and were immediately stored at -80°C until analysis. CSF levels of GFAP and S100B were determined with commercial ELISA kits (BioVendor Research and Diagnostic Products, Candler, NC, USA). Data were analyzed using JMP Version 10.0 software (SAS Institute, Inc., Cary, NC, USA). Comparisons between the data of patients and controls were evaluated by Wilcoxon signed-rank tests. Two-tailed p values < 0.05 were statistically significant. The diagnostic accuracy of the biomarkers, the ROC curves, and the AUC were evaluated by the method of Delong et al. Biomarker cut-off points were determined using the Youden index ($J = \max$ [sensitivity + specificity − 1]). [31, 32]

We examined the CSF levels of astrocytic markers in controls ranging in age from 1 month to 3 years (Figure 3). CSF levels of GFAP were high in infants and decreased with age, indicating the presence of age dependence; this mimicked the changes in total tau protein in CSF [29]. The age dependence in CSF levels of GFAP is in good accord with the previous report, in which GFAP levels in healthy preterm and full-term infants were higher than that in children and young adults [33, 34]. In contrast, there was no apparent age-dependent change in CSF levels of S100B. Considering such differences in developmental changes in the CSF levels of GFAP and S100B, we proposed the glial index (S100B/GFAP), which may specifically reflect the age-dependent variation in astrocytic markers. CSF levels of GFAP and S100B and the glial index in patients with acute pediatric neurologic diseases are summarized in Figure 4. With regard to meningitis patients, the average CSF level of GFAP in controls (n = 17) was 0.776 (SD 0.531) ng/mL, whereas it was 0.346 (SD 0.389) ng/mL in patients with viral meningitis (n = 6) and 2.375 (SD 3.893) ng/mL in patients with bacterial meningitis (n = 19). The average CSF level of S100B in controls was 33.17 (SD 35.03) pg/mL, whereas it was 49.73 (SD 34.66) pg/mL in patients with viral meningitis (n = 5) and 182.13 (SD 315.65) pg/mL in patients with bacterial meningitis (n = 20). The CSF levels of both astrocytic markers in the patients with bacterial meningitis were higher than in controls or patients with viral meningitis. The average glial index in controls (n = 16) was 186.5 (SD 526.2), whereas it was 543.2 (SD 871.8), in patients with viral meningitis (n = 5) and 112.5 (SD 103.5) in patients with bacterial meningitis (n = 19). Interestingly, the glial index was increased in patients with viral meningitis; such increase may be related to a mild decrease in the CSF level of GFAP itself. The combination of astrocytic markers and/or glial index may be useful for early differentiation of bacterial and viral meningitis. With regard to AESD and SE, the average CSF level of GFAP in controls (n = 17) was 0.776 (SD 0.531) ng/mL, whereas it was 0.321 (SD 0.576) ng/mL in patients with SE (n = 21) and 0.320 (SD 0.431) ng/mL in patients with AESD (n = 23). The level of S100B in controls (n = 16) was 33.17 (SD 35.03) pg/mL, whereas it was 71.51 (SD 54.98) pg/mL in patients with SE (n = 20) and 87.49 (SD 85.17) pg/mL in patients with AESD (n = 23). The average glial index in controls (n = 16) was 186.5 (SD 626.3), whereas it was 944.4 (SD 918.8), in patients with SE (n = 20) and 885.3 (SD 1216.7) in patients with AESD (n = 23). There was a significant difference between controls and patients with AESD and between controls and patients with SE; however, the difference between patients with SE and AESD was not significant. The results of the ROC analysis are summarized in Figure 5.

In comparing the AESD patients to controls, the AUC of GFAP was 0.76 (sensitivity, 0.70; specificity, 0.83; cut-off index, 0.272 ng/mL), that of S100B was 0.71 (sensitivity, 0.56; specificity, 0.87; cut-off index, 68.45 pg/mL), and that of the glial index was 0.89 (sensitivity, 0.96; specificity, 0.19; cut-off index, 63.8).

In comparing the AESD patients to the SE patients, the AUC of GFAP was 0.44, that of S100B was 0.53, and that of the glial index was 0.57, although neither the sensitivity, specificity, nor the cut-off index was determined.

Early diagnosis of AESD is required, because it tends to cause severe consequences [22-24]; the CSF samples we examined were isolated at the acute disease stage within 10 days after the onset of AESD, in this analysis. Surprisingly, the GFAP levels of patients with SE or AESD were lower than that of controls.

Although the exact mechanisms underlying such reductions in CSF GFAP levels in the acute phase are not clear, it is possible that the elaborate tuning of GFAP expression and function during the postnatal development of glial cells in the CNS may be damaged in the acute stage of AESD and/or SE.

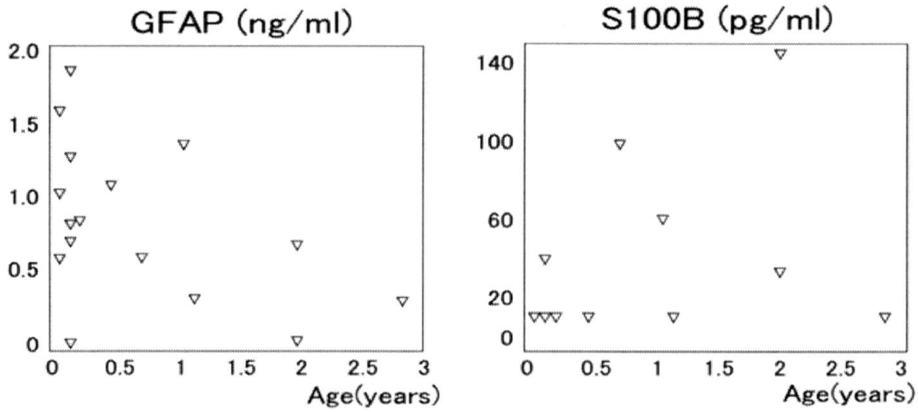

Abbreviations are as follows: GFAP, glial fibrillary acidic protein; S100B, S100 calcium-binding protein B.

Figure 3. Relationship between the age and the levels of astrocytic markers in the cerebrospinal fluid in controls.

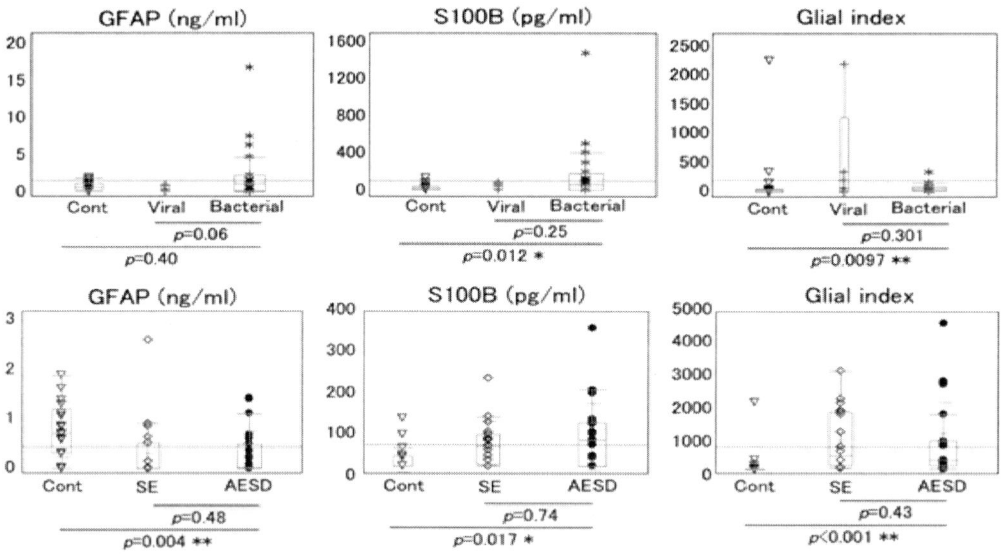

Abbreviations are as follows: Cont, control; Viral, viral meningitis; Bacterial, bacterial meningitis; SE, status epilepticus; AESD, acute encephalopathy with biphasic seizures and late reduced diffusion.

Figure 4. The levels of the astrocytic markers and glial index in the patients with meningitis, AESD, and status epilepticus.

In contrast, the CSF levels of S100B in SE and AESD patients were higher than in controls. CSF levels of S100B may reflect the degree of acute damage in the brain tissue, because S100B is a functional protein that is implicated in the modification of enzyme activities in glial cells. The contrasting changes in the CSF levels of GFAP and S100B led to an increase in the glial index in both SE and AESD patients. Similarly, in the ROC analysis comparing AESD patients to controls, the AUC of the glial index was high compared to that of either GFAP or S100B. The glial index can be a reliable marker in early screening for

AESD. However, there was no significant difference in either the CSF levels of astrocytic markers or the glial index between the SE and AESD patients.

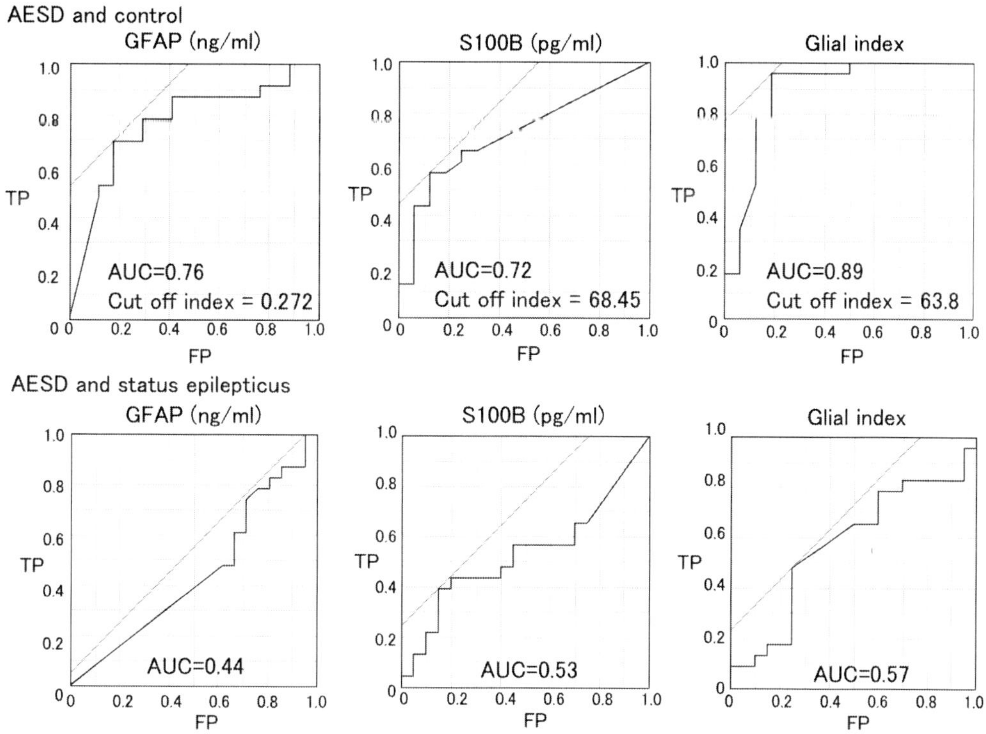

Abbreviations are as follows: AESD, acute encephalopathy with biphasic seizures and late reduced diffusion; ROC, receiver operatorating characteristic; AUC, area under the curve; TP, true positive; FP, false positive.

Figure 5. ROC analysis on the astrocytic markers and the glial index in AESD.

Furthermore, in the ROC analysis comparing the AESD patients to the SE patients, the AUC for either astrocytic marker or the glial index was low. Accordingly, neither the CSF levels of GFAP or S100B nor the glial index is likely to give clues for differentiating AESD from SE. As mentioned previously, MR spectroscopy suggested the possible involvement of excitotoxicity in the brains of AESD patients [24]. Paroxysmal depolarization shifts can be initiated by release of glutamate in astrocytes in experimental seizure models, indicating an important role of astrocyte dysfunction in epileptogenesis [35]. Astrocyte cultures that are infected in vitro with HHV-6 lead to the dysregulation of glutamate uptake, which is associated with the decreased expression of glutamate transporters; thus, it is possible that astrocyte dysfunction is involved in viral-induced brain injuries [36]. The involvement of HHV-6 in epileptogenesis has been suggested by the study of tissues resected from patients with intractable epilepsy [37]. Since HHV-6 frequently causes AESD [29], the changes in the CSF levels of astrocytic markers in this analysis indicate the involvement of astrocyte dysfunction caused by HHV-6 infection in AESD.

REFERENCES

[1] Oberheim, NA; Goldman, SA; Nedergaard, M. Heterogeneity of astrocytic form and function. *Methods Mol Biol* 2012, 814, 23-45.

[2] Middeldorp, J; Hol, EM. GFAP in health and disease. *Prog Neurobiol* 2011, 93, 421-443.

[3] Sedaghat, F; Notopoulos, A. S100 protein family and its application in clinical practice. *Hippokratia* 2008, 12, 198-204

[4] Sen, J; Belli, A. S100B in Neuropathologic States: The CRP of the Brain? *J Neurosci Res*, 2007, 85, 1373-1380

[5] Bartosik-Psujek, H; Psujek, M; Jaworski, J; Stelmasiak, Z. Total tau and S100b proteins in different types of multiple sclerosis and during immunosuppressive treatment with mitoxantrone. *Acta Neurol Scand* 2011, 123, 252-256.

[6] Takano R; Misu, T; Takahashi, T; Sato, S; Fujihara, K; Itoyama, Y. Astrocytic damage is far more severe than demyelination in NMO: a clinical CSF biomarker study. *Neurology* 2010, 75, 208-216.

[7] Fukuyama, R; Izumoto, T; Fushiki, S. The cerebrospinal fluid level of glial fibrillary acidic protein is increased in cerebrospinal fluid from Alzheimer's disease patients and correlates with severity of dementia. *Eur Neurol* 2001, 46, 35-38.

[8] Shobha, K; Alladi, PA; Nalini, A; Sathyaprabha, TN; Raju, TR. Exposure to CSF from sporadic amyotrophic lateral sclerosis patients induces morphological transformation of astroglia and enhances GFAP and S100beta expression. *Neurosci Lett* 2010, 473, 56-61.

[9] Oz, G; Hutter, D; Tkac, I; Clark, HB, Gross, MD; Jiang, H; Eberly, LE, Bushara, KO; Gomez, CM. Neurochemical alterations in spinocerebellar ataxia type 1 and their correlations with clinical status. *Mov Disord* 2010, 25, 1253-1261.

[10] Herrmann, M; Vos, P; Wunderlich, MT; de Bruijn, CH; Lamers, KJ. Release of glial tissue -specific proteins after acute stroke: a comparative analysis of serum concentrations of protein S-100B and glial fibrillary acidic protein. *Stroke* 2000, 31, 2670-2677.

[11] Vos, PE; van Gils, M; Beems, T; Zimmerman, C; Verbeek, MM. Increased GFAP and S100b but not NSE serum levels after subarachnoid haemorrhage are associated with clinical severity. *Eur J Neurol* 2006, 13, 632–638.

[12] Jung, K; Goerdt, C; Lange, P; Blocher, J; Djukic, M; Gerber, J; Spreer, A; Nau, R; Otto, M; Schmidt, H. The use of S100B and Tau protein concentrations in the cerebrospinal fluid for the differential diagnosis of bacterial meningitis: a retrospective analysis. *Eur Neurol* 2011, 66,128-132.

[13] Berger, RP; Pierce, MC; Wisniewski, SR; Adelson, PD; Clark, RS; Ruppel, RA; Kochanek, PM. Neuron-specific enolase and S100B in cerebrospinal fluid after severe traumatic brain injury in infants and children. *Pediatrics* 2002, 109, E31.

[14] Fraser, DD; Close, TE; Rose, KL; Ward, R; Mehl, M; Farrell, C; Lacroix, J; Creery, D; Kesselman, M; Stanimirovic, D; Hutchinson, JS; Canadian Critical Care Translational Biology Group. Severe traumatic brain injury in children elevates glial fibrillary acidic protein in cerebrospinal fluid and serum. *Pediatr Crit Care Med* 2011, 12, 319-324.

[15] Blennow, M; Hagberg, H; Rosengren, L. Glial fibrillary acidic protein in the cerebrospinal fluid: a possible indicator of prognosis in full-term asphyxiated newborn infants? *Pediatr Res* 1995, 37, 260-264.

[16] Beems, T; Simons, KS; Van Geel, WJ; De Reus, HP; Vos, PE; Verbeek, MM. Serum- and CSF-concentrations of brain specific proteins in hydrocephalus. *Acta Neurochir (Wien)* 2003, 145, 37-43.

[17] Kyllerman, M; Rosengren, L; Wiklund, LM; Holmberg, E. Increased levels of GFAP in the cerebrospinal fluid in three subtypes of genetically confirmed Alexander disease. *Neuropediatrics* 2005, 36, 319-323.

[18] Kristjansdottir, R; Uvebrant, P; Rosengren, L. Glial fibrillary acidic protein and neurofilament in children with cerebral white matter abnormalities. *Neuropediatrics* 2001, 32, 307-312.

[19] Gavhed, D; Akefeldt, SO; Osterlundh, G; Laurencikas, E; Hjorth, L; Blennow, K; Rosengren, L; Henter, JI. Biomarkers in the cerebrospinal fluid and neurodegeneration in Langerhans cell histiocytosis. *Pediatr Blood Cancer* 2009, 53, 1264-1270.

[20] Osterlundh, G; Kjellmer, I; Lannering, B; Rosengren, L; Nilsson, UA; Marky, I. Neurochemical markers of brain damage in cerebrospinal fluid during induction treatment of acute lymphoblastic leukemia in children. *Pediatr Blood Cancer* 2008, 50, 793–798.

[21] Mizuguchi M, Yamanouchi H, Ichiyama T, Shiomi M. Acute encephalopathy associated with influenza and other viral infections. *Acta Neurol Scand Suppl* 2007, 186, 45–56.

[22] Takanashi J. Two newly proposed infectious encephalitis /encephalopathy syndromes. *Brain Dev* 2006, 31, 521-528.

[23] Komatsu, M; Okumura, A; Matsui, K; Kitamura, T; Sato, T; Shimizu, T; Watanabe, K. Clustered subclinical seizures in a patient with acute encephalopathy with biphasic seizures and late reduced diffusion. *Brain Dev* 2010, 32, 472-476.

[24] Takanashi, J; Tada, H; Terada, H; Barkovich, AJ. Excitotoxicity in acute encephalopathy with biphasic seizures and late reduced diffusion. *AJNR Am J Neuroradiol* 2009, 30, 132-135.

[25] Ichiyama, T; Suenaga, N; Kajimoto, M; Tohyama, J; Isumi, H; Kubota, M; Mori, M; Furukawa, S. Serum and CSF levels of cytokines in acute encephalopathy following prolonged febrile seizures. *Brain Dev* 2008, 30, 47-52.

[26] Ichiyama, T; Ito, Y; Kubota, M; Yamazaki, T; Nakamura, K; Furukawa S. Serum and cerebrospinal fluid levels of cytokines in acute encephalopathy associated with human herpesvirus-6 infection. *Brain Dev* 2009, 31, 731–738.

[27] Ehlers, S; Kyllerman, M; Rosengren, L. Analysis of glial fibrillary acidic protein in the cerebrospinal fluid of children investigated for encephalopathy. *Neuropediatrics* 1994, 25, 129-33.

[28] Gurnett, CA; Landt, M; Wong, M. Analysis of cerebrospinal fruid glial fibrillary acidic protein after seizures in children. *Epilepsia* 2003, 44, 1455-1458

[29] Tanuma, N; Miyata, R; Kumada, S; Kubota, M; Takanashi, J; Okumura, A, Hamano, S; Hayashi, M. The axonal damage marker tau protein in the cerebrospinal fluid is increased in patients with acute encephalopathy with biphasic seizures and late reduced diffusion. *Brain Dev* 2010, 32, 435-439.

[30] Shiihara, T; Miyake, T; Izumi, S; Watanabe, M; Kamayachi, K; Kodama, K; Nabetani, M; Ikemiyagi, M; Yamaguchi, Y; Sawaura, N. Serum and cerebrospinal fluid S100B, neuron-spccific enolace, and total tau protein in acute encephalopathy with biphasic seizure and late reduced diffusion: a diagnostic validity. *Pediatr Int* 2012, 54, 52-55.

[31] DeLong, ER; DeLong, DM; Clarke-Pearson, DL. Comparing the areas under two or more correlated receiver operating characteristic curves: a nonparametric approach. *Biometrics* 1988, 44, 837-845.

[32] Youden, WJ. Index for rating diagnostic tests. *Cancer* 1950, 3, 32-35.

[33] Rosengren, LE; Wikkelso, C; Hagberg, L. A sensitive ELISA for glial fibrillary acidic protein: application in CSF of adults. *J Neurosci Methods* 1994, 51, 197-204

[34] Rosengren, LE; Ahlsen, G; Belfrage, M; Gillberg, C; Haglid, KG; Hamberger, L. A sensitive ELISA for glial fibrillary acidic protein: application in CSF of children. *J Neurosci Methods* 1992, 44, 113-119

[35] Tian, GF; Azmi, H; Takano, T; Xu, Q; Peng, W; Lin, J; Oberheim, N, Lou, N, Wang, X, Zielke, HR, Kang, J; Nedergaard, M.. An astrocytic basis of epilepsy. *Nat Med* 2005, 11, 973–981.

[36] Fotheringham, J; Williams, EL; Akhyani, N; Jacobson, S. Human herpesvirus 6 (HHV-6) induces dysregulation of glutamate uptake and transporter expression in astrocytes. *J Neuroimmune Pharmacol* 2008, 3, 105-116.

[37] Theodore, WH; Epstein, L; Gaillard, WD; Shinnar, S; Wainwright, MS; Jacobson, S. Human herpes virus 6B: a possible role in epilepsy? *Epilepsia* 2008, 49, 1828-1837.

In: Glial Cells
Editors: Charanjit Kaur and Eng-Ang Ling
ISBN: 978-1-62618-448-0
© 2013 Nova Science Publishers, Inc.

Chapter 6

REGULATION OF GLIAL METABOLISM AND IMMUNE RESPONSES BY INSULIN

Manpreet Bahniwal, Jonathan P. Little and Andis Klegeris*
Department of Biology, University of British Columbia Okanagan Campus, Kelowna, BC, Canada

ABSTRACT

Insulin resistance and/or deficiency in the brain is increasingly being recognized for its contribution to the pathogenesis of Alzheimer's disease (AD). Research efforts in the last decade have demonstrated deficits of insulin and the insulin-signaling cascade in AD brain. Moreover, metabolic disorders, including obesity and type 2 diabetes mellitus, characterized by a state of peripheral insulin resistance are associated with an increased risk of AD. Growing evidence in this field of research supports the hypothesis that AD represents a metabolic disorder, characterized by progressive impairment in insulin signaling and cerebral glucose utilization. In fact, some researchers have termed the brain insulin-resistant state of AD as 'type 3 diabetes'. Consequently, insulin therapies aimed at restoring cognitive decline and preventing further memory loss are being designed for treatment of AD. A vast majority of research on insulin therapies has focused on the direct effects of insulin on neuronal survival, synaptic plasticity and energy production. A multitude of different mechanisms have been proposed to explain insulin-mediated neuroprotection including inhibition of oxidative stress, activation of survival and anti-apoptotic genes, modulation of different neurotransmitter receptors etc. with no mention of possible contributions of glial cells. There are at least ten times more glial cells than neurons in the central nervous system (CNS). Moreover, glial cells are known to express the insulin receptor and a functionally active insulin-signaling cascade. Nevertheless, the effect of insulin on metabolic and immune responses of glial cells is currently unknown. Chronic neuroinflammation mediated by activated glial cells of the brain is known to play a critical role in progression of neurodegenerative disorders such as AD. The activation of glial cells is triggered by the constant presence of pathological formations such as amyloid β protein (Aβ) containing neuritic plaques. Under chronic

* Corresponding author. Department of Biology, University of British Columbia Okanagan Campus, 3333 University Way, Kelowna, BC, Canada V1V 1V7. Tel.: +1 250 807 9557; fax: +1 250 807 8005. E-mail address: andis.klegeris@ubc.ca (A. Klegeris).

neuroinflammatory conditions, persistently activated glia, mainly microglia and astrocytes lose their neuroprotective functions and release a host of pro-inflammatory and toxic mediators, thus contributing to neuronal loss and cognitive decline. In such a scenario, it is important to investigate how insulin administration could affect the inflammatory status of glial cells that are already in a state of activation. Research on peripheral counterparts of microglia (i.e., peripheral monocytes and macrophages) is inconclusive of whether insulin has a pro- or anti-inflammatory effect on peripheral immune responses. Current interest in insulin therapy as a potential therapeutic strategy for treatment of AD warrants extensive research into the modulation of glial cell responses by insulin.

1. Introduction

Glial cells, including microglia and astrocytes play a vital role in support and protection of neurons in the central nervous system (CNS) (Tambuyzer et al., 2009; Polazzi and Monti, 2010; Tremblay et al., 2011; Ransom and Ransom, 2012). In chronic neurodegenerative disorders such as Alzheimer's disease (AD), glia may lose their neuroprotective functions and contribute to increased neuroinflammation and neurotoxicity by releasing a host of pro-inflammatory and toxic mediators (Block et al., 2007; Parpura et al., 2012; Smith et al., 2012; Steele and Robinson, 2012). As such, characterizing pro-inflammatory pathways in glial cells, and identifying potential anti-inflammatory therapies, is an emerging area of research in AD and other neurodegenerative conditions. Glial cells express receptors for a variety of different metabolic hormones including leptin (Hosoi et al., 2000; Dallaporta et al., 2009), adiponectin (Guillod-Maximin et al., 2009) and insulin (Grunberger et al., 1986; Montiel et al., 1989). Moreover, glial cells are capable of regulating neuroendocrine events in response to hormonal messages (Garcia-Segura and McCarthy, 2004). However, there is very limited research investigating the effects of metabolic hormones on glial cell physiology. Of particular interest among these hormones is insulin, which is conventionally recognized as a critical regulator of metabolism in peripheral tissues.

The purpose of this review is to summarize published evidence concerning the effects of insulin on metabolic and immune functions of glial cells. Traditionally, the brain was assumed to be insensitive to the effects of insulin. However, recent research has established that peripheral insulin crosses the blood-brain barrier (BBB) via an active receptor-mediated transport system (Banks, 2004). The importance of insulin in the brain is increasingly being recognized as it plays a significant role in glucose metabolism, synaptic transmission, memory, cognition and modulation of energy homeostasis (Hallschmid and Schultes, 2009; Banks et al., 2012; Duarte et al., 2012). Insulin signals through the insulin receptor, a disulphide-linked transmembrane receptor, distributed in a widespread but selective pattern in the brain (Weyhenmeyer, 1984; Unger et al., 1991b).

Similar to other metabolic hormones, research investigating the roles of insulin in the brain thus far has mainly focused on insulin signaling in neurons. Recently, intranasal insulin therapy has shown promising results in patients with mild cognitive impairment and AD (Reger et al., 2008; Craft et al., 2012). This therapeutic approach is based on evidence that insulin levels in the cerebrospinal fluid (CSF) are reduced in AD (Craft et al., 1998) and therefore the resulting impairment of insulin signaling may contribute to pathophysiology of AD (Neumann et al., 2008; de la Monte, 2012; Duarte et al., 2012). Even though the above effects could be mediated by actions of insulin on neurons, the role of glial cells in insulin signaling cannot be ruled out. Literature concerning the metabolic effects of insulin on glial cells including microglia and astrocytes is rudimentary. Moreover, only limited information is available about the effect of insulin on the inflammatory status of glial cells in chronic neuroinflammatory conditions. Numerous studies suggest that insulin at high concentrations can act as a pro-inflammatory signal in peripheral macrophages. On the other hand, anti-inflammatory effects of insulin on peripheral immune responses have also been reported. Therefore, the overall effect of insulin on immune function in the periphery is still controversial. Since microglia and peripheral monocytes/macrophages belong to the same lineage, insulin may act in a similar manner on this subtype of glial cells. Therefore, the immunomodulatory effects of insulin in peripheral monocytes will be reviewed and discussed in the context of glial-mediated neuroinflammation in AD.

2. Glia of the CNS

Glia were first defined in 1856 by the German pathologist Rudolf Virchow as the 'glue' of the nervous system (Jacobsen, 1991). Traditionally, glial cells were believed to play only a supportive role in the nervous system, providing structural support to neurons. However, over the last two decades, significant amount of research has indicated that glial cells, besides acting as the non-neuronal support cells, serve important functions in the regulation of brain development, metabolism, synaptic transmission and neuronal communication (Garcia-Segura and McCarthy, 2004; Ndubaku and de Bellard, 2008). Even though neurons are the key functional unit of the brain involved in information transmission, glial cells have emerged as dynamic partners in the functioning of the nervous system. Glial cells actively contribute to migration and proliferation of neurons; myelination of axons; synapse formation; synaptic plasticity; and clearance of neurotransmitters (Ndubaku and de Bellard, 2008; Tambuyzer et al., 2009; Ransom and Ransom, 2012). Moreover, growing evidence points to the involvement of glial cells in pathology of various neurological (Kurosinski and Gotz, 2002; Parpura et al., 2012) and psychiatric disorders (Rajkowska and Miguel-Hidalgo, 2007). Therefore, the perception of glial cells has changed from passive bystanders of the nervous system to active participants in neural function and development.

2.1. Types of Glia

Glial cells are classified into two main categories: microglia and macroglia. Microglia, the resident tissue macrophages in the CNS, represent the innate immune system of the brain (Tambuyzer et al., 2009). They belong to the mononuclear phagocyte system and comprise 5-20% of all glial cells in the CNS (Lawson et al., 1990; Lawson et al., 1992). Microglia are capable of mediating pro-inflammatory and anti-inflammatory signals to protect the brain from bacteria, viruses and other foreign agents (Tambuyzer et al., 2009; Kettenmann and Verkhratsky, 2011). They remove cellular debris and play important roles in repair and remodeling of the CNS (Hanisch and Kettenmann, 2007; Napoli and Neumann, 2009). Macroglia include a heterogenous group of cells subdivided into four types: ependymal cells, oligodendrocytes, Schwann cells and astroglia (Kettenmann and Verkhratsky, 2011). Ependymal cells form the lining of the ventricles of the CNS, while Schwann cells and oligodendrocytes form the myelin sheath of the axons in the peripheral nervous system and CNS respectively (Kettenmann and Ransom, 2005). Astroglia comprise a variety of different cell types including astrocytes, Muller cells in the retina and tanycytes in the hypothalamus, grouped together due to common expression of the cytoskeletal protein - glial fibrillary acidic protein (GFAP) (Garcia-Segura and McCarthy, 2004). Astrocytes are the most abundant and versatile cells among all glial cells, involved in an array of important functions including maintenance of the BBB, regulation of extracellular ion concentrations, recycling of glutamate, release of energy substrates for neurons, glycogen storage, glutathione synthesis and modulation of synaptic transmission (Araque et al., 1999; Kurosinski and Gotz, 2002; Caudle, 2006; Ransom and Ransom, 2012).

2.2. Glia in Neuroinflammation

Chronic neuroinflammation mediated by pathological activation of glial cells in the brain is widely recognized for its critical contribution to AD-associated neuronal loss and synaptic dysfunction (Blasko et al., 2004; Frank-Cannon et al., 2009; Cameron and Landreth, 2010). In general, an acute inflammatory response triggered by foreign pathogens or toxic insults is beneficial to the CNS, since it provides protection and minimizes further damage (Laroux, 2004). However, chronic inflammation is a self-perpetuating process that causes extensive, collateral damage to healthy cells surrounding the site of inflammation. Brain inflammation in AD is characterized by persistent activation of glial cells, mainly microglia and astrocytes in response to various pathological formations such as amyloid β protein (Aβ) containing plaques or malfunctioning endogenous signals (Block et al., 2007; Krause and Muller, 2010; Steele and Robinson, 2012). Such activation of glial cells results in excessive production of free radical species, complement activation and upregulation of key pro-inflammatory mediators leading to neuronal damage and death (Mandrekar-Colucci and Landreth, 2010; Smith et al., 2012). The resulting neuronal damage can in turn activate more microglia, leading to a cycle of inflammation and cell death that continues even in the absence of the initial trigger (Pais et al., 2008). Therefore, therapeutic strategies aimed at reducing glial cell activation and/or switching the phenotype of glial cells from pro- to anti-inflammatory may decrease neuroinflammation and thus prove beneficial in treatment of AD.

2.3. Role of Glia in Neuroendocrinology

Research investigating the hormonal regulation of the nervous system has primarily focused on neuronal systems with little to no mention of the involvement of glial cells. Hormones act on cell surface or intracellular receptors to induce a cascade of signaling pathways in the target cells, ultimately leading to a desired cellular response. Glial cells, similar to neurons, express receptors for a variety of different hormones including steroid hormones (Cadepond et al., 2002), thyroid hormone (Mohacsik et al., 2011), insulin (Grunberger et al., 1986), glucagon (Chowen et al., 1999) and leptin (Dallaporta et al., 2009). Therefore, hormones in the CNS (Garcia-Segura and McCarthy, 2004) exert their actions equally on both glia and neurons. Glial cells are capable of transmitting hormonal signals to neurons through physical and chemical (e.g., via release of a growth factor) interactions thus mediating hormonal actions in the CNS (Garcia-Segura and McCarthy, 2004; Su et al., 2012). Glial cells not only metabolize hormones to generate the active metabolite (Garcia-Segura et al., 1996), but also modulate the secretion of hormones in the case of hypothalamic neurons (Miyata and Hatton, 2002; Theodosis, 2002). The communication between neurons and glia is important for development, cognition, synaptic plasticity and regulation of behavioral patterns such as sleep and appetite (Fields and Stevens-Graham, 2002; Garcia-Segura and McCarthy, 2004).

Due to complexity of neuron-glia cross communication, it is difficult to pinpoint the exact cell type involved in mediating the effects of a particular hormone in the CNS. Certain hormones may act directly on microglia and astrocytes to modulate the release of neurotrophic and neurotoxic molecules and/or alter glial inflammatory responses. For example, progesterone provides neuroprotection by stimulating the release of the brain-derived neurotrophic factor (BDNF) from glial cells (Su et al., 2012). *In vitro* and *in vivo* studies indicate that estradiol reduces chronic activation of microglia, decreases production of several pro-inflammatory mediators and enhances microglial Aβ uptake (Arevalo et al., 2010). Estradiol is also known to exert anti-inflammatory effects on reactive astrocytes including decrease in expression of nitric oxide and pro-inflammatory cytokines such as tumor necrosis factor (TNF)-α and interleukin (IL)-6 (Micevych et al., 2010). Therefore, neuroprotection conferred by estradiol in neurodegenerative conditions such as AD may be partly mediated by its anti-inflammatory effects on glial cells. In addition, estradiol increases expression of a number of glial-specific genes including the glutamine synthetase, an enzyme that converts glutamate to glutamine (Blutstein et al., 2006). Therefore, hormonally responsive glial cells could be responsible for estradiol-mediated modulation of glutamate neurotransmission (Blutstein et al., 2009). Regulation of myelin formation and brain development by the thyroid hormone triiodothyronine is also mediated by its actions on glial cells including oligodendrocytes (Rodriguez-Pena, 1999) and Schwann cells (Mercier et al., 2001). Moreover, neurons may transmit hormonal signals to glial cells, which in turn could transmit the signal to other neurons and lead to a specific response. For example, estradiol acts on the enzyme cyclooxygenase (COX)-2 in neurons to induce prostaglandin E_2 synthesis; which in turn signals glutamate release from astrocytes, which is important for inducing dendritic spine synapse formation in the pre-optic area (Amateau and McCarthy, 2002). In conclusion, glial cells play a vital role in modulation of various neuroendocrine events. It is therefore pivotal that research investigating hormonal signaling in the CNS recognizes the possible involvement of glial cells in mediating hormonal actions.

3. Insulin in the Brain

Of all the hormones and trophic factors relevant to the CNS, the hormone insulin has caught the most attention of researchers in the last few years (Craft et al., 2012; Duarte et al., 2012). Human insulin is a 51-amino acid (5808 Da) peptide hormone produced by β-cells in the islets of Langerhans of the pancreas (Harfenist and Craig, 1952). It belongs to the insulin-related family of structurally related proteins that includes insulin-like growth factor (IGF)-1 and IGF-2 (Chan et al., 1992). In response to rising blood glucose levels, insulin secreted by the pancreas stimulates uptake of glucose by liver, muscle and adipose tissue, thereby lowering blood glucose levels. Insulin has pleiotropic effects on carbohydrate and fat metabolism that extend beyond the lowering of blood glucose including decreased gluconeogenesis; increased glycogen synthesis; decreased lipolysis; and increased lipid synthesis and esterification of fatty acids (Flakoll et al., 2004). Traditionally, insulin was believed to be a peripheral hormone with no ability to affect the CNS. In fact, brain was considered to be an insulin insensitive organ (Bachelard, 1981; Seaquist et al., 2001). It is now known that insulin is present in the brain (Margolis and Altszuler, 1967; Schechter et al., 1992) and that the brain is sensitive to the effects of insulin, just not to the same extent as other metabolic tissues such as the liver and the muscle (McCall, 2004). Moreover, research in the last two decades has highlighted new roles of insulin in the CNS including the ability to affect distinct cognitive functions (Kern et al., 2001; Benedict et al., 2004), memory formations (Park et al., 2000) and mood (Hallschmid et al., 2008). In addition, insulin may act as an adiposity signal informing the brain of the amount of fat tissue (Woods and Seeley, 2001). Peripheral hyperglycemia leads to activation of insulin signaling in the glucosensing neurons of the hypothalamus; which causes hyperpolarization of these neurons and reduces their firing rate (Pocai et al., 2005). Activation of insulin signaling in the hypothalamus is integrated with meal-related signals like cholecystokinin and ghrelin to regulate food intake and energy metabolism (Morton et al., 2006). Intracerebroventricular administration of insulin reduces body fat by inhibiting food intake and promoting energy expenditure (Woods et al., 1979). Hypothalamic insulin signaling is also known to regulate gluconeogenesis in the liver (Obici et al., 2002). Impairment of insulin signaling in the hypothalamus leads to decreased sensitivity of the liver to circulating insulin and hence stimulates glucose production (Buettner and Camacho, 2008; Ono et al., 2008). Among other roles, insulin has been proposed to promote neurogenesis, inhibit neuronal apoptosis, improve synaptic plasticity and modulate synaptic transmission within the CNS (Hallschmid and Schultes, 2009; Banks et al., 2012; Duarte et al., 2012).

3.1. Origin of CNS Insulin

There is some evidence to support *de novo* synthesis of insulin in the brain (Schechter et al., 1996; Hoyer, 2003). Cultured neurons from the rat brain can synthesize insulin (in a biphasic manner similar to β cells of the pancreas) in response to potassium and calcium ion mediated stimulation (Clarke et al., 1986). However, most of the insulin in the brain is of a peripheral origin (Banks et al., 1997b; Banks, 2004; Laron, 2009). Insulin is believed to cross the BBB via a receptor-mediated saturable transport system (Miller et al., 1994; Banks et al., 1997a; Banks, 2004; Duarte et al., 2012). Another possible route of insulin entry into the brain is the circumventricular region, which is a specialized area of the brain that has a leaky BBB and is in contact with the CSF (Porte et al., 1998; Duarte et al., 2012). It is widely accepted that insulin is present in the CNS and can reach relatively high concentrations (Margolis and Altszuler, 1967; Schechter et al., 1992). However, the exact insulin concentration in the brain is still controversial and is believed to change during brain development (Schechter et al., 1992). In response to intravenous insulin infusions (plasma insulin increase from a mean basal level of ~77 pM to a mean level of ~1750 pM), the CSF insulin concentration increases from a mean basal level of ~6 pM to a mean of ~18 pM (Wallum et al., 1987). Thus, CSF insulin levels seem to be tuned in to the peripheral levels of insulin. However, the rate of increase in CSF insulin levels becomes proportionately smaller at higher plasma insulin levels suggesting that the relationship is non-linear (Margolis and Altszuler, 1967; Kahn, 1995). In contrast to CSF insulin levels, insulin concentrations in individualized brain regions are estimated to be 10 to 100 fold greater than in the plasma (Schulingkamp et al., 2000).

3.2. Brain Insulin Resistance in AD

Epidemiological studies have identified metabolic disorders such as obesity, type 2 diabetes mellitus and insulin resistance as significant risk factors for AD (Ronnemaa et al., 2008; Lu et al., 2009; Profenno et al., 2010). In this context, insulin resistance has been proposed as the mechanistic link between metabolic disorders and AD (Neumann et al., 2008; de la Monte, 2012; Duarte et al., 2012). Hyperinsulinemia is a compensatory mechanism in response to insulin resistance. In conditions of chronic peripheral hyperinsulinemia, as observed in obesity and insulin resistance states, the CSF to plasma ratio of insulin is reduced owing to the impaired transport of insulin into the brain, leading to low levels of insulin in the brain (Stein et al., 1987; Kaiyala et al., 2000; Kern et al., 2006). Interestingly, deficits in insulin signaling and reduced brain insulin levels have been noted in age-related neurodegenerative disorders such as AD. Down-regulation of the insulin receptor and several of its key signaling molecules is observed in patients with AD leading to reduced levels of insulin receptor binding and decreased responsiveness to insulin stimulation (Jolivalt et al., 2008; Liu et al., 2011). Brain insulin-resistant state in AD is associated with impaired cognition and memory (Neumann et al., 2008; de la Monte, 2012; Duarte et al., 2012). This has led some researchers to propose that AD represents 'type 3 diabetes' in the brain (de la Monte and Wands, 2008). Insulin regulates a plethora of different genes and downstream signaling pathways in the CNS. Therefore, deficits in insulin signaling may help explain the oxidative stress, mitochondrial dysfunction and activation of pro-inflammatory and pro-apoptotic pathways observed in AD, and have also been linked to the accumulation of Aβ plaques and hyperphosphorylation of tau (de la Monte and Wands, 2008; Neumann et al., 2008; de la Monte, 2012; Duarte et al., 2012). Intranasal insulin administration could override the impaired BBB transport of insulin into the brain; thus delivering insulin directly to the brain without affecting blood glucose levels. A recent pilot clinical trial has demonstrated that intranasal insulin therapy improves cognition in patients with mild to moderate AD (Craft et al., 2012). Long-term clinical trials are now focusing on the use of insulin to improve memory and cognition in AD. However, as mentioned before, no information is available on the effects of insulin on glial cells of the brain. It is possible that insulin's effects on memory and cognition are partially mediated by glial cells. Moreover, without any information on how different doses of insulin could affect glial cell physiology and the resulting cross talk between glia and neurons, it is difficult to conclusively establish the mechanisms by which brain insulin administration acts. In addition, in chronic neuroinflammatory conditions such as AD, it is important to investigate how insulin administration could affect the inflammatory status of both microglia and astrocytes that are already in a state of chronic activation.

4. INSULIN RECEPTOR

The insulin receptor is a heterotetrameric glycoprotein belonging to the tyrosine kinase family of growth factor receptors. It is composed of two extracellular ligand-binding α subunits (120-135 kDa), linked by disulphide bonds to two membrane-spanning β (92-97 kDa) subunits (Lee and Pilch, 1994). Two isoforms of the insulin receptor exist due to alternative splicing of the transcript: insulin receptor isoform A and insulin receptor isoform B (Seino and Bell, 1989). The adipose tissue has the highest expression of the insulin receptor, followed by about 30% relative expression in the liver, heart and lungs, and about 10% in the brain, muscle and kidney (Bailyes et a*l*., 1997). Insulin receptor isoform B accounts for 80% of the total insulin receptor expression in the liver and 60% of the total insulin receptor expression in the muscle and adipose tissue (Benecke et al., 1992). In general, insulin receptor isoform B is primarily involved in metabolic insulin signaling in differentiated tissues (Belfiore et al., 2009). On the other hand, insulin receptor isoform A is a high-affinity receptor for IGF-2 and its upregulation is associated with increased IGF-2 signaling (Frasca et al., 1999).

Localization of insulin receptors in the brain was first studied *in vitro* (Baskin et al., 1986; Hill et al., 1986) and *in vivo* by autoradiography techniques (van Houten et al., 1979). However, differences in insulin receptor expression by various brain cell types could not be distinguished using such techniques. Moreover, due to cross-reactivity of insulin with the IGF-1 receptor, it was difficult to determine the relative contribution of each receptor to the effects of insulin in regions of overlap between the two receptors (Unger et al., 1991a). Using immunocytochemistry with antibodies designed specifically against the insulin receptor, it was found to be expressed in a widespread but selective pattern in the brain including the hypothalamus, cerebral cortex, hippocampus, olfactory bulb, cerebellum and striatum (Weyhenmeyer, 1984; Unger et al., 1991b). The expression level is developmentally regulated and it is more enriched in neurons compared to glial cells (Unger et al., 1991a). Electron microscopy techniques revealed that insulin receptors are located along the cell processes and are also concentrated at postsynaptic terminals (Unger et al., 1991a).

Insulin binding studies have shown differences in the binding characteristics and subunit structure of the brain insulin receptor compared to insulin receptors in peripheral metabolic tissues including the adipose tissue and liver: a lower molecular weight of the α subunit that lacks neuraminidase sensitivity (115 kDa instead of 130 kDa); a 2-5 times higher affinity for IGF-1 and IGF-2; and absence of negative cooperativity (Gammeltoft et al., 1985; Lowe et al., 1986). However, the molecular weight of the β subunit (~ 94 kDa) and the tyrosine kinase activity is similar between insulin receptors from different tissues. Studies using cultured neuronal and glial cells from neonatal rats established that the brain-specific insulin receptor is expressed by neurons (Lowe et al., 1986). On the other hand, the structural and binding characteristics of insulin receptors expressed by glial cells of the brain as well as peripheral immune cells (e.g., monocytes and macrophages) are similar to that of peripheral metabolic tissues (Lowe et al., 1986). Glial insulin receptors from human cerebral gliomas are sensitive to neuraminidase treatment and are down-regulated in response to high insulin concentrations (Grunberger et al., 1986). Therefore, two types of insulin receptors are expressed in the mammalian brain – lower density peripheral-type insulin receptor expressed by glial cells and the higher density neuronal-type insulin receptor expressed by neurons. In its initial stages, peripheral hyperinsulinemia (e.g., in conditions of obesity or insulin resistance) may lead to periods of high insulin concentrations in the brain (Neumann et al., 2008).

As mentioned above, the neuronal insulin receptors lack negative cooperativity. However, the glial insulin receptor may be down-regulated in response to high insulin levels in the brain (Grunberger et al., 1986; Baskin et al., 1987).

As discussed earlier, down-regulation of the insulin receptor and its various signaling molecules is observed in AD (Jolivalt et al., 2008; Liu et al., 2011). Therefore, down-regulation of the glial insulin receptor may comprise one of the mechanisms of hyperinsulinemia-induced insulin resistance in AD.

5. Comparison of Insulin Signaling in Neurons, Monocytes/Macrophages and Glial Cells

Insulin signaling in various metabolic and vascular tissues shares many of the common signaling molecules and cascades, with some subtle differences. Classical metabolic insulin signaling is well characterized in insulin-sensitive metabolic tissues such as the liver, skeletal muscle and adipose tissue (Saltiel and Kahn, 2001; Pansuria et al., 2012). Signaling cascades employed by insulin in the CNS are very similar to those in the peripheral metabolic tissues (Banks et al., 2012; Duarte et al., 2012).

Although the glial cells express the insulin receptor and its signaling molecules at a lower level compared to neurons, insulin signaling in glial cells could contribute to some of the effects of insulin in the brain. In order to understand the importance of insulin signaling in microglia, we turn our attention to their peripheral counterparts: monocytes and macrophages. Monocytes are immune cells that form an integral part of the innate immune system and are produced by hematopoietic stem cell precursors known as monoblasts (Tambuyzer et al., 2009). In tissues, monocytes differentiate into tissue-resident macrophages (e.g., microglia are brain-resident macrophages). Monocytes, macrophages and brain microglia all belong to the mononuclear phagocyte system and share the same lineage. Therefore, insulin signaling in these peripheral immune cells could shed some light on the effects of insulin on glial cells, especially microglia.

On the other hand, insulin signaling in neurons could explain some of the differences between the effects of insulin in the periphery and the CNS.

5.1. Classical Insulin-Signaling Pathways

In all insulin target tissues, the binding of insulin to the α subunits of the insulin receptor leads to autophosphorylation of the β subunits at multiple tyrosine kinase residues (Nystrom and Quon, 1999; Saltiel and Kahn, 2001), followed by phosphorylation of insulin receptor substrate proteins (IRS) 1-4 (White, 2002). Binding of the active IRS to the p85 regulatory subunit of phosphatidylinositol 3-kinase (PI3K) leads to activation of the catalytic subunit of PI3K (Shepherd et al., 1998; Cantley, 2002) as well as the growth factor receptor-bound protein 2 (Grb-2) (Skolnik et al., 1993). This leads to downstream activation of two signaling pathways: the PI3K/Akt pathway and the Ras/mitogen-activated protein kinase (MAPK) pathway (Saltiel and Kahn, 2001; Pansuria et al., 2012). Activation of PI3K leads to its translocation to the plasma membrane and formation of downstream signaling molecules that recruit the Ser/Thr kinase Akt to the plasma membrane. Phosphorylation of Akt leads to its activation and detachment from the plasma membrane (Andjelkovic et al., 1997). Activated Akt translocates to the cytosol and nucleus where it phosphorylates various proteins at Ser/Thr residues including caspase 9, glycogen synthase kinase (GSK)-3β and the pro-apoptotic Bad protein (Manning and Cantley, 2007). The phosphorylation of these proteins by Akt leads to their inactivation and therefore leads to inhibition of apoptosis. Moreover, the PI3K-Akt activation stimulates translocation of the glucose transporter (GLUT)-4 protein from the cytosol to the plasma membrane and hence regulates glucose metabolism (Berwick et al., 2004; Welsh et al., 2005). GLUT-4 is primarily involved in insulin-mediated glucose uptake by classical insulin-sensitive tissues (Huang and Czech, 2007). Activation of the Ras/MAPK signaling pathway following binding of insulin to the insulin receptor occurs via Grb2, which leads to activation of Ras and recruitment of the Raf kinase (Skolnik et al., 1993). This pathway causes activation of MAPK kinase (MAP2K) and extracellular signal-regulated kinase (ERK1/2) leading to activation of various transcription factors that regulate growth, mitogenesis, proliferation and inflammation (Yoon and Seger, 2006).

5.2. Insulin Signaling in Neurons

In the CNS, certain selective populations of neurons may express GLUT-4 (Rayner et al., 1994). However, neurons primarily express the high affinity GLUT-3 (Nagamatsu et al., 1992; Rayner et al., 1994). In neurons, activation of the PI3K/Akt pathway may phosphorylate nuclear-factor kappa B (NFkB) and thus provide protection against oxidative stress and apoptosis (Duarte et al., 2012). The PI3K/Akt pathway activation also phosphorylates the survival transcription factor cAMP response element-binding (CREB), which increases intracellular ATP levels, hexokinase activity and mitochondrial membrane potential to improve glucose metabolism (Huang et al., 2005).

Impaired insulin signaling and insulin resistance in AD causes down-regulation of the PI3K/Akt signaling components, ultimately leading to multiple dysregulations in the downstream signaling pathways. For example, decreased PI3K/Akt-mediated phosphorylation (and therefore inactivation) of GSK-3β due to deficits in insulin signaling leads to hyperphosphorylation of the microtubule-associated tau protein. Self-aggregation of hyperphosphorylated tau generates insoluble fibrillar structures that cause synaptic dysfunction and neurodegeneration in AD (Iqbal and Grundke-Iqbal, 2008). However, the Ras/MAPK pathway is less affected in an insulin-resistant state (Rensing et al., 2011; Duarte et al., 2012). Traditionally, it was believed that these two signaling pathways function separately with the PI3K/Akt pathway controlling metabolism and the Ras/MAPK signaling pathway regulating mitogenic effects (Groop et al., 2005). However, there is some evidence of cross talk mediated by Raf (Levinthal and DeFranco, 2004). Moreover, the Ras/MAPK pathway was originally considered as anti-apoptotic in neurons due to phosphorylation of the Bad protein (Hetman et al., 1999; Johnson-Farley et al., 2006). However, activation of the Ras/MAPK pathway is also known to cause neuronal cell death after oxidative stress (Purves et al., 2001) and NMDA receptor-mediated excitotoxicity (Haddad, 2005). The anti-apoptotic effects of insulin seem to be mediated primarily by the PI3K/Akt pathway in neurons (Huang et al., 2005; Yu et al., 2006; Duarte et al., 2008). In addition, p38 MAPK-mediated stimulation of anti-oxidant defense mechanisms and glucose transport in peripheral tissues is not observed in neurons (Geiger et al., 2005).

5.3. Insulin Signaling in Peripheral Monocytes/Macrophages

The PI3K/Akt (Welham et al., 1997; Liang et al., 2004) and Ras/MAPK (Buscher et al., 1995) insulin signaling pathways are known to be active in monocytes and macrophages. Insulin has been shown to increase viability and protein synthesis in macrophages (Han et al., 2006). Insulin increases activity of glucose-metabolizing enzymes such as hexokinase, citrate synthase and antioxidant enzymes such as Cu/Zn superoxide dismutase in rat macrophages (Rosa et al., 1992; Pereira et al., 1995). Interestingly, T lymphocytes do not express the insulin receptor under normal circumstances (Stentz and Kitabchi, 2004); but express the insulin receptor following antigen presentation leading to activation of the PI3K/Akt signaling (Helderman, 1984; Stentz and Kitabchi, 2004). It is not clear whether insulin has effects on antigen processing and presentation in macrophages; it does, however, seem to affect their phagocytic and redox activity (Bar et al., 1977; Ghezzo et al., 1983). There is also some *in vitro* evidence to suggest that physiological concentrations of insulin may alter their specific immunological functions including antibody-dependent cell-mediated cytotoxicity (Bar et al., 1977). Activation of the PI3K/Akt pathway by insulin inhibits apoptosis in differentiated THP-1 macrophages by increasing the expression of the anti-apoptotic gene Bcl-x (Iida et al., 2002). Since IRS-1 isoform is undetectable in monocytes and macrophages (Liang et al., 2004), IRS-2 seems to be the primary insulin-receptor substrate isoform in monocytes and macrophages (Welham et al., 1997). Moreover, decreased phosphorylation of the insulin receptor and deficits in downstream signaling are observed in monocytes from obese subjects (Bar et al., 1976) and macrophages from obese, insulin resistant mice (Liang et al., 2004). Whether similar defects in insulin signaling could be observed in brain macrophages is unknown.

5.4. Insulin Signaling in Glia

Limited literature is available regarding the specific insulin signaling cascades in brain glial cells. Insulin stimulates the phosphorylation of exogenous substrates by the glial insulin receptor isolated from human cerebral gliomas by activation of the tyrosine kinase activity of the β subunits (Grunberger et al., 1986). Moreover, insulin receptors have been characterized in cultured astrocytes (Clarke et al., 1985; Heni et al., 2011) and C6 astrocytoma cells (Montiel et al., 1989). In cultured astrocytic rodent glial cells, insulin stimulates protein, RNA and DNA synthesis as measured by valine, uridine and thymidine incorporation into proteins, RNA and DNA respectively (Clarke et al., 1985). Such stimulation of macromolecular synthesis also seems to occur via the insulin receptor of glial cells. Insulin is capable of regulating differentiation, phenotypic appearance and GFAP expression of astroglial cells in organotypic cultures of mouse cerebellum (Toran-Allerand et al., 1991). A recent study demonstrated that insulin treatment in normal human astrocytes derived from the fetal brain led to a dose-dependent increase in Akt phosphorylation and PI3K activity (Heni et al., 2011).

Therefore, the insulin-signaling cascade is functional in human astrocytes. Moreover, insulin stimulated cell proliferation and glycogen storage in astrocytes (Heni et al., 2011). Unlike in monocytes and macrophages, both IRS-1 and IRS-2 are expressed in astrocytes (Heni et al., 2011).

Müller cells, the principal glia of the retina, are also known to express glial-type insulin receptor, IRS-1 and a functional insulin-signaling cascade (Ola et al., 2011). Moreover, insulin, in combination with fibroblast growth factor (FGF)-2 is known to cause de-differentiation and proliferation of Muller glia (Fischer et al., 2002; Fischer and Reh, 2003). However, insulin-mediated stimulation of Muller glia and microglia-like cells in the retina seems to increase susceptibility of retinal neurons to an excitotoxic insult (Fischer et al., 2009). To the best of our knowledge, specific insulin signaling components in microglial cells have not been reported.

Overall, it is evident that, similar to peripheral insulin-sensitive tissues, activation of the insulin receptor and downstream insulin signaling pathways occur in the neurons of the CNS as well as the peripheral immune cells such as monocytes and macrophages. However, specific insulin signaling in glia has not been studied extensively.

6. Regulation of Brain Glucose Metabolism by Insulin

Brain glucose metabolism was believed to be insensitive to the effects of insulin. Early abnormalities in glucose uptake and utilization parallel the worsening of dementia in AD (Hoyer, 2004).

Some researchers believe that this impairment in glucose metabolism is a consequence of impaired insulin signaling transduction (Hoyer, 2004; Neumann et al., 2008). However, the regulation of glucose metabolism by insulin in the brain is still controversial. Some studies suggest that there is no change in the rate of brain glucose metabolism in response to increasing concentrations of circulating insulin (Cranston et al., 1998; Hasselbalch et al., 1999).

Conversely, other studies indicate that regional increases in brain glucose utilization may occur in response to hyperinsulinemia (Lucignani et al., 1987). Moreover, due to kinetics of insulin transport from the plasma to CSF, there is a 60-150 min lag period before CSF insulin concentrations increase following plasma increases in insulin levels (Schwartz et al., 1990). Therefore, it is possible that some studies failed to show an effect of insulin administration on brain glucose metabolism due to shorter run-in periods. Using 18-fluorodeoxyglucose and positron emission tomography (FDG-PET) in healthy human volunteers, Bingham et al. (2002) concluded that whole brain glucose uptake is maximally stimulated at basal insulin concentrations. Fasting insulin levels stimulated global glucose metabolism, primarily in the cortical areas and to a lesser extent in the cerebellum.

The co-localization of insulin, the insulin receptor and GLUT-4 expressed by certain neuronal populations in selective regions of the brain suggests that neuronal glucose uptake could be regulated by insulin (Alquier et al., 2006). Also, cerebellar GLUT-4 expression is modulated by changes in circulating insulin levels (Vannucci et al., 1998).

6.1. Insulin Regulates Glial Glucose Metabolism

It is believed that insulin may stimulate glucose uptake and regulate glucose metabolism only in glia and not in neurons (Werner et al., 1989; Duarte et al., 2012). Bingham et al. (2002) suggest that the direct effect of insulin on glucose uptake in the cerebral cortex might involve the recruitment of the glial GLUT-1 to the plasma membrane and subsequent uptake of glucose by glial cells since the main neuronal GLUT-3 is insulin insensitive. Insulin is known to increase GLUT-1 mRNA steady state levels in glial cells (Werner et al., 1989). Binding of insulin to its receptor stimulates uptake of 2-deoxy-D-glucose in peripheral monocytes (Daneman et al., 1992) as well as glial cells cultured from the rat brain (Clarke et al., 1984). However, insulin does not stimulate uptake of glucose by mouse macrophages (Liang et al., 2004).

These differences may be explained by differential expression of GLUT isoforms by different immune cells. Monocytes, macrophages and glial cells of the brain do not express the insulin-sensitive GLUT-4 (Malide et al., 1998). Instead, they express the partially insulin-sensitive GLUT-1 and insulin-insensitive GLUT-3 and GLUT-5 (Fu et al., 2004). Lipopolysaccharide stimulation is known to increase GLUT-1 and decrease GLUT-3 expression in monocytes (Fu et al., 2004).

Conversely, differentiation of THP-1 monocytic cells to macrophages leads to decreased GLUT-1 and increased GLUT-3 and GLUT-5 expression (Fu et al., 2004).

6.2. Glial Glycogen Stores Are Sensitive to Insulin

Glial cells may provide an alternative energy source to neurons in response to insulin stimulation of the brain (Schulingkamp et al., 2000; Duarte et al., 2012). One of the actions of insulin involves the inhibition of norepinephrine reuptake by neurons leading to increased norepinephrine in the synaptic cleft (Boyd et al., 1986). Norepinephrine causes activation of the glial β-adrenoceptors leading to increased cAMP levels which enhance the extrusion of glucose from the glycogen stores of glial cells, primarily astrocytes (Wozniak et al., 1993). This glucose is then available as an alternative energy source for neurons. Glycogen is mainly stored in the muscle and liver and to a lesser extent in astrocytes (McCall, 2004). However, the glycogen stores of astrocytes could be as high as 10 μmol/g (Choi and Gruetter, 2003; Oz et al., 2003); substantially greater than what had been previously estimated (McCall, 2004). Moreover, glycogen stores of astrocytes are sensitive to the effects of insulin-induced hypoglycemia and are mobilized to provide glucose within 6-8 h of hypoglycemia (Choi et al., 2003).

7. Effects of Insulin on Peripheral and Central Inflammation

Recent studies investigating the effect of exogenous and endogenous insulin on atherosclerotic processes including foam cell formation, smooth muscle cell proliferation and coagulation have challenged the well-established anti-inflammatory effects of insulin. It has been proposed that hyperinsulinemia can act in a pro-inflammatory and pro-atherogenic factor, thus contributing to atherosclerosis in diabetes and other insulin-resistant states (DeFronzo, 2010; Rensing et al., 2011). Conversely, others believe that such cardiovascular complications are a result of the insulin resistant state and not hyperinsulinemia *per se* (Garg et al., 2003; Dandona et al., 2007a). High insulin concentrations are compensatory to insulin resistance (Rensing et al., 2011). Disruptions in the PI3K/Akt insulin signaling pathway due to insulin resistance lead to impaired glucose uptake by metabolic tissues and high glucose concentrations in the blood. Consequently, more insulin is produced by the pancreas leading to a state of hyperinsulinemia.

Literature concerning insulin-mediated regulation of immune responses of peripheral monocytes and macrophages derives from the research investigating the effects of hyperinsulinemia on atherosclerosis and mortalities related to adverse cardiovascular events. Macrophages play an important role in initiating foam cell formation and contribute to inflammation, ultimately leading to atherosclerosis (Takahashi et al., 2002; Moore and Tabas, 2011). Macrophages from obese and type 2 diabetic patients are insulin resistant and show increased expression of various inflammatory markers (Liang et al., 2004). Inhibition of macrophage apoptosis by insulin is believed to contribute to instability of atherosclerotic plaques *in vivo* (Iida et al., 2002). Moreover, high concentrations of insulin suppress high-density lipoprotein-mediated cholesterol efflux from macrophages by inhibiting various enzymes involved in this process, thereby contributing to foam cell formation (Yamashita et al., 2010).

7.1. Anti-Inflammatory Effects of Insulin in the Periphery

Widely accepted anti-inflammatory effects of insulin were first observed in human umbilical vein endothelial cells, in which insulin caused a dose dependent increase in the expression of the endothelial nitric oxide synthase (Aljada and Dandona, 2000) and release of nitric oxide (Zeng and Quon, 1996). Physiological concentrations of insulin are known to decrease expression of various pro-inflammatory mediators including intercellular adhesion molecule (ICAM)-1, monocyte chemotactic protein (MCP)-1 and the pro-inflammatory transcription factor, NFkB in human aortic endothelial cells (Aljada et al., 2000; Aljada et al., 2001). Studies in animal models of rats and pigs have demonstrated suppression of endotoxin-induced pro-inflammatory transcription factors and gene expression by insulin (Brix-Christensen et al., 2004; Jeschke et al., 2004). In addition, insulin suppresses macrophage migration-inhibitory factor (MIF) expression by adipocytes (Sakaue et al., 1999), TNF-α generation by peritoneal exudate cells (Satomi et al., 1985) and carrageenan-induced inflammation in rats (Ottlecz et al., 1977). *In vivo* experiments involving low-dose insulin infusions in obese subjects provided solid evidence for an anti-inflammatory effect of insulin. Insulin was shown to reduce reactive oxygen species (ROS) generation and $p47^{phox}$ and NFkB expression in mononuclear cells (Dandona et al., 2001). Moreover, insulin infusions, while maintaining normoglycemia, decreased plasma concentrations of ICAM-1, MCP-1, matrix metalloproteinase (MMP)-2, MMP-9 and plasminogen activator inhibitor-1 (Dandona et al., 2001; Aljada et al., 2002). Insulin leads to a 40% reduction in plasma C-reactive protein (CRP) and serum amyloid A concentrations in patients with acute myocardial infarction (Chaudhuri et al., 2004). Moreover, anti-inflammatory, anti-oxidant and anti-thrombotic effects of low-dose insulin infusions, which are independent of decreases in glucose concentrations, have also been observed in intensive care unit patients and patients undergoing coronary artery bypass (Dandona et al., 2007a; Dandona et al., 2007b).

7.2. Pro-Inflammatory Effects of Insulin

The effects of insulin on inflammatory status of monocytes and macrophages could delineate some of the possible effects of insulin on glial cell immune responses.

High insulin concentrations *in vitro* (10^{-7}M) cause a dose-dependent increase in mRNA expression and secretion of pro-inflammatory cytokines TNF-α (Iida et al., 2001) and IL-8 (Wurm et al., 2008) in THP-1 derived macrophages and primary human monocytes, respectively. Similar insulin concentrations lead to augmentation of MMP-9 expression in THP-1 monocytic cells (Fischoeder et al., 2007). MMP-9 induction facilitates accelerated chemotaxis of monocytes and macrophages (Kappert et al., 2008). These effects of high insulin concentrations on inflammatory mediators in monocytes and macrophages are mediated by the Ras/MAPK insulin signaling pathway and are not suppressed by inhibition of the PI3K/Akt pathway or p38 MAPK.

Hyperinsulinemia is also known to induce NADPH oxidase-dependent superoxide production in human monocytes and murine macrophages via insulin receptor-mediated activation of PI3K and protein kinase C (San Jose et al., 2009). Activation of the NADPH oxidase turns on the ERK 1/2, p38 MAPK and NFkB signaling pathways leading to proliferation of the cells and activation of MMP-9 (San Jose et al., 2009).

Interestingly, activation of THP-1 derived macrophages by LPS (6 h), followed by insulin treatment (10^{-7}M) for 1 h and 24 h leads to significantly higher production of TNF-α and IL-6 by insulin-treated cells compared to cells treated with LPS alone (Brundage et al., 2008). On the other hand, 24 h pre-treatment of THP-1 derived macrophages with insulin (10^{-7}M) attenuates the production of TNF-α and IL-8, when the cells are subsequently challenged with LPS (Cuschieri et al., 2008).

Another study showed that insulin alone did not affect production of IL-6 and TNF-α in THP-1 monocytes (Bunn et al., 2010). However, insulin combined with the saturated non-esterified fatty acid palmitate led to more IL-6 and TNF-α production compared to palmitate alone (Bunn et al., 2010). This synergistic action of insulin on the release of pro-inflammatory cytokines was mediated by the RAS/MAPK signaling pathway. Using HuH7 hepatocytes, Iwasaki et al. (2009) showed that insulin may exert short term anti-inflammatory and long term pro-inflammatory effects. Insulin alone (10^{-9} M) did not affect NFkB mediated transcription of pro-inflammatory genes. However, simultaneous treatment of HuH7 hepatocytes with insulin and TNF-α led to a dual response: short-term (6h) suppression and long-term (36 h) stimulation of NFKB mediated transcription.

The former effect was mediated by the PI3K/Akt signaling pathway, while the latter was mediated by the Ras/MAPK signaling and led to a seven-fold increase in TNF-α-stimulated NFkB-dependent transcription by insulin. Insulin infusions in healthy adults to reach plasma insulin levels typical of insulin resistance, while maintaining euglycemia led to increased plasma and CSF levels of pro-inflammatory cytokines such as IL-1α, IL-1β, TNF-α and IL-6 as well as increased plasma and CSF levels of Aβ42 (Fishel et al., 2005). Accumulation of Aβ42 in the brain contributes to neurotoxicity in AD (de la Monte, 2012). Therefore, peripheral hyperinsulinemia may not only contribute to peripheral and central inflammation but may also lead to accumulation of Aβ42, thus contributing to AD pathogenesis.

As discussed earlier, low-dose insulin concentrations exert anti-inflammatory effects on monocyte and macrophage-mediated inflammation. Conversely, high insulin concentrations seem to act in a pro-inflammatory manner.

The effect of different insulin concentrations on immune responses of glial cells, especially microglia and astrocytes has not been studied. However, we can hypothesize that similar to monocytes and macrophages, an insulin concentration threshold exists that may determine the pro-inflammatory vs. anti-inflammatory effects of insulin on glial cell immune responses.

Moreover, based on the evidence presented above, the effects of insulin on monocytes and macrophages not only depend on the concentration and time of incubation with insulin, but also on the presence of other stimulatory agents. Therefore, insulin may exacerbate glial cell mediated neuroinflammation in chronic inflammatory conditions such as AD due to presence of several other inflammatory triggers and the ongoing cycle of inflammation.

8. Effects of Insulin on Memory and Learning: Possible Role of Glia

It is well known that insulin plays important roles in the CNS development including stimulation of nerve growth, neuronal protein synthesis and synapse formation (Banks et al., 2012; Duarte et al., 2012). Moreover, insulin administration, while maintaining normal blood glucose levels, is known to improve memory and learning in rats (Babri et al., 2007; Haj-ali et al., 2009) and humans, in both healthy and disease states (Benedict et al., 2004; Reger et al., 2008; Craft et al., 2012). The effects of insulin on synaptic plasticity, cognition and memory formation are possibly mediated by its ability to modulate synaptic transmission and receptor activity in neurons and/or glial cells, especially in the hippocampus (Duarte et al., 2012).

As discussed earlier, insulin influences actions of catecholamines by inhibiting synaptic reuptake of norepinephrine (Boyd et al., 1986; Raizada et al., 1988) and stimulating neuronal uptake of serotonin (Duarte et al., 2012). Insulin modulates expression of the glutamate N-methyl-D-aspartate (NMDA) receptors, which play a critical role in learning, memory and synaptic plasticity (Newcomer and Krystal, 2001; Nakazawa et al., 2003). Insulin administration recruits NMDA receptors to the membrane surface, increases NMDA channel activity and therefore modulates long-term potentiation (Liao and Leonard, 1999; Skeberdis et al., 2001). Furthermore, insulin augments γ-aminobutyric acid (GABA)-receptor mediated synaptic inhibition, important for learning-associated neuronal functions (Wan et al., 1997; Ma et al., 2003). Such effects of insulin on receptor modulation have primarily been studied in neurons. However, functional NMDA receptors are also expressed by brain macroglia including astrocytes, Muller glia and oligodendrocytes (Verkhratsky and Kirchhoff, 2007). Moreover, NDMA receptors of cortical astrocytes are activated upon synaptic transmission and play an important role in neuron-glia signal transmission (Lalo et al., 2006). Metabotropic and ionotropic GABA receptors of microglia, astrocytes and oligodendrocytes are activated by neuronal signaling mechanisms and all these cell types may signal back to neurons by releasing GABA (Velez-Fort et al., 2012). In addition, activation of glial receptors by GABA is known to influence neuronal activity, differentiation and neuroprotective mechanisms (Velez-Fort et al., 2012). As such, insulin-mediated improvements in memory and cognition could involve modulation of receptor activity and synaptic transmission of glial cells. Interestingly, insulin modulates expression of certain glial enzymes and transporters involved in glutamate neurotransmission. Insulin increases the total and surface expression of the astroglial cell-specific glutamate transporter subtype 2, GLT1 in cultured astrocytes (Ji et al., 2011). GLT1 is important for clearance of glutamate from the synaptic cleft in the CNS and protects from excitotoxicity that develops after damage to the CNS. Expression of glutamine synthetase, a key enzyme involved in glutamate metabolism in Muller glia is regulated by insulin (Ola et al., 2011). Insulin treatment causes a dose and time-dependent decrease in glutamine synthetase expression. Therefore, it is important to investigate possible involvement of glial cells in neuromodulatory and neuroprotective effects of insulin in the CNS.

Conclusion

Short-term clinical trials of intranasal insulin therapies show promise in improvement of memory and cognition in patients with mild to moderate AD (Craft et al., 2012). Insulin is known to reach high concentrations in the brain where it could play many roles apart from regulating glucose metabolism including synaptic plasticity, memory formation, cognition, neurotransmission and neuroprotection (Banks et al., 2012; Duarte et al., 2012). However, based on evidence reviewed above, the effects of insulin on glial cells have not been studied extensively. Glial cells express the insulin receptor and insulin signaling components (Grunberger et al., 1986; Montiel et al., 1989; Heni et al., 2011). Moreover, high concentrations of insulin down-regulate the insulin receptor expression in glial cells (Grunberger et al., 1986; Baskin et al., 1987). Therefore, periods of central hyperinsulinemia resulting from peripheral hyperinsulinemia may lead to impairment of the glial insulin receptors and a state of insulin resistance in glial cells. There is evidence to suggest that insulin regulates glucose metabolism in glial cells (Clarke et al., 1984; Werner et al., 1989). However, the regulation of glial immune responses by insulin is not well studied. Evidence collected by studies investigating the pro- vs. anti-inflammatory effects of insulin on peripheral monocytes and macrophages is inconclusive. In general, high insulin concentrations exert pro-inflammatory effects on peripheral immune responses, especially in a setting of insulin resistance and ongoing inflammation. A state of chronic neuroinflammation (Blasko et al., 2004; Frank-Cannon et al., 2009; Cameron and Landreth, 2010) and insulin resistance (Neumann et al., 2008; de la Monte, 2012) is evident in the AD brain. Moreover, deficits in the PI3K/Akt pathway are observed thereby increasing the relative contribution of the Ras/MAPK pathway to insulin signaling in the insulin-resistant AD brain. Peripheral studies indicate that the Ras/MAPK insulin signaling may be responsible for the pro-inflammatory effects of hyperinsulinemia. Whether high doses of insulin could act through the intact Ras/MAPK pathway to contribute to glia-mediated neuroinflammation in the insulin-resistant AD brain is not known. It is apparent that effects of different doses of insulin on the inflammatory status of chronically activated microglia and astrocytes must be investigated to understand the therapeutic window for the beneficial effects of insulin. If insulin administration at therapeutically relevant concentrations is found to exert anti-inflammatory effects on glial-mediated neuroinflammation, some of the beneficial effects of insulin in AD could be mediated by its effects on inflammation in addition to modulation of different glial receptor activities.

Acknowledgment

This work was supported by grants from the Natural Sciences and Engineering Research Council of Canada and the Jack Brown and Family Alzheimer's Disease Research Foundation.

References

Aljada, A. and Dandona, P. (2000) Effect of insulin on human aortic endothelial nitric oxide synthase. *Metabolism*, 49, 147-150.

Aljada, A., Ghanim, H., Mohanty, P., Kapur, N. and Dandona, P. (2002) Insulin inhibits the pro-inflammatory transcription factor early growth response gene-1 (Egr)-1 expression in mononuclear cells (MNC) and reduces plasma tissue factor (TF) and plasminogen activator inhibitor-1 (PAI-1) concentrations. *J Clin Endocrinol Metab*, 87, 1419-1422.

Aljada, A., Ghanim, H., Saadeh, R. and Dandona, P. (2001) Insulin inhibits NFkappaB and MCP-1 expression in human aortic endothelial cells. *J Clin Endocrinol Metab*, 86, 450-453.

Aljada, A., Saadeh, R., Assian, E., Ghanim, H. and Dandona, P. (2000) Insulin inhibits the expression of intercellular adhesion molecule-1 by human aortic endothelial cells through stimulation of nitric oxide. *J Clin Endocrinol Metab*, 85, 2572-2575.

Alquier, T., Leloup, C., Lorsignol, A. and Penicaud, L. (2006) Translocable glucose transporters in the brain - Where are we in 2006? *Diabetes*, 55, S131-S138.

Amateau, S.K. and McCarthy, M.M. (2002) A novel mechanism of dendritic spine plasticity involving estradiol induction of prostaglandin-E2. *J Neurosci*, 22, 8586-8596.

Andjelkovic, M., Alessi, D.R., Meier, R., Fernandez, A., Lamb, N.J., Frech, M., Cron, P., Cohen, P., Lucocq, J.M. and Hemmings, B.A. (1997) Role of translocation in the activation and function of protein kinase B. *J Biol Chem*, 272, 31515-31524.

Araque, A., Parpura, V., Sanzgiri, R.P. and Haydon, P.G. (1999) Tripartite synapses: glia, the unacknowledged partner. *Trends Neurosci*, 22, 208-215.

Arevalo, M.A., Santos-Galindo, M., Bellini, M.J., Azcoitia, I. and Garcia-Segura, L.M. (2010) Actions of estrogens on glial cells: Implications for neuroprotection. *Biochim Biophys Acta*, 1800, 1106-1112.

Babri, S., Badie, H.G., Khamenei, S. and Seyedlar, M.O. (2007) Intrahippocampal insulin improves memory in a passive-avoidance task in male wistar rats. *Brain Cogn*, 64, 86-91.

Bachelard, H. (1981) Cerebral metabolism and hypoglycaemia. In Marks, V., Rose, F.C. (eds) *Hypoglycaemia*. Blackwell, Oxford, pp. 51-68.

Bailyes, E.M., Nave, B.T., Soos, M.A., Orr, S.R., Hayward, A.C. and Siddle, K. (1997) Insulin receptor/IGF-I receptor hybrids are widely distributed in mammalian tissues:

quantification of individual receptor species by selective immunoprecipitation and immunoblotting. *Biochem J*, 327 (Pt 1), 209-215.

Banks, W.A. (2004) The source of cerebral insulin. *Eur J Pharmacol*, 490, 5-12.

Banks, W.A., Jaspan, J.B., Huang, W. and Kastin, A.J. (1997a) Transport of insulin across the blood-brain barrier: saturability at euglycemic doses of insulin. *Peptides*, 18, 1423-1429.

Banks, W.A., Jaspan, J.B. and Kastin, A.J. (1997b) Selective, physiological transport of insulin across the blood-brain barrier: novel demonstration by species-specific radioimmunoassays. *Peptides*, 18, 1257-1262.

Banks, W.A., Owen, J.B. and Erickson, M.A. (2012) Insulin in the brain: There and back again. *Pharmacol Ther.* [doi:10.1016/j.pharmthera.2012.07.006, published online ahead of print July 17 2012].

Bar, R.S., Gorden, P., Roth, J., Kahn, C.R. and De Meyts, P. (1976) Fluctuations in the affinity and concentration of insulin receptors on circulating monocytes of obese patients: effects of starvation, refeeding, and dieting. *J Clin Invest*, 58, 1123-1135.

Bar, R.S., Kahn, C.R. and Koren, H.S. (1977) Insulin inhibition of antibody-dependent cytoxicity and insulin receptors in macrophages. *Nature*, 265, 632-635.

Baskin, D.G., Davidson, D., Corp, E.S., Lewellen, T. and Graham, M. (1986) An inexpensive microcomputer digital imaging system for densitometry: quantitative autoradiography of insulin receptors with 125I and LKB Ultrofilm. *J Neurosci Methods*, 16, 119-129.

Baskin, D.G., Figlewicz, D.P., Woods, S.C., Porte, D., Jr. and Dorsa, D.M. (1987) Insulin in the brain. *Annu Rev Physiol*, 49, 335-347.

Belfiore, A., Frasca, F., Pandini, G., Sciacca, L. and Vigneri, R. (2009) Insulin receptor isoforms and insulin receptor/insulin-like growth factor receptor hybrids in physiology and disease. *Endocr Rev*, 30, 586-623.

Benecke, H., Flier, J.S. and Moller, D.E. (1992) Alternatively spliced variants of the insulin receptor protein. Expression in normal and diabetic human tissues. *J Clin Invest*, 89, 2066-2070.

Benedict, C., Hallschmid, M., Hatke, A., Schultes, B., Fehm, H.L., Born, J. and Kern, W. (2004) Intranasal insulin improves memory in humans. *Psychoneuroendocrinology*, 29, 1326-1334.

Berwick, D.C., Dell, G.C., Welsh, G.I., Heesom, K.J., Hers, I., Fletcher, L.M., Cooke, F.T. and Tavare, J.M. (2004) Protein kinase B phosphorylation of PIKfyve regulates the trafficking of GLUT4 vesicles. *J Cell Sci*, 117, 5985-5993.

Blasko, I., Stampfer-Kountchev, M., Robatscher, P., Veerhuis, R., Eikelenboom, P. and Grubeck-Loebenstein, B. (2004) How chronic inflammation can affect the brain and support the development of Alzheimer's disease in old age: the role of microglia and astrocytes. *Aging Cell*, 3, 169-176.

Block, M.L., Zecca, L. and Hong, J.S. (2007) Microglia-mediated neurotoxicity: uncovering the molecular mechanisms. *Nat Rev Neurosci*, 8, 57-69.

Blutstein, T., Baab, P.J., Zielke, H.R. and Mong, J.A. (2009) Hormonal modulation of amino acid neurotransmitter metabolism in the arcuate nucleus of the adult female rat: a novel action of estradiol. *Endocrinology*, 150, 3237-3244.

Blutstein, T., Devidze, N., Choleris, E., Jasnow, A.M., Pfaff, D.W. and Mong, J.A. (2006) Oestradiol up-regulates glutamine synthetase mRNA and protein expression in the hypothalamus and hippocampus: implications for a role of hormonally responsive glia in amino acid neurotransmission. *J Neuroendocrinol*, 18, 692-702.

Boyd, F.T., Jr., Clarke, D.W. and Raizada, M.K. (1986) Insulin inhibits specific norepinephrine uptake in neuronal cultures from rat brain. *Brain Res*, 398, 1-5.

Brix-Christensen, V., Andersen, S.K., Andersen, R., Mengel, A., Dyhr, T., Andersen, N.T., Larsson, A., Schmitz, O., Orskov, H. and Tonnesen, E. (2004) Acute hyperinsulinemia restrains endotoxin-induced systemic inflammatory response: an experimental study in a porcine model. *Anesthesiology*, 100, 861-870.

Brundage, S.I., Kirilcuk, N.N., Lam, J.C., Spain, D.A. and Zautke, N.A. (2008) Insulin increases the release of proinflammatory mediators. *J Trauma*, 65, 367-372.

Buettner, C. and Camacho, R.C. (2008) Hypothalamic control of hepatic glucose production and its potential role in insulin resistance. *Endocrinol Metab Clin North Am*, 37, 825-840.

Bunn, R.C., Cockrell, G.E., Ou, Y., Thrailkill, K.M., Lumpkin, C.K., Jr. and Fowlkes, J.L. (2010) Palmitate and insulin synergistically induce IL-6 expression in human monocytes. *Cardiovasc Diabetol*, 9, 73.

Buscher, D., Hipskind, R.A., Krautwald, S., Reimann, T. and Baccarini, M. (1995) Ras-dependent and -independent pathways target the mitogen-activated protein kinase network in macrophages. *Mol Cell Biol*, 15, 466-475.

Cadepond, F., Massaad, C., Trousson, A., Grenier, J., Groyer, G., Baulieu, E. and Schumacher, M. (2002) Steroid receptors in various glial cell lines expression and functional studies. *Ann NY Acad Sci*, 973, 484-487.

Cameron, B. and Landreth, G.E. (2010) Inflammation, microglia, and Alzheimer's disease. *Neurobiol Dis*, 37, 503-509.

Cantley, L.C. (2002) The phosphoinositide 3-kinase pathway. *Science*, 296, 1655-1657.

Caudle, R.M. (2006) Memory in astrocytes: a hypothesis. *Theor Biol Med Model*, 3, 2.

Chan, S.J., Nagamatsu, S., Cao, Q.P. and Steiner, D.F. (1992) Structure and evolution of insulin and insulin-like growth factors in chordates. *Prog Brain Res*, 92, 15-24.

Chaudhuri, A., Janicke, D., Wilson, M.F., Tripathy, D., Garg, R., Bandyopadhyay, A., Calieri, J., Hoffmeyer, D., Syed, T., Ghanim, H., Aljada, A. and Dandona, P. (2004) Anti-inflammatory and profibrinolytic effect of insulin in acute ST-segment-elevation myocardial infarction. *Circulation*, 109, 849-854.

Choi, I.Y. and Gruetter, R. (2003) In vivo 13C NMR assessment of brain glycogen concentration and turnover in the awake rat. *Neurochem Int*, 43, 317-322.

Choi, I.Y., Seaquist, E.R. and Gruetter, R. (2003) Effect of hypoglycemia on brain glycogen metabolism in vivo. *J Neurosci Res*, 72, 25-32.

Chowen, J.A., de Fonseca, F.R., Alvarez, E., Navarro, M., Garcia-Segura, L.M. and Blazquez, E. (1999) Increased glucagon-like peptide-1 receptor expression in glia after mechanical lesion of the rat brain. *Neuropeptides*, 33, 212-215.

Clarke, D.W., Boyd, F.T., Jr., Kappy, M.S. and Raizada, M.K. (1984) Insulin binds to specific receptors and stimulates 2-deoxy-D-glucose uptake in cultured glial cells from rat brain. *J Biol Chem*, 259, 11672-11675.

Clarke, D.W., Boyd, F.T., Jr., Kappy, M.S. and Raizada, M.K. (1985) Insulin stimulates macromolecular synthesis in cultured glial cells from rat brain. *Am J Physiol*, 249, C484-489.

Clarke, D.W., Mudd, L., Boyd, F.T., Jr., Fields, M. and Raizada, M.K. (1986) Insulin is released from rat brain neuronal cells in culture. *J Neurochem*, 47, 831-836.

Craft, S., Baker, L.D., Montine, T.J., Minoshima, S., Watson, G.S., Claxton, A., Arbuckle, M., Callaghan, M., Tsai, E., Plymate, S.R., Green, P.S., Leverenz, J., Cross, D. and

Gerton, B. (2012) Intranasal insulin therapy for Alzheimer disease and amnestic mild cognitive impairment: a pilot clinical trial. *Arch Neurol*, 69, 29-38.

Craft, S., Peskind, E., Schwartz, M.W., Schellenberg, G.D., Raskind, M. and Porte, D., Jr. (1998) Cerebrospinal fluid and plasma insulin levels in Alzheimer's disease: relationship to severity of dementia and apolipoprotein E genotype. *Neurology*, 50, 164-168.

Cranston, I., Marsden, P., Matyka, K., Evans, M., Lomas, J., Sonksen, P., Maisey, M. and Amiel, S.A. (1998) Regional differences in cerebral blood flow and glucose utilization in diabetic man: the effect of insulin. *J Cereb Blood Flow Metab*, 18, 130-140.

Cuschieri, J., Bulger, E., Grinsell, R., Garcia, I. and Maier, R.V. (2008) Insulin regulates macrophage activation through activin A. *Shock*, 29, 285-290.

Dallaporta, M., Pecchi, E., Pio, J., Jean, A., Horner, K.C. and Troadec, J.D. (2009) Expression of leptin receptor by glial cells of the nucleus tractus solitarius: possible involvement in energy homeostasis. *J Neuroendocrinol*, 21, 57-67.

Dandona, P., Aljada, A., Mohanty, P., Ghanim, H., Hamouda, W., Assian, E. and Ahmad, S. (2001) Insulin inhibits intranuclear nuclear factor kappaB and stimulates IkappaB in mononuclear cells in obese subjects: evidence for an anti-inflammatory effect? *J Clin Endocrinol Metab*, 86, 3257-3265.

Dandona, P., Chaudhuri, A., Ghanim, H. and Mohanty, P. (2007a) Proinflammatory effects of glucose and anti-inflammatory effect of insulin: relevance to cardiovascular disease. *Am J Cardiol*, 99, 15B-26B.

Dandona, P., Chaudhuri, A., Mohanty, P. and Ghanim, H. (2007b) Anti-inflammatory effects of insulin. *Curr Opin Clin Nutr Metab Care*, 10, 511-517.

Daneman, D., Zinman, B., Elliott, M.E., Bilan, P.J. and Klip, A. (1992) Insulin-stimulated glucose transport in circulating mononuclear cells from nondiabetic and IDDM subjects. *Diabetes*, 41, 227-234.

de la Monte, S.M. (2012) Brain insulin resistance and deficiency as therapeutic targets in Alzheimer's disease. *Curr Alzheimer Res*, 9, 35-66.

de la Monte, S.M. and Wands, J.R. (2008) Alzheimer's disease is type 3 diabetes-evidence reviewed. *J Diabetes Sci Technol*, 2, 1101-1113.

DeFronzo, R.A. (2010) Insulin resistance, lipotoxicity, type 2 diabetes and atherosclerosis: the missing links. The Claude Bernard Lecture 2009. *Diabetologia*, 53, 1270-1287.

Duarte, A.I., Moreira, P.I. and Oliveira, C.R. (2012) Insulin in central nervous system: more than just a peripheral hormone. *J Aging Res*, 2012, 384017.

Duarte, A.I., Santos, P., Oliveira, C.R., Santos, M.S. and Rego, A.C. (2008) Insulin neuroprotection against oxidative stress is mediated by Akt and GSK-3beta signaling pathways and changes in protein expression. *Biochim Biophys Acta*, 1783, 994-1002.

Fields, R.D. and Stevens-Graham, B. (2002) New insights into neuron-glia communication. *Science*, 298, 556-562.

Fischer, A.J., McGuire, C.R., Dierks, B.D. and Reh, T.A. (2002) Insulin and fibroblast growth factor 2 activate a neurogenic program in Muller glia of the chicken retina. *J Neurosci*, 22, 9387-9398.

Fischer, A.J. and Reh, T.A. (2003) Potential of Muller glia to become neurogenic retinal progenitor cells. *Glia*, 43, 70-76.

Fischer, A.J., Scott, M.A., Ritchey, E.R. and Sherwood, P. (2009) Mitogen-activated protein kinase-signaling regulates the ability of Muller glia to proliferate and protect retinal neurons against excitotoxicity. *Glia*, 57, 1538-1552.

Fischoeder, A., Meyborg, H., Stibenz, D., Fleck, E., Graf, K. and Stawowy, P. (2007) Insulin augments matrix metalloproteinase-9 expression in monocytes. *Cardiovasc Res*, 73, 841-848.

Fishel, M.A., Watson, G.S., Montine, T.J., Wang, Q., Green, P.S., Kulstad, J.J., Cook, D.G., Peskind, E.R., Baker, L.D., Goldgaber, D., Nie, W., Asthana, S., Plymate, S.R., Schwartz, M.W. and Craft, S. (2005) Hyperinsulinemia provokes synchronous increases in central inflammation and beta-amyloid in normal adults. *Arch Neurol*, 62, 1539-1544.

Flakoll, P.J., Jensen, M.D. and Cherrington, A.D. (2004) Physiologic action of insulin. In LeRoith, D., Taylor, S.I., Olefsky, J.M. (eds) *Diabetes Mellitus: A fundamental and clinical text*. Lippincott Williams and Wilkins Pennsylvania.

Frank-Cannon, T.C., Alto, L.T., McAlpine, F.E. and Tansey, M.G. (2009) Does neuroinflammation fan the flame in neurodegenerative diseases? *Mol Neurodegener*, 4, 47.

Frasca, F., Pandini, G., Scalia, P., Sciacca, L., Mineo, R., Costantino, A., Goldfine, I.D., Belfiore, A. and Vigneri, R. (1999) Insulin receptor isoform A, a newly recognized, high-affinity insulin-like growth factor II receptor in fetal and cancer cells. *Mol Cell Biol*, 19, 3278-3288.

Fu, Y., Maianu, L., Melbert, B.R. and Garvey, W.T. (2004) Facilitative glucose transporter gene expression in human lymphocytes, monocytes, and macrophages: a role for GLUT isoforms 1, 3, and 5 in the immune response and foam cell formation. *Blood Cells Mol Dis*, 32, 182-190.

Gammeltoft, S., Fehlmann, M. and Van Obberghen, E. (1985) Insulin receptors in the mammalian central nervous system: binding characteristics and subunit structure. *Biochimie*, 67, 1147-1153.

Garcia-Segura, L.M., Chowen, J.A. and Naftolin, F. (1996) Endocrine glia: roles of glial cells in the brain actions of steroid and thyroid hormones and in the regulation of hormone secretion. *Front Neuroendocrinol*, 17, 180-211.

Garcia-Segura, L.M. and McCarthy, M.M. (2004) Minireview: Role of glia in neuroendocrine function. *Endocrinology*, 145, 1082-1086.

Garg, R., Tripathy, D. and Dandona, P. (2003) Insulin resistance as a proinflammatory state: mechanisms, mediators, and therapeutic interventions. *Curr Drug Targets*, 4, 487-492.

Geiger, P.C., Wright, D.C., Han, D.H. and Holloszy, J.O. (2005) Activation of p38 MAP kinase enhances sensitivity of muscle glucose transport to insulin. *Am J Physiol Endocrinol Metab*, 288, E782-788.

Ghezzo, F., Garbarino, G. and Ioverno, L. (1983) Insulin modulates human mononuclear adherent cell fibrinolytic and phagocytic activities. *Scand J Haematol*, 30, 379-383.

Groop, P.H., Forsblom, C. and Thomas, M.C. (2005) Mechanisms of disease: Pathway-selective insulin resistance and microvascular complications of diabetes. *Nat Clin Pract Endocrinol Metab*, 1, 100-110.

Grunberger, G., Lowe, W.L., Jr., McElduff, A. and Glick, R.P. (1986) Insulin receptor of human cerebral gliomas. Structure and function. *J Clin Invest*, 77, 997-1005.

Guillod-Maximin, E., Roy, A.F., Vacher, C.M., Aubourg, A., Bailleux, V., Lorsignol, A., Penicaud, L., Parquet, M. and Taouis, M. (2009) Adiponectin receptors are expressed in hypothalamus and colocalized with proopiomelanocortin and neuropeptide Y in rodent arcuate neurons. *J Endocrinol*, 200, 93-105.

Haddad, J.J. (2005) N-methyl-D-aspartate (NMDA) and the regulation of mitogen-activated protein kinase (MAPK) signaling pathways: a revolving neurochemical axis for therapeutic intervention? *Prog Neurobiol*, 77, 252-282.

Haj-ali, V., Mohaddes, G. and Babri, S.H. (2009) Intracerebroventricular insulin improves spatial learning and memory in male Wistar rats. *Behav Neurosci*, 123, 1309-1314.

Hallschmid, M., Benedict, C., Schultes, B., Born, J. and Kern, W. (2008) Obese men respond to cognitive but not to catabolic brain insulin signaling. *Int J Obes (Lond)*, 32, 275-282.

Hallschmid, M. and Schultes, B. (2009) Central nervous insulin resistance: a promising target in the treatment of metabolic and cognitive disorders? *Diabetologia*, 52, 2264-2269.

Han, S., Liang, C.P., DeVries-Seimon, T., Ranalletta, M., Welch, C.L., Collins-Fletcher, K., Accili, D., Tabas, I. and Tall, A.R. (2006) Macrophage insulin receptor deficiency increases ER stress-induced apoptosis and necrotic core formation in advanced atherosclerotic lesions. *Cell Metab*, 3, 257-266.

Hanisch, U.K. and Kettenmann, H. (2007) Microglia: active sensor and versatile effector cells in the normal and pathologic brain. *Nat Neurosci*, 10, 1387-1394.

Harfenist, E.J. and Craig, L.C. (1952) The molecular weight of insulin *J Am Chem Soc*, 74, 3087-3089.

Hasselbalch, S.G., Knudsen, G.M., Videbaek, C., Pinborg, L.H., Schmidt, J.F., Holm, S. and Paulson, O.B. (1999) No effect of insulin on glucose blood-brain barrier transport and cerebral metabolism in humans. *Diabetes*, 48, 1915-1921.

Helderman, J.H. (1984) Acute regulation of human lymphocyte insulin receptors. Analysis by the glucose clamp. *J Clin Invest*, 74, 1428-1435.

Heni, M., Hennige, A.M., Peter, A., Siegel-Axel, D., Ordelheide, A.M., Krebs, N., Machicao, F., Fritsche, A., Haring, H.U. and Staiger, H. (2011) Insulin promotes glycogen storage and cell proliferation in primary human astrocytes. *PLoS One*, 6, e21594.

Hetman, M., Kanning, K., Cavanaugh, J.E. and Xia, Z. (1999) Neuroprotection by brain-derived neurotrophic factor is mediated by extracellular signal-regulated kinase and phosphatidylinositol 3-kinase. *J Biol Chem*, 274, 22569-22580.

Hill, J.M., Lesniak, M.A., Pert, C.B. and Roth, J. (1986) Autoradiographic localization of insulin receptors in rat brain: prominence in olfactory and limbic areas. *Neuroscience*, 17, 1127-1138.

Hosoi, T., Okuma, Y. and Nomura, Y. (2000) Expression of leptin receptors and induction of IL-1beta transcript in glial cells. *Biochem Biophys Res Commun*, 273, 312-315.

Hoyer, S. (2003) Memory function and brain glucose metabolism. *Pharmacopsychiatry*, 36 Suppl 1, S62-67.

Hoyer, S. (2004) Glucose metabolism and insulin receptor signal transduction in Alzheimer disease. *Eur J Pharmacol*, 490, 115-125.

Huang, S. and Czech, M.P. (2007) The GLUT4 glucose transporter. *Cell Metab*, 5, 237-252.

Huang, T.J., Verkhratsky, A. and Fernyhough, P. (2005) Insulin enhances mitochondrial inner membrane potential and increases ATP levels through phosphoinositide 3-kinase in adult sensory neurons. *Mol Cell Neurosci*, 28, 42-54.

Iida, K.T., Shimano, H., Kawakami, Y., Sone, H., Toyoshima, H., Suzuki, S., Asano, T., Okuda, Y. and Yamada, N. (2001) Insulin up-regulates tumor necrosis factor-alpha production in macrophages through an extracellular-regulated kinase-dependent pathway. *J Biol Chem*, 276, 32531-32537.

Iida, K.T., Suzuki, H., Sone, H., Shimano, H., Toyoshima, H., Yatoh, S., Asano, T., Okuda, Y. and Yamada, N. (2002) Insulin inhibits apoptosis of macrophage cell line, THP-1 cells, via phosphatidylinositol-3-kinase-dependent pathway. *Arterioscler Thromb Vasc Biol*, 22, 380-386.

Iqbal, K. and Grundke-Iqbal, I. (2008) Alzheimer neurofibrillary degeneration: significance, etiopathogenesis, therapeutics and prevention. *J Cell Mol Med*, 12, 38-55.

Jacobsen, M. (1991) *Developmental neurobiology*. Plenum Press, New York.

Jeschke, M.G., Klein, D., Bolder, U. and Einspanier, R. (2004) Insulin attenuates the systemic inflammatory response in endotoxemic rats. *Endocrinology*, 145, 4084-4093.

Ji, Y.F., Xu, S.M., Zhu, J., Wang, X.X. and Shen, Y. (2011) Insulin increases glutamate transporter GLT1 in cultured astrocytes. *Biochem Biophys Res Commun*, 405, 691-696.

Johnson-Farley, N.N., Travkina, T. and Cowen, D.S. (2006) Cumulative activation of akt and consequent inhibition of glycogen synthase kinase-3 by brain-derived neurotrophic factor and insulin-like growth factor-1 in cultured hippocampal neurons. *J Pharmacol Exp Ther*, 316, 1062-1069.

Jolivalt, C.G., Lee, C.A., Beiswenger, K.K., Smith, J.L., Orlov, M., Torrance, M.A. and Masliah, E. (2008) Defective insulin signaling pathway and increased glycogen synthase kinase-3 activity in the brain of diabetic mice: parallels with Alzheimer's disease and correction by insulin. *J Neurosci Res*, 86, 3265-3274.

Kahn, C.R. (1995) Glucose homeostasis and insulin action. In Becker, K.L. (ed) *Principles and Practice of Endocrinology and Metabolism*. J.B. Lippincott, Philadelphia, pp. 1198-1202.

Kaiyala, K.J., Prigeon, R.L., Kahn, S.E., Woods, S.C. and Schwartz, M.W. (2000) Obesity induced by a high-fat diet is associated with reduced brain insulin transport in dogs. *Diabetes*, 49, 1525-1533.

Kappert, K., Meyborg, H., Clemenz, M., Graf, K., Fleck, E., Kintscher, U. and Stawowy, P. (2008) Insulin facilitates monocyte migration: a possible link to tissue inflammation in insulin-resistance. *Biochem Biophys Res Commun*, 365, 503-508.

Kern, W., Benedict, C., Schultes, B., Plohr, F., Moser, A., Born, J., Fehm, H.L. and Hallschmid, M. (2006) Low cerebrospinal fluid insulin levels in obese humans. *Diabetologia*, 49, 2790-2792.

Kern, W., Peters, A., Fruehwald-Schultes, B., Deininger, E., Born, J. and Fehm, H.L. (2001) Improving influence of insulin on cognitive functions in humans. *Neuroendocrinology*, 74, 270-280.

Kettenmann, H. and Ransom, B.R. (2005) *Neuroglia*. Oxford University Press, New York

Kettenmann, H. and Verkhratsky, A. (2011) [Neuroglia--living nerve glue]. *Fortschr Neurol Psychiatr*, 79, 588-597.

Krause, D.L. and Muller, N. (2010) Neuroinflammation, microglia and implications for anti-inflammatory treatment in Alzheimer's disease. *Int J Alzheimers Dis*, 2010, 732806.

Kurosinski, P. and Gotz, J. (2002) Glial cells under physiologic and pathologic conditions. *Arch Neurol*, 59, 1524-1528.

Lalo, U., Pankratov, Y., Kirchhoff, F., North, R.A. and Verkhratsky, A. (2006) NMDA receptors mediate neuron-to-glia signaling in mouse cortical astrocytes. *J Neurosci*, 26, 2673-2683.

Laron, Z. (2009) Insulin and the brain. *Arch Physiol Biochem*, 115, 112-116.

Laroux, F.S. (2004) Mechanisms of inflammation: the good, the bad and the ugly. *Front Biosci*, 9, 3156-3162.

Lawson, L.J., Perry, V.H., Dri, P. and Gordon, S. (1990) Heterogeneity in the distribution and morphology of microglia in the normal adult mouse brain. *Neuroscience*, 39, 151-170.

Lawson, L.J., Perry, V.H. and Gordon, S. (1992) Turnover of resident microglia in the normal adult mouse brain. *Neuroscience*, 48, 405-415.

Lee, J. and Pilch, P.F. (1994) The insulin receptor: structure, function, and signaling *Am J Physiol*, 266, C319-C334.

Levinthal, D.J. and DeFranco, D.B. (2004) Transient phosphatidylinositol 3-kinase inhibition protects immature primary cortical neurons from oxidative toxicity via suppression of extracellular signal-regulated kinase activation. *J Biol Chem*, 279, 11206-11213.

Liang, C.P., Han, S., Okamoto, H., Carnemolla, R., Tabas, I., Accili, D. and Tall, A.R. (2004) Increased CD36 protein as a response to defective insulin signaling in macrophages. *J Clin Invest*, 113, 764-773.

Liao, G.Y. and Leonard, J.P. (1999) Insulin modulation of cloned mouse NMDA receptor currents in Xenopus oocytes. *J Neurochem*, 73, 1510-1519.

Liu, Y., Liu, F., Grundke-Iqbal, I., Iqbal, K. and Gong, C.X. (2011) Deficient brain insulin signalling pathway in Alzheimer's disease and diabetes. *J Pathol*, 225, 54-62.

Lowe, W.L., Jr., Boyd, F.T., Clarke, D.W., Raizada, M.K., Hart, C. and LeRoith, D. (1986) Development of brain insulin receptors: structural and functional studies of insulin receptors from whole brain and primary cell cultures. *Endocrinology*, 119, 25-35.

Lu, F.P., Lin, K.P. and Kuo, H.K. (2009) Diabetes and the risk of multi-system aging phenotypes: a systematic review and meta-analysis. *PLoS One*, 4, e4144.

Lucignani, G., Namba, H., Nehlig, A., Porrino, L.J., Kennedy, C. and Sokoloff, L. (1987) Effects of insulin on local cerebral glucose utilization in the rat. *J Cereb Blood Flow Metab*, 7, 309-314.

Ma, X.H., Zhong, P., Gu, Z., Feng, J. and Yan, Z. (2003) Muscarinic potentiation of GABA(A) receptor currents is gated by insulin signaling in the prefrontal cortex. *J Neurosci*, 23, 1159-1168.

Malide, D., Davies-Hill, T.M., Levine, M. and Simpson, I.A. (1998) Distinct localization of GLUT-1, -3, and -5 in human monocyte-derived macrophages: effects of cell activation. *Am J Physiol*, 274, E516-526.

Mandrekar-Colucci, S. and Landreth, G.E. (2010) Microglia and inflammation in Alzheimer's disease. *CNS Neurol Disord Drug Targets*, 9, 156-167.

Manning, B.D. and Cantley, L.C. (2007) AKT/PKB signaling: navigating downstream. *Cell*, 129, 1261-1274.

Margolis, R.U. and Altszuler, N. (1967) Insulin in the cerebrospinal fluid. *Nature*, 215, 1375-1376.

McCall, A.L. (2004) Cerebral glucose metabolism in diabetes mellitus. *Eur J Pharmacol*, 490, 147-158.

Mercier, G., Turque, N. and Schumacher, M. (2001) Rapid effects of triiodothyronine on immediate-early gene expression in Schwann cells. *Glia*, 35, 81-89.

Micevych, P., Bondar, G. and Kuo, J. (2010) Estrogen actions on neuroendocrine glia. *Neuroendocrinology*, 91, 211-222.

Miller, D.W., Keller, B.T. and Borchardt, R.T. (1994) Identification and distribution of insulin receptors on cultured bovine brain microvessel endothelial cells: possible function in insulin processing in the blood-brain barrier. *J Cell Physiol*, 161, 333-341.

Miyata, S. and Hatton, G.I. (2002) Activity-related, dynamic neuron-glial interactions in the hypothalamo-neurohypophysial system. *Microsc Res Tech*, 56, 143-157.

Mohacsik, P., Zeold, A., Bianco, A.C. and Gereben, B. (2011) Thyroid hormone and the neuroglia: both source and target. *J Thyroid Res*, 2011, 215718.

Montiel, F., Ortiz-Caro, J., Villa, A., Pascual, A. and Aranda, A. (1989) Presence of insulin receptors in cultured glial C6 cells. Regulation by butyrate. *Biochem J*, 258, 147-155.

Moore, K.J. and Tabas, I. (2011) Macrophages in the pathogenesis of atherosclerosis. *Cell*, 145, 341-355.

Morton, G.J., Cummings, D.E., Baskin, D.G., Barsh, G.S. and Schwartz, M.W. (2006) Central nervous system control of food intake and body weight. *Nature*, 443, 289-295.

Nagamatsu, S., Kornhauser, J.M., Burant, C.F., Seino, S., Mayo, K.E. and Bell, G.I. (1992) Glucose transporter expression in brain. cDNA sequence of mouse GLUT3, the brain facilitative glucose transporter isoform, and identification of sites of expression by in situ hybridization. *J Biol Chem*, 267, 467-472.

Nakazawa, K., Sun, L.D., Quirk, M.C., Rondi-Reig, L., Wilson, M.A. and Tonegawa, S. (2003) Hippocampal CA3 NMDA receptors are crucial for memory acquisition of one-time experience. *Neuron*, 38, 305-315.

Napoli, I. and Neumann, H. (2009) Microglial clearance function in health and disease. *Neuroscience*, 158, 1030-1038.

Ndubaku, U. and de Bellard, M.E. (2008) Glial cells: old cells with new twists. *Acta Histochem*, 110, 182-195.

Neumann, K.F., Rojo, L., Navarrete, L.P., Farias, G., Reyes, P. and Maccioni, R.B. (2008) Insulin resistance and Alzheimer's disease: molecular links and clinical implications. *Curr Alzheimer Res*, 5, 438-447.

Newcomer, J.W. and Krystal, J.H. (2001) NMDA receptor regulation of memory and behavior in humans. *Hippocampus*, 11, 529-542.

Nystrom, F.H. and Quon, M.J. (1999) Insulin signalling: metabolic pathways and mechanisms for specificity. *Cell Signal*, 11, 563-574.

Obici, S., Zhang, B.B., Karkanias, G. and Rossetti, L. (2002) Hypothalamic insulin signaling is required for inhibition of glucose production. *Nat Med*, 8, 1376-1382.

Ola, M.S., Hosoya, K. and LaNoue, K.F. (2011) Influence of insulin on glutamine synthetase in the Muller glial cells of retina. *Metab Brain Dis*, 26, 195-202.

Ono, H., Pocai, A., Wang, Y., Sakoda, H., Asano, T., Backer, J.M., Schwartz, G.J. and Rossetti, L. (2008) Activation of hypothalamic S6 kinase mediates diet-induced hepatic insulin resistance in rats. *J Clin Invest*, 118, 2959-2968.

Ottlecz, A., Gecse, A., Koltai, M. and West, G.B. (1977) Involvement of the kinin system in the insulin-induced inhibition of carrageenin oedema in rats. *Monogr Allergy*, 12, 131-137.

Oz, G., Henry, P.G., Seaquist, E.R. and Gruetter, R. (2003) Direct, noninvasive measurement of brain glycogen metabolism in humans. *Neurochem Int*, 43, 323-329.

Pais, T.F., Figueiredo, C., Peixoto, R., Braz, M.H. and Chatterjee, S. (2008) Necrotic neurons enhance microglial neurotoxicity through induction of glutaminase by a MyD88-dependent pathway. *J Neuroinflam*, 5, 43.

Pansuria, M., Xi, H., Li, L., Yang, X.F. and Wang, H. (2012) Insulin resistance, metabolic stress, and atherosclerosis. *Front Biosci (Schol Ed)*, 4, 916-931.

Park, C.R., Seeley, R.J., Craft, S. and Woods, S.C. (2000) Intracerebroventricular insulin enhances memory in a passive-avoidance task. *Physiol Behav*, 68, 509-514.

Parpura, V., Heneka, M.T., Montana, V., Oliet, S.H., Schousboe, A., Haydon, P.G., Stout, R.F., Jr., Spray, D.C., Reichenbach, A., Pannicke, T., Pekny, M., Pekna, M., Zorec, R. and Verkhratsky, A. (2012) Glial cells in (patho)physiology. *J Neurochem*, 121, 4-27.

Pereira, B., Rosa, L.F., Safi, D.A., Bechara, E.J. and Curi, R. (1995) Hormonal regulation of superoxide dismutase, catalase, and glutathione peroxidase activities in rat macrophages. *Biochem Pharmacol*, 50, 2093-2098.

Pocai, A., Lam, T.K., Gutierrez-Juarez, R., Obici, S., Schwartz, G.J., Bryan, J., Aguilar-Bryan, L. and Rossetti, L. (2005) Hypothalamic K(ATP) channels control hepatic glucose production. *Nature*, 434, 1026-1031.

Polazzi, E. and Monti, B. (2010) Microglia and neuroprotection: from in vitro studies to therapeutic applications. *Prog Neurobiol*, 92, 293-315.

Porte, D., Jr., Seeley, R.J., Woods, S.C., Baskin, D.G., Figlewicz, D.P. and Schwartz, M.W. (1998) Obesity, diabetes and the central nervous system. *Diabetologia*, 41, 863-881.

Profenno, L.A., Porsteinsson, A.P. and Faraone, S.V. (2010) Meta-analysis of Alzheimer's disease risk with obesity, diabetes, and related disorders. *Biol Psychiatry*, 67, 505-512.

Purves, T., Middlemas, A., Agthong, S., Jude, E.B., Boulton, A.J., Fernyhough, P. and Tomlinson, D.R. (2001) A role for mitogen-activated protein kinases in the etiology of diabetic neuropathy. *FASEB J*, 15, 2508-2514.

Raizada, M.K., Shemer, J., Judkins, J.H., Clarke, D.W., Masters, B.A. and LeRoith, D. (1988) Insulin receptors in the brain: structural and physiological characterization. *Neurochem Res*, 13, 297-303.

Rajkowska, G. and Miguel-Hidalgo, J.J. (2007) Gliogenesis and glial pathology in depression. *CNS Neurol Disord Drug Targets*, 6, 219-233.

Ransom, B.R. and Ransom, C.B. (2012) Astrocytes: multitalented stars of the central nervous system. *Methods Mol Biol*, 814, 3-7.

Rayner, D.V., Thomas, M.E. and Trayhurn, P. (1994) Glucose transporters (GLUTs 1-4) and their mRNAs in regions of the rat brain: insulin-sensitive transporter expression in the cerebellum. *Can J Physiol Pharmacol*, 72, 476-479.

Reger, M.A., Watson, G.S., Green, P.S., Wilkinson, C.W., Baker, L.D., Cholerton, B., Fishel, M.A., Plymate, S.R., Breitner, J.C., DeGroodt, W., Mehta, P. and Craft, S. (2008) Intranasal insulin improves cognition and modulates beta-amyloid in early AD. *Neurology*, 70, 440-448.

Rensing, K.L., Reuwer, A.Q., Arsenault, B.J., von der Thusen, J.H., Hoekstra, J.B., Kastelein, J.J. and Twickler, T.B. (2011) Reducing cardiovascular disease risk in patients with type 2 diabetes and concomitant macrovascular disease: can insulin be too much of a good thing? *Diabetes Obes Metab*, 13, 1073-1087.

Rodriguez-Pena, A. (1999) Oligodendrocyte development and thyroid hormone. *J Neurobiol*, 40, 497-512.

Ronnemaa, E., Zethelius, B., Sundelof, J., Sundstrom, J., Degerman-Gunnarsson, M., Berne, C., Lannfelt, L. and Kilander, L. (2008) Impaired insulin secretion increases the risk of Alzheimer disease. *Neurology*, 71, 1065-1071.

Rosa, L.F., Cury, Y. and Curi, R. (1992) Effects of insulin, glucocorticoids and thyroid hormones on the activities of key enzymes of glycolysis, glutaminolysis, the pentose-phosphate pathway and the Krebs cycle in rat macrophages. *J Endocrinol*, 135, 213-219.

Sakaue, S., Nishihira, J., Hirokawa, J., Yoshimura, H., Honda, T., Aoki, K., Tagami, S. and Kawakami, Y. (1999) Regulation of macrophage migration inhibitory factor (MIF) expression by glucose and insulin in adipocytes in vitro. *Mol Med*, 5, 361-371.

Saltiel, A.R. and Kahn, C.R. (2001) Insulin signalling and the regulation of glucose and lipid metabolism. *Nature*, 414, 799-806.

San Jose, G., Bidegain, J., Robador, P.A., Diez, J., Fortuno, A. and Zalba, G. (2009) Insulin-induced NADPH oxidase activation promotes proliferation and matrix metalloproteinase activation in monocytes/macrophages. *Free Radic Biol Med*, 46, 1058-1067.

Satomi, N., Sakurai, A. and Haranaka, K. (1985) Relationship of hypoglycemia to tumor necrosis factor production and antitumor activity: role of glucose, insulin, and macrophages. *J Natl Cancer Inst*, 74, 1255-1260.

Schechter, R., Beju, D., Gaffney, T., Schaefer, F. and Whetsell, L. (1996) Preproinsulin I and II mRNAs and insulin electron microscopic immunoreaction are present within the rat fetal nervous system. *Brain Res*, 736, 16-27.

Schechter, R., Whitmire, J., Holtzclaw, L., George, M., Harlow, R. and Devaskar, S.U. (1992) Developmental regulation of insulin in the mammalian central nervous system. *Brain Res*, 582, 27-37.

Schulingkamp, R.J., Pagano, T.C., Hung, D. and Raffa, R.B. (2000) Insulin receptors and insulin action in the brain: review and clinical implications. *Neurosci Biobehav Rev*, 24, 855-872.

Schwartz, M.W., Sipols, A., Kahn, S.E., Lattemann, D.F., Taborsky, G.J., Jr., Bergman, R.N., Woods, S.C. and Porte, D., Jr. (1990) Kinetics and specificity of insulin uptake from plasma into cerebrospinal fluid. *Am J Physiol*, 259, E378-383.

Seaquist, E.R., Damberg, G.S., Tkac, I. and Gruetter, R. (2001) The effect of insulin on in vivo cerebral glucose concentrations and rates of glucose transport/metabolism in humans. *Diabetes*, 50, 2203-2209.

Seino, S. and Bell, G.I. (1989) Alternative splicing of human insulin receptor messenger RNA. *Biochem Biophys Res Commun*, 159, 312-316.

Shepherd, P.R., Withers, D.J. and Siddle, K. (1998) Phosphoinositide 3-kinase: the key switch mechanism in insulin signalling. *Biochem J*, 333 (Pt 3), 471-490.

Skeberdis, V.A., Lan, J., Zheng, X., Zukin, R.S. and Bennett, M.V. (2001) Insulin promotes rapid delivery of N-methyl-D- aspartate receptors to the cell surface by exocytosis. *Proc Natl Acad Sci USA*, 98, 3561-3566.

Skolnik, E.Y., Batzer, A., Li, N., Lee, C.H., Lowenstein, E., Mohammadi, M., Margolis, B. and Schlessinger, J. (1993) The function of GRB2 in linking the insulin receptor to Ras signaling pathways. *Science*, 260, 1953-1955.

Smith, J.A., Das, A., Ray, S.K. and Banik, N.L. (2012) Role of pro-inflammatory cytokines released from microglia in neurodegenerative diseases. *Brain Res Bull*, 87, 10-20.

Steele, M.L. and Robinson, S.R. (2012) Reactive astrocytes give neurons less support: implications for Alzheimer's disease. *Neurobiol Aging*, 33, 423 e421-413.

Stein, L.J., Dorsa, D.M., Baskin, D.G., Figlewicz, D.P., Porte, D., Jr. and Woods, S.C. (1987) Reduced effect of experimental peripheral hyperinsulinemia to elevate cerebrospinal fluid insulin concentrations of obese Zucker rats. *Endocrinology*, 121, 1611-1615.

Stentz, F.B. and Kitabchi, A.E. (2004) De novo emergence of growth factor receptors in activated human CD4+ and CD8+ T lymphocytes. *Metabolism*, 53, 117-122.

Su, C., Cunningham, R.L., Rybalchenko, N. and Singh, M. (2012) Progesterone Increases the Release of Brain-Derived Neurotrophic Factor from Glia via Progesterone Receptor Membrane Component 1 (Pgrmc1)-Dependent ERK5 Signaling. *Endocrinology*, 153, 4389-4400.

Takahashi, K., Takeya, M. and Sakashita, N. (2002) Multifunctional roles of macrophages in the development and progression of atherosclerosis in humans and experimental animals. *Med Electron Microsc*, 35, 179-203.

Tambuyzer, B.R., Ponsaerts, P. and Nouwen, E.J. (2009) Microglia: gatekeepers of central nervous system immunology. *J Leukoc Biol*, 85, 352-370.

Theodosis, D.T. (2002) Oxytocin-secreting neurons: A physiological model of morphological neuronal and glial plasticity in the adult hypothalamus. *Front Neuroendocrinol*, 23, 101-135.

Toran-Allerand, C.D., Bentham, W., Miranda, R.C. and Anderson, J.P. (1991) Insulin influences astroglial morphology and glial fibrillary acidic protein (GFAP) expression in organotypic cultures. *Brain Res*, 558, 296-304.

Tremblay, M.E., Stevens, B., Sierra, A., Wake, H., Bessis, A. and Nimmerjahn, A. (2011) The role of microglia in the healthy brain. *J Neurosci*, 31, 16064-16069.

Unger, J.W., Livingston, J.N. and Moss, A.M. (1991a) Insulin receptors in the central nervous system: localization, signalling mechanisms and functional aspects. *Prog Neurobiol*, 36, 343-362.

Unger, J.W., Moss, A.M. and Livingston, J.N. (1991b) Immunohistochemical localization of insulin receptors and phosphotyrosine in the brainstem of the adult rat. *Neuroscience*, 42, 853-861.

van Houten, M., Posner, B.I., Kopriwa, B.M. and Brawer, J.R. (1979) Insulin-binding sites in the rat brain: in vivo localization to the circumventricular organs by quantitative radioautography. *Endocrinology*, 105, 666-673.

Vannucci, S.J., Koehler-Stec, E.M., Li, K., Reynolds, T.H., Clark, R. and Simpson, I.A. (1998) GLUT4 glucose transporter expression in rodent brain: effect of diabetes. *Brain Res*, 797, 1-11.

Velez-Fort, M., Audinat, E. and Angulo, M.C. (2012) Central role of GABA in neuron-glia interactions. *Neuroscientist*, 18, 237-250.

Verkhratsky, A. and Kirchhoff, F. (2007) NMDA Receptors in glia. *Neuroscientist*, 13, 28-37.

Wallum, B.J., Taborsky, G.J., Jr., Porte, D., Jr., Figlewicz, D.P., Jacobson, L., Beard, J.C., Ward, W.K. and Dorsa, D. (1987) Cerebrospinal fluid insulin levels increase during intravenous insulin infusions in man. *J Clin Endocrinol Metab*, 64, 190-194.

Wan, Q., Xiong, Z.G., Man, H.Y., Ackerley, C.A., Braunton, J., Lu, W.Y., Becker, L.E., MacDonald, J.F. and Wang, Y.T. (1997) Recruitment of functional GABA(A) receptors to postsynaptic domains by insulin. *Nature*, 388, 686-690.

Welham, M.J., Bone, H., Levings, M., Learmonth, L., Wang, L.M., Leslie, K.B., Pierce, J.H. and Schrader, J.W. (1997) Insulin receptor substrate-2 is the major 170-kDa protein phosphorylated on tyrosine in response to cytokines in murine lymphohemopoietic cells. *J Biol Chem*, 272, 1377-1381.

Welsh, G.I., Hers, I., Berwick, D.C., Dell, G., Wherlock, M., Birkin, R., Leney, S. and Tavare, J.M. (2005) Role of protein kinase B in insulin-regulated glucose uptake. *Biochem Soc Trans*, 33, 346-349.

Werner, H., Raizada, M.K., Mudd, L.M., Foyt, H.L., Simpson, I.A., Roberts, C.T., Jr. and LeRoith, D. (1989) Regulation of rat brain/HepG2 glucose transporter gene expression by insulin and insulin-like growth factor-I in primary cultures of neuronal and glial cells. *Endocrinology*, 125, 314-320.

Weyhenmeyer, J.A. (1984) Localization of insulin receptors in primary cultures of fetal rat brain by immunocytochemistry. *Monogr Neural Sci*, 10, 140-157.

White, M.F. (2002) IRS proteins and the common path to diabetes. *Am J Physiol Endocrinol Metab*, 283, E413-422.

Woods, S.C., Lotter, E.C., McKay, L.D. and Porte, D., Jr. (1979) Chronic intracerebroventricular infusion of insulin reduces food intake and body weight of baboons. *Nature*, 282, 503-505.

Woods, S.C. and Seeley, R.J. (2001) Insulin as an adiposity signal. *Int J Obes Relat Metab Disord*, 25 Suppl 5, S35-38.

Wozniak, M., Rydzewski, B., Baker, S.P. and Raizada, M.K. (1993) The cellular and physiological actions of insulin in the central nervous system. *Neurochem Int*, 22, 1-10.

Wurm, S., Neumeier, M., Weigert, J., Wanninger, J., Gerl, M., Gindner, A., Schaffler, A., Aslanidis, C., Scholmerich, J. and Buechler, C. (2008) Insulin induces monocytic CXCL8 secretion by the mitogenic signalling pathway. *Cytokine*, 44, 185-190.

Yamashita, M., Tamasawa, N., Matsuki, K., Tanabe, J., Murakami, H., Matsui, J. and Suda, T. (2010) Insulin suppresses HDL-mediated cholesterol efflux from macrophages through inhibition of neutral cholesteryl ester hydrolase and ATP-binding cassette transporter G1 expressions. *J Atheroscler Thromb*, 17, 1183-1189.

Yoon, S. and Seger, R. (2006) The extracellular signal-regulated kinase: multiple substrates regulate diverse cellular functions. *Growth Factors*, 24, 21-44.

Yu, X.R., Jia, G.R., Gao, G.D., Wang, S.H., Han, Y. and Cao, W. (2006) Neuroprotection of insulin against oxidative stress-induced apoptosis in cultured retinal neurons: involvement of phosphoinositide 3-kinase/Akt signal pathway. *Acta Biochim Biophys Sin (Shanghai)*, 38, 241-248.

Zeng, G. and Quon, M.J. (1996) Insulin-stimulated production of nitric oxide is inhibited by wortmannin. Direct measurement in vascular endothelial cells. *J Clin Invest*, 98, 894-898.

In: Glial Cells
Editors: Charanjit Kaur and Eng-Ang Ling
ISBN: 978-1-62618-448-0
© 2013 Nova Science Publishers, Inc.

Chapter 7

GLIAL CELL INVOLVEMENT IN OSTEOARTHRITIC PAIN

***Frank B. Wydra*[1,2]*, Bryan M. Saltzman*[2]*, Kasra Ahmadinia*[2]*, Jae-Sung Kim*[1] *and Hee-Jeong Im*[1,2,3*]**

[1]Department of Biochemistry,
[2]Department of Orthopedic Surgery,
[3]Department of Internal Medicine (Rheumatology)
Rush University Medical Center, Chicago, IL, US

ABSTRACT

The pathological process of joint degeneration due to osteoarthritis (OA) is well defined in literature today. However, the mechanism in which this destruction correlates to pain production is still under investigation. While the articular cartilage itself is non-innervated, inflammatory and neuropathic pain pathways have been described to be responsible for the pain produced in OA. Another concept called central sensitization has been described to be accountable for the exaggerated amount of pain produced from OA. This central process involves activation of glial cells in the dorsal root ganglion and spinal cord by the affected joint. Activated glial cells increase pro-inflammatory cytokine production as well as excitatory cytokine production. These cytokines lead to depolarization of N-Methyl-D-aspartate (NMDA) receptors in the dorsal horn of the spinal cord contributing to enhancement of pain signaling.

This chapter will describe the background and proposed mechanisms of central sensitization in OA pain pathways and how they differ from neuropathic pain pathways. We will explore current research of the key glial cells, mainly astrocytes and microglia, contributing to central sensitization as well as the cytokines involved in the process. Discussion of therapeutic targets in regards to central processes of pain in OA will be a valuable contributing factor. Lastly, we will propose direction for future research to advance the understanding of pain in OA.

1. Introduction

Osteoarthritis (OA) is one of the most common conditions affecting the aging population and is the largest cause of regional pain in older individuals [1-2]. The pathological process of joint degeneration due to OA is well defined in literature today [3].

However, the mechanism by which this destruction correlates to pain production is still under investigation. The characteristic pain pathway, identified as the nociceptor pathway, is a conduit of nerve fibers relaying action potentials from a peripheral joint to the brain. Acute injuries convey pain signals via this nociceptor pathway. However, in chronic pain states such as OA, inflammation of peripheral tissue can also generate pain via the nociceptive pathway.

Traditionally, pain in OA was described by degeneration of the joint leading to production of various inflammatory cytokines and neuropeptides within the joint [4]. This biochemical reaction activates nociceptors from the peripheral joint and transmits pain signals along afferent nerve fibers to their first relay in the dorsal root ganglion (DRG). From there, the action potential travels along axons and is eventually perceived by the cortex [5]. More recent literature has identified nerve injury, or neuropathic pain, as a contributing factor to the pain perceived in OA [6-7].

However, neither the degree of damage to the joint nor radiographic evidence of OA fully correlates with the amount of pain perceived by the patient [1, 8-9].

Adding to the complexity of the disease, the articular cartilage, which is the primary location of pathology, does not contain nociceptors [10]. Recent investigation has revealed that there are other cells, which may contribute to the pain perceived in OA. Glial cells, mainly microglia and astrocytes, are those cells, which have been implicated in participating in the OA pain pathway [11-12].

2. Glial Cells

Glial cells, or neuroglia, are found in the central nervous system (CNS) and outnumber neurons 10:1. They serve many important functions that are well-documented, among which are regulation of the CNS ionic environment, guidance of growing axonal development, neurotransmitter reuptake from neuronal synapses, and immune surveillance of the CNS [13]. Understanding the neural-glial relationship has only recently evolved to include the notion that glial cells are active modifiers of the neural circuits that mediate chronic pain states, particularly in the pathological condition of OA. Glial cells themselves do not transmit pain signals, as they do not have axons, yet they have been demonstrated to participate in an important mechanism within the dorsal root ganglia (DRG) as well as the dorsal horn of the spinal cord [14-15]. They modify nociceptive transmission and central sensitization after activation from peripheral nerve or tissue injury [16]. They do so via upregulation of mitogen-activated protein kinases (MAPKs), pro-inflammatory cytokines, and pro-inflammatory chemokines [17]. MAPKs specific to this glial mechanism of chronic pain maintenance include extracellular signal-regulated kinases (ERKs), c-Jun N-terminal kinases (JNK), and p38 MAPK [18-19]. The pro-inflammatory cytokines involved include interleukin (IL) -1β, IL-6, IL-18, and tumor necrosis factor (TNF)-α [20]. The chemokine C-C motif ligand (CCL) 2 is also well established in the literature for its part in this chronic pain pathway [21]. The two types of glial cells – microglia and astrocytes – are primarily responsible for the aforementioned involvement in chronic pain states and herein are discussed.

3. Experimental OA Pain Models

Before discussing glial involvement, it is prudent to discuss experimental designs used to research the pathogenesis of OA pain. Much of the literature on OA pain utilizes experimental animal models due to the difficulty of assessing the pathological process in living human subjects. Here we describe three distinctive knee joint OA animal models including intraarticular injection of monosodium iodoacetate (MIA), destabilization of the medial meniscus (DMM), and anterior cruciate ligament transection (ACLT). Additionally, we also depict three experimental back pain animal models including MIA-induced degeneration of the facet joint, facet joint compression, and disc puncture.

3.1. Knee Joint OA Models

3.1.1. Degeneration with Intraarticular Injection of MIA

MIA is an inhibitor of glycolysis that disrupts metabolism of chondrocytes, and when injected into rat joints it has the ability to mimic OA of human joints [22]. Rats injected with the MIA developed allodynia (pain perceived from a typically non-noxious stimulus) in the affected joints. It was also noted that the rats in this experimental model tended to shift their weight-bearing to undamaged joints similar to that seen with human OA subjects. Histologically, pathological changes in joint structure and cartilage damage were also similar to that observed in human OA specimens [22, 23]. The intraarticular injection of MIA model has helped to develop a further understanding of glial involvement in OA pain.

Previously, studies have identified ionized calcium binding adaptor molecule 1 (Iba1) as a protein upregulated in microglial cells when activated in response to inflammation. With immunohistologic staining, ipsilateral spinal cords of rat joints treated with MIA showed a significant increase in Iba1 expression indicating an activation of glial cells in response to MIA. Immunofluorescence and quantitative real-time polymerase chain reaction (PCR) have also been utilized to detect glial fibrillary acidic protein (GFAP), an astrocyte marker in neural tissue. A significant elevation of GFAP was seen in the ipsilateral DRG of rats treated with MIA and levels directly correlated with increased distal allodynia. Minocycline and nimesulide, inhibitors of glial cell activation, when administered showed a significant reduction of allodynia as well as decreased expression of Iba1 and GFAP [24].

A recent study noticed an increase of calcitonin gene-related peptide (CGRP), an indicator of inflammation, within the ipsilateral DRG of rats injected with MIA in a peripheral joint. This same study showed there was an increase in activating transcription factor-3 (ATF3) and growth associated protein-43 (GAP43), indicators of neuronal damage within the DRG [25]. Together, this suggests that both inflammatory and neuropathic pain contribute to pain perceived in OA. Additionally, the study showed an elevation in the number of glial cells in the DRG after injection of MIA indicating that glial cells are recruited to the DRG of an OA joint [25]. Collectively, recent research indicates that MIA successfully reproduces OA changes at both the functional and cellular levels, and that glial cells may be involved in the pathological process of OA.

3.1.2. Destabilization of the Medial Meniscus (DMM)

The DMM model is another in vivo mechanism of OA generation that utilizes the concept that surgical instability - via meniscal or ligamentous damage - provides the framework for OA development through alterations in the normal joint mechanics. As with the MIA model, its use in induction of OA in rat species has proven to be easily reproducible with an adequately slow progression of OA pathological changes. The DMM model relies on the native meniscus' role in dissipating transmitted load from the knee articular surface and providing stability to the knee joint. The mechanism for this model involves surgical sectioning of the medial meniscotibial ligament, with consequent medial displacement of the medial meniscus. Subsequently there is a focus of weight-bearing forces across a newly smaller area of contact between articulating structures than there was previously with the intact meniscus. Ultimately this causes an enhanced mechanical stress on the posteromedial femoral condyle and central tibial plateau during knee flexion of the mouse while weight-bearing, and thus a slow progression to a moderate level of OA at the joint in several weeks time. Notably, this characteristically slow progression to the final disease state in the DMM model is unique in allowing the study of OA at different stages of the disease [26].

As a result of the DMM model of OA pathogenesis, objective changes in joint laxity and bone/cartilage consistency are demonstrated. With regards to laxity of the knee joint after DMM surgery, a statistically significant increase in tibial translation anteriorly is observed, as is the total anterior-posterior range of motion at the tibia. There is significantly lower bone volume fraction of the medial epiphysis of the DMM leg as compared to the contralateral medial epiphysis. Significant cartilage loss was also observed on the medial plateau of the DMM leg when compared to the normal contralateral limb. These changes demonstrate the relationship between joint mechanics and the specific location of OA pathogenesis in the DMM model, and hence its overall utility in studying OA [27].

The fact that mechanical allodynia observed in rat subjects after DMM does not develop in ADAMTS-5 (A Disintegrin and Metalloproteinase with Thrombospondin Motif) knockout mice indicates the importance of this aggrecanase in the development of OA-like joint pathology. Cells from affected tissues in the DMM OA model exhibit increased ADAMTS-4/5 activity, which leads to perineuronal hyalectan proteolysis. The fragments from the ADAMTS-5 catabolic activity (specifically aggrecan, versican, and brevican) activate neurons and glial cells in the DRG and thereby contribute to pain development in this OA model [28].

3.1.3. Anterior Cruciate Ligament Transection (ACLT)

ACL transection is a second in vivo mechanism of OA generation that utilizes surgical instability to cause an OA state due to alterations in the normal joint mechanics. This model is favorable in that it has use in many animal species, including rodents. In this model, surgical induction of knee joint instability is performed by first dislocating the patella medially to allow improved exposure of the femoral-tibial joint so that the ACL may then be transected under direct visualization. Positive anterior drawer test indicates complete transection because of the role that the native ACL plays in preventing anterior translation of the tibia along the femur. A more severe form of OA occurs in the central weight-bearing knee region in this experimental model as compared to the DMM model above. From this model, the posterior tibial plateau is destroyed in some test subjects to the depth of the growth plate, and thus prominent neochondrogenesis, proteoglycan deposition, blood cells, and even bone marrow are evident within the joint. A noted limitation to this model is the degree of difficulty required in the surgery itself, which is reportedly high due to the risk of iatrogenic damage to surrounding structures within the joint [26].

Additionally, recent research with rats that had undergone the ACLT model of OA pathogenesis demonstrated that peptide antagonists of bradykinin receptor B1 (BKB1) slow or stabilize the induction of OA at the joint, and improve hind limb nociceptive tolerance in the animal subjects. Thus, there is evidence that bradykinin - a pro-inflammatory vasodilatory factor - is involved in the generation of pain from the ACLT model [29].

3.2. Back Pain OA Models

3.2.1. Lumbar Facet Joint Degeneration with MIA

Similar to that of the knee, intraarticular injection of MIA into the facet joints of adult Sprague Dewey rats has been used. This model causes a slow structural destruction of the facet joint and produces sufficient pain responses - including hyperalgesia, increased sensitivity to regional mechanical stimuli, and the development of chronic pain - to characterize an OA-like state. The structural alterations include degradation of cartilage, proteoglycan loss, subchondral bone remodeling, and formation of osteophytes at the facet joint. Microbiologically, the MIA injection stimulates immune cell recruitment into the facet joint, indicating a partial role for inflammatory components in the chronic pain resulting from OA in the lower back. However, it is thought that the chronic lower back pain associated with facet joint arthrosis in this model is a predominantly neuropathic process as opposed to an inflammatory process. This is because there is significant pain relief with administration of morphine as well as pregabalin in rat studies with this experimental model, however there is no analgesic effect with administration of non-steroidal anti-inflammatory drugs [30].

3.2.2. Lumbar Facet Joint Compression

The lumbar facet joint compression model examines the relationship between back pain and facet pathology by using male Sprague Dawley rats. In it, the model rats undergo a midline incision over the posterior aspect of their spine and their L5/6 facet joint is exposed. Compression is applied over the facet joint using a modified clamp for 3 minutes (at an average force of 400 grams).

After the compression is released, the incision is closed and the subjects are then allowed to recover. In a control group, the rat subjects undergo the same incision and exposure but no compression is placed over the facet joint. Pain sensation is measured through hind paw tactile sensitivity and pressure sensitivity and can be compared between experimental and control groups [31]. This model is novel in that it allows for analysis of mechanically induced damage to the facet joint versus autoimmune damage [32], cartilage cell apoptosis with collagenase injection [33], or chondrocyte disruption with MIA [30].

3.2.3. Disc Degeneration by Needle Puncture

Degeneration of the intervertebral disc is a known cause of chronic discogenic back pain syndrome [34]. Previous studies in rabbits have elucidated a model for disc degeneration through puncture of the annulus fibrosis [35]. However, since rabbits have minimal response to pain, they may not be the best model to assess discogenic back pain. In order to study the role of chemical modulators involved in discogenic back pain, a novel in vivo model was developed again using adult Sprague Dawley rats [36].

In this particular model, the rats are anesthetized and a ventral midline incision approach is used to access the abdominal cavity. With the abdominal cavity retracted, the lumbar discs are punctured with a microsurgical drill. Puncture of the intervertebral disc induces slow development of disc degeneration and chronic back pain, which are corroborated with both histopathological and radiographic changes.

4. Central Sensitization

With regards to glial involvement in pathological pain, one must discuss the concept of central sensitization. Central sensitization is a phenomenon whereby pain from peripheral inflammation is magnified by components of the CNS, most notably in the DRG [37]. Woolf originally described separate parallel sensory pathways for pain (nociceptor fibers) and touch (mechanoreceptor fibers) that under normal circumstances act independently. Plasticity of the neurons in the DRG allow for modification of these pathways in response to inflammation of a peripheral joint. His research highlights several theories as to how the pain signals are amplified leading to the hyperalgesia commonly associated with OA pain.

These modifications include an amplified stimulus from the peripheral tissue due to inflammation, lessening of the activating threshold of afferent neurons in the DRG, and decreasing the inhibitory input of the CNS to nociceptor fibers located in the DRG. His work suggests that the nociceptor and mechanoreceptor fibers converge and this interaction leads to the allodynia typically seen in OA [14, 38].

5. Microglia

Microglial cells are derived from the myelomonocytic lineage and serve as the macrophages and intrinsic immune cells of the CNS. Their primary role in the immune system is to identify and eliminate either damaged or infected cellular debris within the brain and spinal cord [13]. They are the first elements in the brain to respond to any form of disturbance, and in so doing transform from ‘resting’ to ‘activated’ morphology.

The activated microglia then may migrate, proliferate, or release cytokines and chemokines in an effort to eradicate the insult to the CNS structure. They will additionally respond to neurotransmitters within the CNS, which instruct the activated microglia to perform specific response cascades [15].

As mentioned previously, central sensitization is thought to be a mechanism for both hyperalgesia and allodynia [39]. Microglial cells within the spinal dorsal horn also are imperative to the central sensitization mechanism of chronic pain. Evidence for this notion is seen with the attenuation of both allodynia and hyperalgesia in rat models in response to neuropathic and inflammatory pain sources after the administration of the microglial antagonist minocycline [40-42].

Specifically, neuropathic pain has been demonstrated to increase microglial marker OX42 in rat test subjects, providing evidence for their role in the response mechanism to such stimuli [17]. The microglia release various pro-nociceptive and pro-inflammatory cytokines and chemokines and upregulate such chemokine and tachykinin receptors as C-X3-C motif receptor 1 (CX3CR1) and substance P receptors, respectively, to enhance nerve injury-induced tactile allodynia and potentiate a pro-inflammatory response [11, 15, 43]. Microglial p38 MAPK and P2X4 receptors are activated in the rat spinal dorsal horn as well to mediate neuronal excitation after the rat has incurred peripheral nerve injury. There is a predictable corresponding depression in neuronal excitation levels in the rat spinal dorsal horn with inhibition of microglia. These results indicate the involvement of microglia in the neuropathic pain pathway of rats, and by probable extension in humans as well [17]. However, unlike the astrocyte as is described next in this chapter, microglial cells appear to provide no contributory effects to the inflammatory pain pathway.

Microglial cells are also intimately related to the pathology in chronic low back pain. Low back pain is a common problem among the current population; however, the etiology is poorly understood. Much of the low back pain in the aging population can be attributed to degenerative disk disease (DDD), which is comparable to arthritis of peripheral joints. There is a disparity between the anabolic and catabolic processes within the intervertebral discs leading to loss of proteoglycan content as well as disc height. Adjacent vertebrae subsequently develop osteophytic changes similar to that of other arthritic joints.

Recent research has been directed at preventing disc degeneration in hopes to eliminate pain caused by DDD [44-46]. Studies have shown that glial cells are activated in response to DDD [47].

Upon activation, glial cells upregulate expression of pro-inflammatory products such as TNFα, toll-like receptor (TLR) -4, and monocyte chemotactic protein (MCP) -1 within the DRG and dorsal horn of the spinal cord. These inflammatory products are responsible for augmentation of the pain signal initiated in DDD. Interestingly, expression of $\alpha 2\delta 1$, a subunit of calcium channels involved in the neuropathic pain pathway, is also elevated in the DRG of DDD animal models [47]. This indicates that there is an overlap of inflammatory and neuropathic pain responses to DDD of the spine.

As previously discussed, the facet joint pain model recreates morphological changes and pain of the low back similar to that seen in OA [30]. The facet joint has a close approximation to the DRG of the spinal cord. It has been hypothesized that this close proximity may allow “cross-talk” of the facet joint and the DRG that may enhance pain. Upon facet joint degeneration, there is a significant production of pro-inflammatory cytokines (i.e. TNFα, IL-1, IL-17), enzymes (i.e. cyclooxygenase and nitric oxide synthase), and prostaglandin receptors. Using an ex vivo co-culture model, it has been shown that normal DRG exposed to degenerated facet joint capsules demonstrate a significant upregulation of CGRP and substance P within the DRG [48].

As discussed previously, these components have all been linked to glial cells such as microglia and are implicated in enhancing pain signals of OA via central sensitization.

6. ASTROCYTES

Astrocytes are glial cells of the subtype "macroglial" cells and occur in the CNS as well, particularly within the DRG and surrounding blood vessels of the brain and spinal cord. They are highly abundant and have a significant role in neurotransmission due to their close approximation to neuronal cell bodies and synapses [49]. A protein, connexin-43, allows astrocytes to connect to one another through gap junctions [17]. Many of the functions of these cells are well described in the literature and include such tasks as providing structural support for nervous tissue during neuronal migration, reuptake of neurotransmitters at the sites of neuronal synapses, and contribution to the formation of a blood-brain barrier. Astrocytes additionally proliferate within the CNS to aid in reparation of damaged neural tissue [13]. They contain a number of receptors such as those for substance P, N-Methyl-D-aspartate (NMDA), and glutamate, which allow for activation and contribution to cell communication [50-51]. Upon activation, the ERK and JNK pathways are then activated leading to downstream upregulation of transcription factor nuclear factor kappa beta (NFκB). NFκB allows for production of pro-inflammatory cytokines such as IL-1ß, TNF-α, IL-6, prostaglandin E2 (PGE2), nitric oxide (NO), D-serine, and glutamate [52]. Specifically, it is the binding of substance P on the astrocyte in conjunction with IL-1ß, TNF-α and transforming growth factor (TGF) -1ß that has a synergistic effect on astrocyte production of IL-6 and PGE_2 [53]. These pro-inflammatory cytokines are responsible for the amplification of the pain signal in the neurons of the superficial dorsal horn by either reduction of inhibitory transmission or enhancement of excitatory transmission to potentiate pain signaling [54-55].

It is well-documented that astrocytes are activated just as microglia are in response to peripheral nerve injury, and are thus also involved in central sensitization [14, 56-57]. When stimulated by pathological inflammatory-type pain, astrocytes in the rat dorsal spinal root undergo slight morphologic changes through neuron-to-astrocyte and microglia-to-astrocyte signaling which allow for contribution to neuronal excitation levels. It is suggested that hypersensitivity to inflammatory pain is maintained and mediated by the activation of astrocyte JNK and gap junctions. Inhibition of neuronal excitation by L-α-aminoadipate – an astrocyte antagonist – in rats subjected to inflammatory-type pain stimuli confirms the notion that astrocytes play a major role in the chain of events present in the inflammatory pain pathway [17].

The mechanism by which spinal astrocytes are implicated in the maintenance of chronic pain involves the basic fibroblast growth factor (bFGF or FGF-2)/JNK pathway. When stimulated by neuropathic pain, JNK is activated by bFGF in the astrocytic cell, and subsequently allows for mitosis, growth, differentiation, and gliosis. bFGF activation of JNK furthermore regulates gene transcription in astrocytes to synthesize increased levels of those pro-inflammatory cytokines as described with microglia above (IL-1β, TNF-α, IL-6).

Additionally, bFGF is shown to increase expression of GFAP in the spinal cord, which has been found to correlate clinically with chronic pain [58-59]. However, it is known that astrocytes are not independently responsible for the continued signaling from chronic OA pain stimuli, as chronic pain can be successfully managed without a corresponding decrease in GFAP or astrocyte activity [60]. Ultimately, the changes in spinal astrocytes with chronic pain are present for longer duration than the corresponding changes in microglia, suggesting that the function of astrocytes in chronic pain states is greater than that of their glial counterpart [39].

7. Factors Involving Glial Activation

Glial cells, including microglia, astrocytes, and oligodendrocytes, constitute 70~80 % of the total cellular components in the CNS including brain and spinal cord [13]. Until recently, glial cells were considered to be passive support cells for the neurons. However, emerging data suggest a critical link between glial activity and the neuronal immune responses that implicate inflammation and chronic pain disorders. Pain signal shifts the glia to an activated state as a consequence of signals released by nociceptors and/or stressed and damaged neurons. Once activated, the glial cells release pro-inflammatory cytokines, including IL-1ß, IL-6, and TNF-α. At the later stage, anti-inflammatory cytokines can be generated to help dampen the injury response as a feedback response. Overview of the pain pathway involving glial activity is illustrated in the Figure 1.

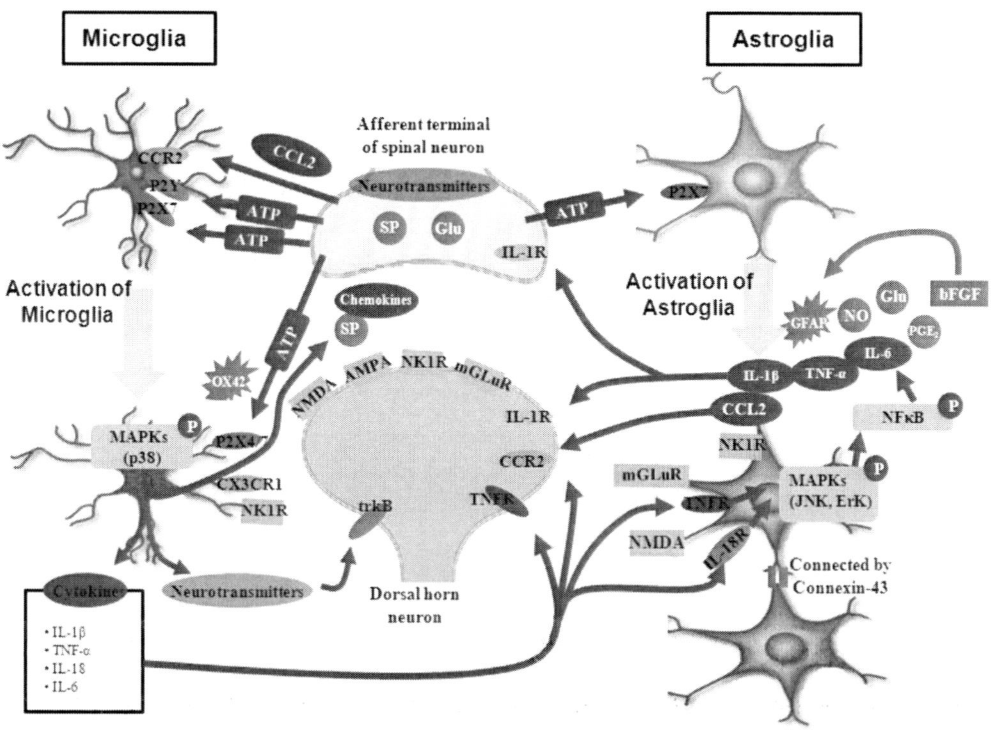

Figure 1. Overview of the OA Pain Pathway.

7.1. Cytokines and Chemokines

Cytokines are soluble proteins produced by a variety of cell types and are critical in the regulation of the growth and activation of immune system cells and in the maintenance of the inflammatory response [13]. High levels of several different inflammatory cytokines and neuropeptides are found in the synovial fluid, synovium, joint capsular tissue, and cartilage of chronic OA pain patients. The activation of peripheral nociceptors in OA pain stimulates the production of inflammatory cytokines. These cytokines may then stimulate the pain mediators' cognate receptors, increasing their role in causing pain perception to the patient with OA [61].

Experimental OA generation in rodent test subjects via MIA-induced chronic knee joint pain results in significant increases in multiple pro-inflammatory cytokines and chemokines, including IL-1α, IL-1β, CCL5 (or RANTES), cytokine-induced neutrophil chemoattractant 2α/β, IL-17, thymus chemokine, TNF-α, L-selectin, and vascular endothelial growth factor (VEGF). Moreover, reduced levels of fractalkine (an acute spinal injury pain-associated chemokine) and granulocyte-macrophage colony-stimulating factor (GM-CSF), as well as the anti-inflammatory factors IL-4 and IL-10, are demonstrated in these rodent test subjects. Although, increased levels of IL-13, an anti-inflammatory factor, are found at the spinal level of MIA-induced OA pain subjects [62]. An increase in this anti-inflammatory factor may indicate a compensatory response for the inflammation of OA.

TNF-α is a cytokine protein constitutively produced by glia, and it rapidly increases expression of α-amino-3-hydroxy-5-methyl-4-isoxazolepropionic acid (AMPA) receptors on the synaptic plasma membrane. This quickly enhances synaptic efficacy and strength at excitatory synapses, and may both contribute to and modulate responses from neural injury [63]. In the late stages of OA-induced pain, TNF-α has substantially increased messenger RNA (mRNA) levels in the spinal cord. The early stages, by contrast, do not exhibit such high levels of TNF-α, suggesting that the chronic pain in OA may be affected by alterations in various cytokine expression levels. Ultimately it appears that nociceptive signals from peripheral OA pain regions are transduced through sensory neurons and the spinal cord to produce high pro-inflammatory cytokines in the CNS [62].

Chemokines are a family of small cytokines who derive their name from the ability to induce directed chemotaxis in nearby responsive cells ("*chemo*tactic cyto*kines*"). They are crucial to the inflammatory response, and are released locally from hematologic cells at sites of inflammation to recruit leukocytes to damaged tissues. With the inclusion of certain chemokines, mechanisms have been described using rodent chronic pain models for two different pain signaling pathways between injured sensory neurons in the peripheral nervous system and spinal cord microglia: CCL2/CCR2 and cathepsin S/CX3CL1 (Fractalkine) CX3CR1. CCL2 is expressed constitutively in cell bodies of small and medium diameter size DRG neurons, where it is stored in neuropeptide-containing and neuropeptide-free vesicles to be released in the dorsal horn of the spinal cord through calcium-dependent mechanisms. The pro-nociceptive effects and increased sensitivity to pain caused by CCL2 are mediated via CCR2 at the spinal level to induce persistent hyperalgesia and allodynia. CCR2 is normally expressed in monocyte/macrophage lineage cells in peripheral locations, but in response to peripheral nerve injury its expression is upregulated on spinal microglia and spinal microglial activation is triggered. The second modulatory pathway for neuropathic pain involves the chemotactic cytokine fractalkine, a full-length transmembrane protein expressed on neuronal membranes. It is thought to mediate the nociceptive signaling in pain generation from neurons to glial cells in the dorsal horn. The lysosomal cysteine protease cathepsin S – released by activated microglia under conditions of persistent pain – proteolytically cleaves fractalkine into its soluble form. This soluble fractalkine may then bind its receptor CX3CR1, found exclusively in the spinal cord on microglial cells, therein causing their activation and release of more microglial substances and forming a positive feedback loop perpetuating the chronic pain state in conditions including OA [11]. Inflammatory cytokines TNF-α and IL-1 upregulate the expression of fractalkine and the CX3CR1 on the glial cells [64].

7.2. Neurotrophic Factors

Glial cell line-derived neurotrophic factor (GDNF) is shown to have potent analgesic effects in neuropathic pain states by preventing and reversing sensory abnormalities from this pathological pain type. This is potentially performed through regulatory effects on the expression of substance P.

As a result, it appears that GDNF has a therapeutic effect on many chronic pain disorders. Research has demonstrated a fast-acting and long-lasting down-regulation of GDNF mRNA expression in the dorsal spinal cord of rats subjected to complete Freund's adjuvant-induced unilateral arthritis (another model mimicking human OA pathology), which negatively correlated with pain-test scores in the rats. This suggests the possibility of a functional relationship between GDNF levels and the maintenance of chronic pain pathways in OA [65].

7.3. Involvement of Protein Kinases

Protein kinases are enzymes that regulate many of the transduction events in eukaryotic cells via phosphorylation of other proteins. There are 4 groups of enzymes under the classification MAP kinases within the serine/threonine family: extracellular signal related kinase (ERK – contains isoforms ERK1, ERK2), p38 MAP kinase (contains α, β, γ, δ isoforms), c-Jun-N-terminal kinase (JNK – 3 isoforms JNK1, JNK2, JNK3), and ERK5. These MAP kinases are unique in comparison to other protein kinases as they are activated only by stimuli producing cellular stress or damage, as is the case with chronic pain conditions like OA. Their activation leads to downstream alterations in gene expression, leading to maintenance of chronic neuropathic and inflammatory pain [66].

Multiple experimental models for OA pathophysiology describe an important role for MAP kinase signaling in the development and continuation of chronic inflammatory pain. As described earlier in this chapter, one model for the development of chronic OA pain is determined in rat models with injection of MIA into the knee joint.

It is MAP kinase proteins that are involved as signaling molecules in this model of OA pain generation, as MIA injection into rat test subjects results in both the appropriate development of chronic pain (measured, for example, as significant decreases in rat hind limb grip strength) [67] and in significantly increased levels of ERK1/2 and p38 MAPK in the dorsal horn of the spinal cord. Importantly, ERK1/2 inhibition causes significant decreases in chronic pain behavior in rat subjects, demonstrating its importance to the presence and production of chronic pain. Microglial cells, as described previously, are well-known to be involved in the OA pain mechanism. They are predictably found to be activated in significantly increased numbers in the joints exposed to MIA, as they are the source of the enhanced levels of the p38 MAPK [66].

7.4. ATP and Downstream Pathways

Adenosine triphosphate, or ATP, is a downstream product of cellular respiration and used as a coenzyme by cells mainly as a source of energy. ATP is also known to be released from nerve terminals in the DRG in response to OA joint degeneration. Microglial cells react to the elevated extracellular ATP levels via a P2 receptor, most convincingly the P2X7 receptor [68]. Spinal microglia also upregulates their P2 receptor expression in response to nerve injury enhancing pain signaling [18]. Activation of the P2 receptor allows for calcium influx and upregulation of TNF-α mRNA expression and TNF-α release [69]. While ATP alone can stimulate TNF-α release, an absence of calcium results in lower concentrations of TNF-α. ATP has been shown to activate ERK and p38 in the absence of extracellular calcium in astrocytes and microglial cells. It has been postulated that calcium exhibits its effects downstream of the MAP kinases [66].

ATP-activated P2 channels also decrease levels of intracellular potassium allowing for cleavage of pro-IL-1β to activated IL-1β, a pro-inflammatory cytokine [70-71]. ATP-activated P2 receptors also cause increased glial cell production of ATP leading to activation of surrounding glial cells and therefore amplifying the pain signal [72].

7.5. Prostaglandin E_2 (PGE_2)

Prostaglandins are products of fatty acids and can act locally as a paracrine hormone affecting local signaling pathways. The enzyme cyclooxygenase (COX) is responsible for the conversion of arachidonic acid to PGH_2, a precursor to multiple subtypes of Prostaglandins. Prostaglandins have many different roles ranging from bronchoconstriction to platelet aggregation. PGE_2, a product of PGH_2 modified by the enzyme PGE synthase, has been implicated in OA pain. Interestingly, IL-1β and TNF-α have been shown to increase the activity of the COX enzyme as well as nitric oxide synthase (NOS) in astrocytes leading to increased production of PGE_2 and NO [73-74]. NO further increases COX activity in astroglial cells, which in turn enhances further production of PGE_2. NO further increases COX activity in astroglial cells, which in turn enhances further production of PGE_2. This abundant production of PGE_2 increases calcium influx in astrocytes leading to a downstream production of glutamate, the excitatory neurotransmitter of the CNS [75]. Although the details are yet uncertain, glutamate production by astrocytes leads to increased calcium uptake in surrounding sensory neurons of the DRG further activating these neurons and enhancing the pain signal of OA.

7.6. Adaptor Proteins

Signal transducing adaptor proteins, or simply adaptor proteins, assist the primary proteins in any signal transduction pathway. Since they do not have any enzymatic ability, they are able only to support other protein-protein interactions. Myeloid differentiation primary response gene 88 (MyD88) is one adapter protein that functions as an important mediator in OA progression. is one adapter protein that functions as an important mediator in OA progression. It functions to connect TLRs and IL-1 receptors (IL-1Rs) with downstream signaling molecules. TLRs, particularly TLR-2 and TLR-4 have been linked to chronic inflammatory and pain processes that involve inflammatory response and degradation of peripheral joint tissues such as fibroblast-like synovial cells and articular cartilage in knee joints through activation of pro-inflammatory cytokine production such as TNFα, IL-1, IL-6, and IL-8 [76]. This inflammatory response is thought to activate surrounding glial cells further propagating the pain transmission. Importantly, research has shown that inhibition of the MyD88 pathway may be a treatment option for inflammatory cartilage disease [77].

8. Current Therapeutic Options

As discussed throughout the course of this chapter, central sensitization has been documented as an underlying mechanism for pain in OA patients. Intense, constant nociceptive and inflammatory input from OA-affected knees leads to chronic pain via increased temporal summation of excitatory neurogenic pain signals and impaired diffuse noxious inhibitory control. One therapeutic technique currently under examination for the treatment of OA chronic pain is the transcutaneous electrical nerve stimulation (TENS), which utilizes the aforementioned electrical properties of nerves during pain generation to dampen the resultant perceived discomfort [78].

TENS is a non-pharmacological, safe, and inexpensive mechanism of analgesia based on the "Gate Control Theory" of pain perception [79] in which the stimulation of large (A-beta) cutaneous afferent fibers activate inhibitory interneurons in the dorsal horn thereby dampening transmission from A-delta and C-fibers.

Its use to relieve OA pain in the knee as a multi-week burst intervention has been recommended in numerous clinical guidelines. Current ongoing research is being done to better understand the effect that TENS has on pain inhibition in OA knee patients. One limitation already described with the TENS mechanism of pain control is for those patients with knee OA who are already centrally sensitized; such patients may experience a paradoxical increase in pain from the TENS electrical stimulation.

Thus, identification of a subgroup of OA patients who are at the start of therapy still non-centrally-sensitized would be the proper population to benefit from burst TENS therapy. Because the TENS units are small, inexpensive, and easy-to-use at home, their use would provide a simple yet effective asset to the presently limited clinical toolbox of OA therapy options [78].

Finally, efficacy has been previously demonstrated for glial inhibitors in decreasing exaggerated mechanical and neuropathic pain states in various pain models. For example, minocycline – a selective inhibitor of microglial activation – has been found to attenuate allodynia from acute and persistent models of pain facilitation in rats [40]. With the knowledge that activated microglial cells are a major initiator of enhanced pain responses, agents like minocycline that are able to inhibit microglial activation may provide a promising therapeutic option for OA pain.

9. Direction of Future Research

As with any medical condition affecting a large proportion of the population, the goal with obtaining a better scientific understanding of the root pathology is ultimately to utilize such knowledge to generate therapeutic options and combat said pathology. Many of the aforementioned cell types, cytokines, and protein kinases pose potential places in the OA pain pathway where intervention may prevent the development of chronic pain perception.

For instance, further research to gain improved understanding of the molecular alterations during activation of microglia and astrocytes after peripheral nerve injury or inflammation may lead to the development of therapeutic pharmacology for chronic pain control. MAPK, chemokines, and cytokines are other therapeutic targets for possible pharmacologic inhibitors to prevent development of joint degeneration and consequent chronic pain in OA patients. Additionally, while it is known which cytokines are elevated in OA-induced pain states, future research may be directed on the rate-limiting targets being signaled by such cytokines. This may prove invaluable to controlling pain production with targeted analgesic drugs specific to OA-type discomfort. In the more immediate setting, additional research on which exact patient subgroups will benefit from the already proven TENS therapy will help to refine a population of patients that will have the greatest outcome with an already proven therapeutic option [78]. Of note, while many studies have been performed to look at the role of microglia in chronic OA pain generation, there is an identified limitation to studying microglia in an in vitro setting. Microglial cells are inherently found in the human CNS in a resting state. Any change in environment, such as culturing the microglia for experimentation or isolation of the microglia from subject tissue, will cause rapid activation of the microglia. Thus, in vitro experimentation of microglia is performed on activated microglia as would not be characteristically found in native tissue. Future research should be directed to study the behavior of microglia in vivo in living subjects to better approximate their function in situ [15].

References

[1] Dieppe PA, Lohmander LS. Pathogenesis and management of pain in osteoarthritis. *Lancet*. 2005, 365(9463): 965 – 973.

[2] Linaker CH, Walker-Bone K, Palmer K, Cooper C. Frequency and impact of regional musculoskeletal disorders. *Baillieres Best Pract. Res. Clin. Rheumatol.* 1999, 13(2): 197-215.

[3] Swift A. Osteoarthritis 1: Physiology, risk factors and causes of pain. *Nurs Times*. 2012, 108(7): 12-15.

[4] Im HJ, Li X, Muddasani P, Kim GH, Davis F, Rangan J, Forsyth CB, Ellman M, Thonar EJ. Basic fibroblast growth factor accelerates matrix degradation via a neuro-endocrine pathway in human adult articular chondrocytes. *J. Cell Physiol.* 2008, 215(2): 452-463.

[5] Felson DT. The sources of pain in knee osteoarthritis. *Curr. Opin. Rheumatol.* 2005, 17(5): 624-628.

[6] Ivanavicius SP, Ball AD, Heapy CG, Westwood FR, Murray F, Read SJ. Structural pathology in a rodent model of osteoarthritis is associated with neuropathic pain: increased expression of ATF-3 and pharmacological characterization. *Pain*. 2007, 128(3): 272-282.

[7] Ohtori S, Orita S, Yamashita M, Ishikawa T, Ito T, Shigemura T, Nishiyama H, Konno S, Ohta H, Takaso M, Inoue G, Equchi Y, Ochiai N, Kishida S, Kuniyoshi K, Aoki Y, Arai G, Miyagi M, Kamoda II, Suzkuki M, Nakamura J, Furuya T, Kubota G, Sakuma Y, Oikawa Y, Suzuki M, Sasho T, Nakagawa K, Toyone T, Takahashi K. Existence of a neuropathic pain component in patients with osteoarthritis of the knee. *Yonsei. Med. J.* 2012, 53(4): 801-805.

[8] Jordan JM, Helmick CG, Renner JB, Luta G, Dragomir AD, Woodard J, Fang F, Schwartz TA, Abbate LM, Callahan LF, Kalsbeek WD, Hochberg MC. Prevalence of knee symptoms and radiographic and symptomatic knee osteoarthritis in African Americans and Caucasians: the Johnston County Osteoarthritis Project. *J. Rheumatol.* 2007, 34(1): 172-180.

[9] Arendt-Neilson L, Nie H, Laursen MB, Laursen BS, Madeleine P, Simonsen OH, Graven-Nielsen T. Sensitization in patients with painful knee osteoarthritis. *Pain*. 2010, 149(3): 573-581.

[10] Dye SF, Vaupel GL, Dye CC. Conscious neurosensory mapping of the internal structures of the human knee without intraarticular anesthesia. *Am. J. Sports Med.* 1998, 26(6): 773-777.

[11] Abbadie C, Bhangoo S, De Koninck Y, Malcangio M, Melik-Parsadaniantz S, White FA. Chemokines and pain mechanisms. *Brain Research Reviews*. 2009, 60: 125-134.

[12] McMahon SB, Malcangio M. Current challenges in glia-pain biology. *Neuron*. 2009, 64(1): 46-54.

[13] Waxman, S.G. *Clinical Neuroanatomy, 26th edition*. New Haven, CT: The McGraw-Hill Companies, Inc., 2010.

[14] Milligan ED, Watkins LR: Pathological and protective roles of glia in chronic pain. *Nat. Rev. Neurosci.* 2009, 10:23–36.

[15] Pocock JM, Kettenmann H. Neurotransmitter receptors on microglia. *TRENDS in Neurosciences*. 2007, 30(10): 527-535.

[16] Scholz J, Woolf CJ: The neuropathic pain triad: neurons, immune cells and glia. *Nat. Neurosci.* 2007, 10:1361–1368.

[17] Ikeda H, Kiritoshi T, Kazuyuki M. Contribution of microglia and astrocytes to the central sensitization, inflammatory neuropathic pain in the juvenile rat. *Molecular Pain*. 2012, 8: 43.

[18] Ji RR, Gereau RW 4th, Malcangio M, Strichartz GR: MAP kinase and pain. *Brain Res. Rev*. 2009, 60: 135-148.

[19] Tsuda M, Ueno H, Kataoka A, Tozaki-Saitoh H, Inoue K: Activation of dorsal horn microglia contributes to diabetes-induced tactile allodynia via extracellular signal-regulated protein kinase signaling. *Glia*. 2008, 56: 378-386.

[20] Inoue K. The function of microglia through purinergic receptors: neuropathic pain and cytokine release. *Pharmacol. Ther*. 2006, 109: 210-226.

[21] Gao YJ, Ji RR. Chemokines, neuronal-glial interactions, and central processing of neuropathic pain. *Pharmacol. Ther*. 2010, 126: 56-68.

[22] Guzman RE, Evans MG, Bove S, Morenko B, Kilgore K. Mono-iodoacetate-induced histologic changes in subchondral bone and articular cartilage of rat femorotibial joints: an animal model of osteoarthritis. *Toxicol. Pathol.* 2003, 31(6): 619-624.

[23] Combe R, Bramwell S, Field MJ. The monosodium iodoacetate model of osteoarthritis: a model of chronic nociceptive pain in rats? *Neurosci. Lett.* 2004, 370(2-3): 236-240.

[24] Sagar DR, Burston JJ, Hathway GJ, Woodhams SG, Pearson RG, Bennett AJ, Kendall DA, Scammell BE, Chapman V. The contribution of spinal glial cells to chronic pain behaviour in the monosodium iodoacetate model of osteoarthritic pain. *Mol. Pain.* 2011, 7: 88.

[25] Orita S, Ishikawa T, Miyagi M, Ochiai N, Inoue G, Eguchi Y, Kamoda H, Arai G, Toyone T, Aoki Y, Kubo T, Takahashi K, Ohtori S. Pain-related sensory innervations in monoiodoacetate-induced osteoarthritis in rat knees that gradually develops neuronal injury in addition to inflammatory pain. *BMC Musculoskelet Disord.* 2011, 12: 134.

[26] Glasson SS, Blanchet TJ, Morris EA. The surgical destabilization of the medial meniscus (DMM) model of osteoarthritis in the 129/SvEv mouse. *OsteoArthritis and Cartilage.* 2007, 15: 1061-1069.

[27] Moodie JP, Stok KS, Muller R, Vincent TL, Shefelbine SJ. Multimodal imaging demonstrates concomitant changes in bone and cartilage after destabilisation of the medial meniscus and increased joint laxity. *Osteoarthritis and Cartilage.* 2011, 19: 163-170.

[28] Malfait AM, Ritchie J, Gil AS, Austin JS, Hartke J, Qin W, Tortorella MD, Mogil JS. ADAMTS-5 deficient mice do not develop mechanical allodynia associated with osteoarthritis following medial meniscal destabilization. *Osteoarthritis and Cartilage.* 2010, 18: 572-580.

[29] Kaufman GN, Zaouter C, Valteau B, Sirois P, Moldovan F. Nociceptive tolerance is improved by bradykinin receptor B1 antagonism and joint morphology is protected by both endothelin type A and bradykinin receptor B1 antagonism in a surgical model of osteoarthritis. *Arthritis Research and Therapy.* 2011, 13: R76.

[30] Kim JS, Kroin JS, Buvanendran A, Li X, van Wijnen AJ, Tuman KJ, Im HJ. Characterization of a new animal model for evaluation and treatment of back pain due to lumbar facet joint osteoarthritis. *Arthritis and Rheumatism.* 2011, 63(10): 2966-2973.

[31] Henry JL, Yashpal K, Vernon H, Kim J, Im HJ. Lumbar facet joint compressive injury induces lasting changes in local structure, nociceptive scores, and inflammatory mediators in a novel rat model. *Pain Research and Treatment.* 2012, 1-12.

[32] Tachihara H, Kikuchi SI, Konno SI, Sekiguchi M. Does facet joint inflammation induce radiculopathy? An investigation using a rat model of lumbar facet joint inflammation. *Spine.* 2007, 32(4): 406-412.

[33] Yeh TT, Wen ZH, Lee HS et al. Intra-articular injection of collagenase induced experimental osteoarthritis of the lumbar facet joint in rats. *European Spine Journal.* 2008, 17(5): 734-742.

[34] Hurri H, Karppinen J. Discogenic pain. *Pain.* 2004, 112: 225-228.

[35] Kim KS, Yoon ST, Li J, Park JS, Hutton WC. Disc degeneration in the rabbit: a biochemical and radiological comparison between four disc injury models. *Spine.* 2005, 30: 33-37.

[36] Kim JS, Kroin JS, Li X, An HS, Buvanendran A, Yan D, Tuman KJ, van Wijnen AJ, Chen D, Im HJ. The rat intervertebral disc degeneration model: relationships between biological and structural alterations and pain. *Arthritis Res. Ther.* 2011, 13(5):R165.

[37] Woolf CJ. Evidence for a central component of post-injury pain hypersensitivity. *Nature*. 1983, 306(5944): 686-688.

[38] Woolf CJ. Central sensitization: implications for the diagnosis and treatment of pain. *Pain*. 2011, 152(3): S2-15.

[39] Ji RR, Kohno T, Moore KA, Woolf CJ: Central sensitization and LTP: do pain and memory share similar mechanisms?. *Trends Neurosci.* 2003, 26:696–705.

[40] Ledeboer A, Sloane EM, Milligan ED, Frank MG, Mahony JH, Maier SF, Watkins LR. Minocycline attenuates mechanical allodynia and pro-inflammatory cytokine expression in rat models of pain facilitation. *Pain* 2005, 15:71–83.

[41] Mika J, Osikowicz M, Rojewska E, Korostynski M, Wawrzczak-Bargiela A, Przewlocki R, Przewlocka B. Differential activation of spinal microglial and astroglial cells in a mouse model of peripheral neuropathic pain. *Eur. J. Pharmacol.* 2009, 623:65–72.

[42] Raghavendra V, Tanga F, DeLeo JA: Inhibition of microglial activation attenuates the development but not existing hypersensitivity in a rat model of neuropathy. *J. Pharmacol. Exp. Ther.* 2003, 306:624–630.

[43] Ji R, Kawasaki Y, Zhuang Z, Wen Y, Decosterd I. Possible role of spinal astrocytes in maintaining chronic pain sensitization: review of current evidence with focus on bFGF/JNK pathway. *Neuron Glia. Biol.* 2006 November, 2(4): 259-269.

[44] Ellman MB, Kim JS, An HS, Kroin JS, Li X, Chen D, Yan D, Buechter DD, Nakayama K, Liu B, Morgan S, Im HJ. The pathophysiologic role of the protein kinase Cpathway in the intervertebral discs of rabbits and mice: in vitro, ex vivo, and in vivo studies. *Arthritis Rheum.* 2012, 64(6): 1950-1959.

[45] Kim JS, Ellman MB, An HS, van Wijnen AJ, Borgia JA, Im HJ. Insulin-like growth factor 1 synergizes with bone morphogenetic protein 7-mediated anabolism in bovine intervertebral disc cells. *Arthritis Rheum*. 2010, 62(12): 3706-3715.

[46] Li X, Phillips FM, An HS, Ellman M, Thonar EJ, Wu W, Park D, Im HJ. The action of resveratrol, a phytoestrogen found in grapes, on the intervertebral disc. *Spine*. 2008, 33(24): 2587-95.

[47] Kim JS, Kroin JS, Li X, An HS, Buvanendran A, Yan D, Tuman KJ, van Wijnen AJ, Chen D, Im HJ. The rat intervertebral disk degeneration pain model: relationships between biological and structural alterations and pain. *Arthritis Res. Ther.* 2011, 13(5): R165.

[48] Kim J, Ali MH, Wydra F, Li X, An HS, Cs-Szabo G, van Wijnen AJ, Cavanaugh JM, Im HJ. Characterization of degenerative human facet joints and facet joint capsular tissues. *Arthritis and Rheumatism*. 2012, In Review.

[49] Haydon PG. GLIA: Listening and talking to the synapse. *Nat. Rev. Neurosci.* 2001; 2(3): 185-193.

[50] Porter JT, McCarthy KD. Astrocytic neurotransmitter receptors in situ and in vivo. *Prog. Neurobiol.* 1997; 51(4): 439-455.

[51] Mantyh PW, Johnson DJ, Boehmer CG, Catton MD, Vinters HV, Maggio JE, Too HP, Vigna SR. Substance P receptor binding sites are expressed by glia in vivo after neuronal injury. *Proc. Natl. Acad. Sci. U.S.A.* 1989; 86(13): 5193-5197.

[52] Stellwagen D, Malenka RC. Synaptic scaling mediated by glial TNF-α. *Nature*. 2006; 440(7087): 1054-1059.

[53] Palma C, Minghetti L, Astolfi M, Ambrosini E, Silberstein FC, Manzini S, Levi G, Aloisi F. Functional characterization of substance P receptors on cultured human spinal cord astrocytes: synergism of substance P with cytokines in inducing interleukin-6 and prostaglandin E2 production. *Glia*. 1997; 21(2): 183-193.

[54] St-Jacques B, Ma W. Role of prostaglandin E2 in the synthesis of the pro-inflammatory cytokine interleukin-6 in primary sensory neurons: an in vivo and in vitro study. *J. Neurochem*. 2011; 118(5): 841-854.

[55] Nakagawa T, Kaneko S. Spinal astrocytes as therapeutic targets for pathological pain. *J. Pharmacol. Sci*. 2010, 114: 347-353.

[56] McMahon SB, Malcangio M: Current challenges in glia-pain biology. *Neuron* 2009,64:46–54.

[57] Scholz J, Woolf CJ: The neuropathic pain triad: neurons, immune cells and glia. *Nat Neurosci.* 2007, 10:1361–1368.

[58] Colburn RW, DeLeo JA, Rickman AJ, Yeager MP, Kwon P, Hickey WF. Dissociation of microglial activation and neuropathic pain behaviors following peripheral nerve injury in the rat. Journal of Neuroimmunology 1997;79:163–175.

[59] Colburn RW, Rickman AJ, DeLeo JA. The effect of site and type of nerve injury on spinal glial activation and neuropathic pain behavior. Experimental Neurology 1999;157:289–304.

[60] Zhuang ZY, Wen YR, Zhang DR, Borsello T, Bonny C, Strichartz GR, et al. A peptide c-Jun N-terminal kinase (JNK) inhibitor blocks mechanical allodynia after spinal nerve ligation: respective roles of JNK activation in primary sensory neurons and spinal astrocytes for neuropathic pain development and maintenance. *Journal of Neuroscience* 2006a;26:3551–3560.

[61] Longo DL, Fauci AS, Kasper DL, Hauser SL, Jameson JL, Loscalzo J. *Harrison's Principles of Internal Medicine, 18th edition*. New Haven, CT: The McGraw-Hill Companies, Inc., 2012.

[62] Im H, Kim J, Li X, Kotwal N, Sumner DR, van Wijnen AJ, Davis FJ, Yan D, Levine B, Henry JL, Desevre J, Kroin JS. Alteration of sensory neurons and spinal response to an experimental osteoarthritis pain model. *Arthritis and Rheumatism*. 2010, 62(10): 2995-3005.

[63] Beattie EC, Stellwagen D, Morishita W, Bresnahan JC, Keun Ha B, Von Zastrow M, Beattie MS, Malenka RC. Control of synaptic strength by glial TNFα. *Science*. 2002, 295: 2282-2285.

[64] Maciejewski-Lenoir D, Chen S, Feng L, Maki R, Bacon KB. Characterization of fractalkine in rat brain cells: migratory and activation signals for CX3CR1-expressing microglia. *J. Immunol*. 1999, 163(3): 1628-1635.

[65] Fang M, Wang Y, He QH, Sun YX, Deng LB, Wang XM, Han JS. Glial cell line-derived neurotrophic factor contributes to delayed inflammatory hyperalgesia in adjuvant rat pain model. *Neuroscience*. 2003, 117: 503-512.

[66] Crown ED. The role of mitogen activated protein kinase signaling in microglia and neurons in the initiation and maintenance of chronic pain. *Experimental Neurology*. 2012, 234: 330-339.

[67] Lee Y, Pai M, Brederson JD, Wilcox D, Hsieh G, Jarvis MF, Bitner RS. Monosodium iodoacetate-induced joint pain is associated with increased phosphorylation of mitogen activated protein kinases in the rat spinal cord. *Mol. Pain*. 2011; 7: 39.

[68] Hide I, Tanaka M, Inoue A, Nakajima K, Kohsaka S, Inoue K, Nakata Y. Extracellular ATP triggers tumor necrosis factor-alpha release from rat microglia. *J Neurochem*. 2000, 75(3): 965-972.

[69] Takuma K, Matsuda T, Hashimoto H, Kitanaka J, Asano S, Kishida Y, Baba A. Role of Na(+)-Ca2+ exchanger in agonist-induced Ca2+ signaling in cultured rat astrocytes. *J. Neurochem*. 1996, 67(5): 1840-1845.

[70] Ferrari D, Villalba M, Chiozzi P, Falzoni S, Ricciardi-Castagnoli P, Di Virgilio F. Mouse microglial cells express a plasma membrane pore gated by extracellular ATP. *J. Immunol*. 1996, 156(4): 1531-1539.

[71] Ferrari D, Chiozzi P, Falzoni S, Dal Susino M, Melchiorri L, Baricordi OR, Di Virgilio F. Extracellular ATP triggers IL-1 beta release by activating the purinergic P2Z receptor of human macrophages. *J. Immunol*. 1997, 159(3): 1451-1458.

[72] Coull JA, Beggs S, Boudreau D, Boivin D, Tsuda M, Inoue K, Gravel C, Salter MW, De Koninck Y. BDNF from microglia causes the shift in neuronal anion gradient underlying neuropathic pain. *Nature*. 2005, 438(7070): 1017-1021.

[73] Salvemini D, Misko TP, Masferrer JL, Seibert K, Currie MG, Needleman P. Nitric oxide activates cyclooxygenase enzymes. *Proc. Natl. Acad. Sci. U.S.A.* 1993, 90(15): 7240-7244.

[74] Mollace V, Colasanti M, Muscoli C, Lauro GM, Iannone M, Rotiroti D, Nistico G. The effect of nitric oxide on cytokine-induced release of PGE2 by human cultured astroglial cells. *Br. J. Pharmacol*. 1998, 124(4): 742-746.

[75] Bezzi P, Carmignoto G, Pasti L, Vesce S, Rossi D, Rizzini BL, Pozzan T, Volterra A. Prostaglandins stimulate calcium-dependent glutamate release in astrocytes. *Nature*. 1998, 391(6664): 281-285.

[76] Ellman MB, Kim J, An HS, Chen D, Ranjan KC, An J, Dittakavi T, van Wijnen AJ, Cs-Szabo G, Li X, Xiao G, An S, Kim S, Im H. Toll-like receptor adaptor signaling molecule MyD88 on intervertebral disk homeostasis: in vitro, ex vivo studies. *Gene*. 2012, 505: 283-290.

[77] Abdollahi-Roodsaz S, van de Loo FA, Koenders MI, Helsen MM, Walgreen B, van den Bersselaar LA, Arntz OJ, Takahashi N, Joosten LA, van den Berg WB. Destructive role of myeloid differentiation factor 88 and protective role of TIR-containing adaptor inducing interferon beta in IL-17-dependent arthritis. *Arthritis Rheum*. 2011; 64: 1838–1847.

[78] Beckwee D, De Hertogh W, Lievens P, Bautmans I, Vaes P. Effect of TENS on pain in relation to central sensitization in patients with osteoarthritis of the knee: study protocol of a randomized controlled trial. *Trials*. 2012, 13: 21.

[79] Melzack R, Wall PD: Pain mechanisms: a new theory. *Science* 1965, 150(699):971-979.

In: Glial Cells
Editors: Charanjit Kaur and Eng-Ang Ling
ISBN: 978-1-62618-448-0
© 2013 Nova Science Publishers, Inc.

Chapter 8

BK$^+$ CHANNELS CONTRIBUTE TO THE CELLULAR ACTIVATION OF MICROGLIA: A BIG CHANNEL IN SMALL GLIA

***Yoshinori Hayashi*[1] *and Hiroshi Nakanishi*[1,2*]**
[1]Department of Aging Science and Pharmacology,
Faculty of Dental Sciences, KyushuUniversity, Fukuoka, Japan
[2]Japan Science and Technology Agency, Core Research for Evolutional Science and Technology, Tokyo, Japan

ABSTRACT

Ca^{2+}-activated K^+ (K_{Ca}) channels are classified into three major subtypes based on conductance size: BK, IK and SK. Increases in intracellular Ca^{2+} induce channel opening, resulting in K^+ efflux that maintains a driving force for subsequent Ca^{2+} influx. Therefore, K_{Ca} channels in excitable cells such as neurons work as breaks to prevent excessive excitation. In contrast, K_{Ca} channels in non-excitable cells such as T-cells and microglia work as accelerators to induce cellular activation, proliferation and migration. There is increasing evidence that hyperactive microglia play pathological roles in neurodegenerative diseases, neuropsychiatric disorders and chronic pain. Recently, optically pure S-ketaminehas been shown to preferentially suppress nerve injury-induceddevelopment of tactile allodynia and hyperactivation of spinal microglia through the blockade of BK channels in microglia. We herein describe the current understanding of the biophysiological properties, proposed functions and modulatory molecules of BK channels in microglia.

INTRODUCTION

Ion channels are selective filters in the brain that organize specific function, cellular signaling and metabolism via flux of specific ions. Ion channels exhibit individual open-close

* Corresponding author: E-mail: nakan@ent.kyushu-u.ac.jp (HN).

state kinetics. Potassium channels determine the resting membrane potential and modulate the shape, duration and frequency of action potentials. Among potassium channels, specific channels, called Ca^{2+}-activated K^+ (K_{Ca}) channels, are triggered by the intracellular Ca^{2+}concentration. K_{Ca} channels are classified into three principle subtypes based on biophysical single channel conductance: BK (KCa1.1), IK (KCa3.1) and SK (KCa2.1, 2.2, 2.3) (Table 1).

BK channels possess a voltage-operated mechanism in addition to the Ca^{2+}-dependent activation. Little is known about the molecular basis for the activation of BK channels in non-excitable cells because coincident increases in the cytosolic Ca^{2+} concentration and membrane depolarization do not constitute the physiological conditions for most non-excitable cells. On the other hand, IK and SK channels are very sensitive to increases in the cytosolic Ca^{2+} concentration and do not require changes in the membrane potential to become activated. Therefore, much attention has been paid to the functions of IK and SK channels in non-excitable cells, including microglia, which are considered to be the most susceptible sensors of brain pathology (Kettenmann et al., 2011).

Recently, however, it has been reported that BK channels can be activated by the physical voltages and Ca^{2+} levels in non-excitable cells (Yan and Aldrich, 2010). A novel auxiliary protein of a voltage-gated ion channels, leucine-rich repeat (LRR)-containing protein 26 (LRRC26), modulates BK channels by causing negative shifts (-140 mV) in voltage dependence and provides a molecular basis for the activation of BK channels bythe physical voltages and Ca^{2+} levels in non-excitable cells. We also recently found that the BK channels in spinal microglia are activated after spinal nerve injury without significant membrane depolarization (Hayashi et al., 2011).

Table 1. Properties of Ca^{2+}-activated K^+ channel subtypes

Property	BK(Kca1.1)	IK(Kca3.1)	SK(Kca2.1, 2.2, 2.3)
Single-channel Conductance (pS)	100-300	10-60	2-20
Voltage sensitivity	Yes	No	No
Blocker	TEA (5 mM) Iberiotoxin Paxilline Charibdtoxin	Charibdtoxin Clotrimazole TRAM-34	TEA (20 mM) Apamine Scyllatoxin Tamapin
Functions in Neuron	Repolarization Fast after-hyperpolarization Neurotransmitter release	After-hyperpolarization (cerebellar Purkinje cells)	Medium duration phase of the after-hyperpolarization
Functions in Non-excitable cells	Processing and secretion of IL-1β (microglia, Schwann cell)	Morphology, Migration (microglia) Proliferation (T cell)	ROS release Cytokine expression (microglia)

In this chapter, we will therefore focus on the biophysiologicalproperties, cellular expression, proposed functions and modulatorymolecules of BK channels in microglia.

The Biopysiological Properties of BK Channels

BK channelsare expressed in almost every tissue and exert a negative feedback for cellular excitability. BK channels control the tone of blood vessels, neuronal excitability, and neurotransmitter release (Salkoff et al., 2006). These phenomenaare partially attributable to large conductance, 100-300 pS, resulting in the robust efflux of potassium through BK channels. Membrane depolarization accelerates the Ca^{2+} influx through the voltage-dependent Ca^{2+} channels and the subsequent activation of BK channels by the intracellular Ca^{2+} and Mg^{2+} concentrations (Salkoff et al., 2006). Therefore, the opening of BK channels effectively repolarizes and terminates action potential generation. Dysfunction of BK channels results in several disorders (Gribkoff et al., 2001; Runden-Pran et al., 2002; Sausbier et al., 2004; Brenner et al., 2005; Du et al., 2005).

BK channels consistoffour pore-forming α subunits and auxiliary β subunits (Salkoff et al., 2006). The α subunit is encoded by the *Slo1*gene, whereasβ subunit encoded mRNA has various splice variants (Salkoff et al., 2006). Currently, four types of β subunits (β1-β4) have been identified, which express tissue-specific and controlchannel functions(Orio et al., 2002; Lee and Cui, 2009).Therefore, BK channel diversity is determined post-translationally in various tissues.The β1 subunit is primarily distributed in the smooth muscle cells. The β2 subunit is highly expressed in the kidneys, pancreas and ovaries and weakly distributed in the testes, small intestine, chromaffin cells and brain, which do not work at physiological conditions (Lesuffleur et al., 2009). The β3 subunit exhibitsa broad tissue expression, including in the brain. Mutation of the β3 gene is associated with epilepsy (Lorenz et al., 2007). The β4 subunit is thought to act as a neuronal subunit and is involved in acute alcoholtolerance and consumption (Martin et al., 2008). BK channels modulate membrane excitability and intracellular Ca^{2+} concentrations, resulting in the organization of release of neurotransmitters and the shape, duration and frequency of action potentials.

Cellular Expression of BK Channels

The expression of K_{Ca} channels in microgliaremains controversial.Some reports have suggested that IK and SK channels are expressed in microglia play roles in the biological activity of microglia (Schilling et al., 2004b; Kaushal et al., 2007). IK channels in microglia regulate morphology (Schilling et al., 2004a), resting membrane potential (Schilling et al., 2004b) and migration (Ifuku et al., 2007).On the other hand, SK channels contribute to respiratory burst (Khanna et al., 2001), neurotoxicity (Schlichter et al., 2010) and the expression of interleukin (IL)-1β, tumor necrosis factor-α, inducible nitric oxide synthase and IL-10(Liu et al., 2012). There is evidence that K_{Ca} currents in the primary cultured microglia are associated with BK or SK channels (Khanna et al., 2001; Eder, 2005; Bouhy et al., 2011). However, BK currents are not detected in acute hippocampal slices (Schilling and Eder, 2007). We obtained similar results showing that normal microglia in the spinal cord obtained with slice preparation exhibitedno or weak BK currents (Hayashi et al., 2011). Interestingly, hyperactive spinal microglia show large BK currents that are not SK channel-derived components (described below). In addition, the α subunit of BK channels is detected in both normal and hyperactivespinal microglia.The K_{Ca} channels in spinal microglia exhibit a preferential expression for experimental conditions. The BK channels in microglia show a preferential expression in *ex vivo* situations (Bordey and Spencer, 2003; Schilling and Eder, 2007) but not in cultured systems (Schilling et al., 2004b; Kaushal et al., 2007). In contrast, the expression of IK channels is primarily detected in reactive astrocytes, but not in macrophages or microglia, in injured spinal cord *in vivo* (Bouhy et al., 2011). On the basis of these observations, it may be concluded that spinal microglia express functional BK channels, but not IK channels, after cellular activation.

Interestingly, intrathecal administration of NS1619 (low concentration: 20μM, 0.072μg/10μl), a BK channel opener, significantly induces neuropathic pain-like behavior. In contrast, high concentrations of NS1619 (5555μM, 20μg/10μg) have no effect. Indeed, the effective dose of NS1619 *in vivo* is approximately 30 μg (Borbouse et al., 2009). Both concentrations of NS1619 can activate microglia; however, only the higher concentration of NS1619 can suppressneuronal activity.

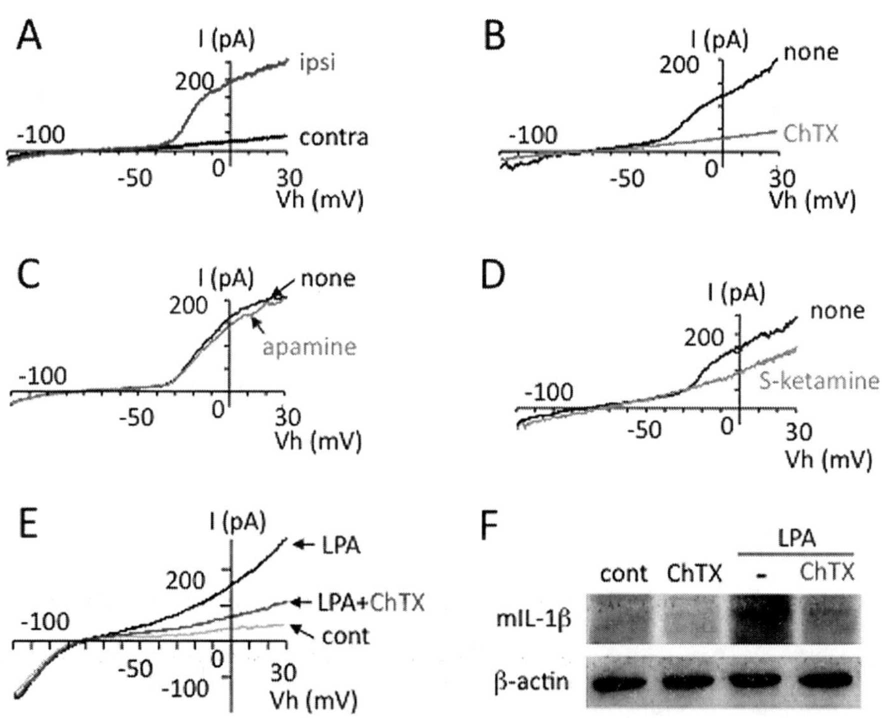

Figure 1. Activation of BK currents in spinal microglia after spinal nerve injury. A: Hyperactivated spinal microglia in the ipsilateral side exhibited outward rectifier activity compared with normal microglia in the contralateral side. B-D: The outward currents were sensitive to ChTX (B) and S-ketamine (D) but not apamine (C). E: Lysophosphatidic acid (LPA), a representative phospholipid derived from injured neurons, significantly activated BK currents in the cultured microglia. F: LPA triggeredmature IL-1β(mIL-1β) production via BK channels in microglia.

These observations might suggest that BK channel properties might be somewhat different in neurons and microglia. In addition, arachidonic acid and its metabolite significantly enhance BK currents in microglia in our preliminary experiments. Arachidonic acid increasesthe open probability of BK channels with β2 or β3, but not β4, subunits by single channel recording (Sun et al., 2007). Therefore, microglia might express β2 or β3 subunits.

THE PROPOSED FUNCTIONS OF BK CHANNELS IN MICROGLIA

BK channels work as brakes in electrical excitable cells; however, they are also expressed in non-excitable cells such as epithelial cells, endothelial cells and glial cells.The BK channelsin the non-excitable cells contribute to several functions such as osmoregulation(Turnheim et al., 1989), cell proliferation (Wiecha et al., 1998), cell migration (Soroceanu et al., 1999), and vascular dilation (Girouard et al., 2010).Recently, we detectedlarge outward currents in the spinal microglia of mice subjected to L4 spinal nerve transection-induced neuropathic pain (Hayashi et al., 2011). The currents were significantly suppressed by tetraethylammonium (TEA, 0.5mM), charybdotoxin (ChTX, 100nM) and iberiotoxin (IbTX,100nM), BK channel blockers, but not by apamin (1μM), an SK channel blocker (Figure 1). Thenerve-injury induced BK currents in spinal microglia were also significantly suppressed by S-ketamine (100 μM). On the other hand, lysophosphatidic acid (LPA, 1 μM) induced BK currents in cultured microglia (Figure 1). The immunoblot analyses for the LPA (1 μM)-induced increased level of mature IL-1β in cultured microglia showed that CThX significantly inhibited LPA-induced production of mature IL-1β (Figure 1F).

Ca^{2+} influx is necessary for the secretion of IL-1β, whereas membrane depolarization is known to inhibit IL-1β, processing and secretion from microglia. Therefore, it is believed that Ca^{2+} influx and the subsequent activation of BK channels play important roles in IL-1β processing and secretion from hyperactive microglia. However, the exact mechanisms by which the membrane hyperpolarization induces IL-1β processing and secretion from microglia remain unclear. Unlike excitable cells, non-excitable cells do not experience the large membrane depolarizations that are associated with action potential propagation and large Ca^{2+} sparks. Activation of Ca^{2+} channels might be attributed to depletion ofinternal Ca^{2+} stores (Ca^{2+} release activated Ca^{2+}channels) (Schilling et al., 2004b) rather than the membrane depolarization. In addition, Ca^{2+} influx is mediated throughnonselective cation channels in microglia (Moller et al., 2001). Interferon-γ, which activates microglia and induces IL-1β production, also triggers elevation of intracellular Ca^{2+} concentrations in human microglia (Franciosi et al., 2002). In some reports, BK channel openers have been found to change intracellular Ca^{2+} concentrationsbypartially affecting internal Ca^{2+} stores (Yamamura et al., 2001; Kraft et al., 2003). There might be a direct link between BK channels and the regulation of intracellular Ca^{2+}concentrations.Activation of BK channels results in the efflux of potassium ions and the subsequent alteration of the resting membrane potential. Indeed, NS1619, a BK channel opener, reduces resting membrane potentials (8.22±2.62 mV) in spinal microglia from naïve mice (our unpublished observation). Efflux of

K^+ is also involved in the activation of caspase-1, the interleukin converting enzyme(Andrei et al., 2004). Interestingly, BK channels contribute toIL-1β maturation and release (Colomar et al., 2003).

Based onthe above observations, the BK channels in microglia are known to regulate cellular functions. After undergoing cellular hyperactivation, spinal microglia exhibit BK currents around the resting membrane potentials (-37.1±4.29 mV), suggesting that the BK channels in the microglia might be functional under pathophysiological situations without membrane depolarization. Therefore, the BK channels in the non-excitable cells are critically involved in the cellular function, not only in the inhibition of membrane depolarization.

MODULATORY MOLECULES OF BK CHANNELS

BK channels are modulated by several factors, including intracellular H^+(Hou et al., 2008a), heme(Tang et al., 2003), carbon monoxide(Williams et al., 2004), ROS(DiChiara and Reinhart, 1997), NO(Hou et al., 2008b) and lipids(Sun et al., 2007). In our pain model, we foundthatLPA is the most potent molecule in the activation of microglial BK channels (Figure 2).

Furthermore, microglia BK channel activation during neuropathic pain is significantly suppressed by S-ketamine, a representative analgesic drug. This effect might be attributed to active binding of the intracellular Ca^{2+} binding domain of BK channels (Denson and Eaton, 1994).

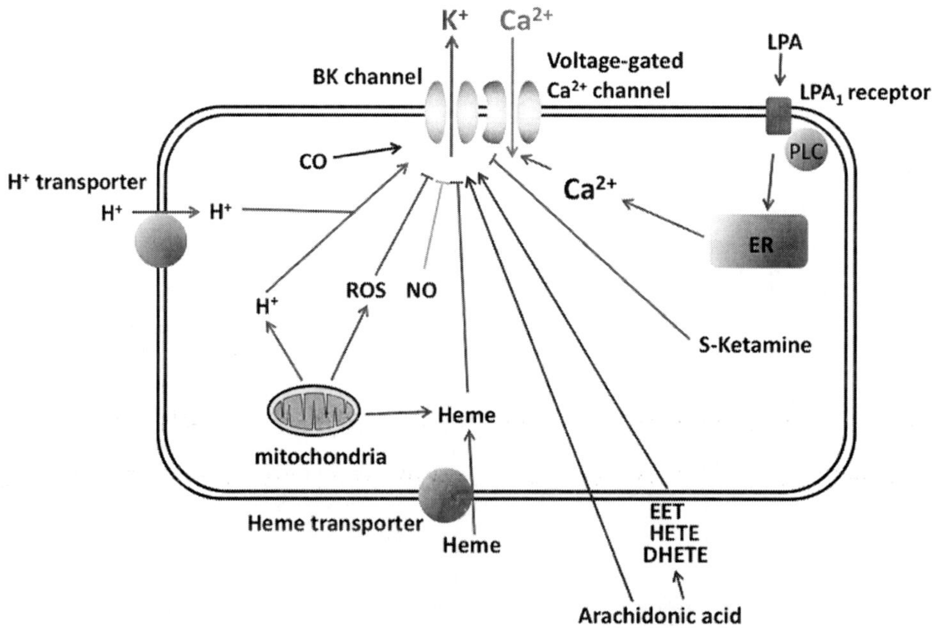

Figure 2. The regulatory molecules of BK channels: LPA (lysophosphatidic acid), PLC (phospholipase), ER (endoplasmic reticulum), EET (epoxyeicosatetraenoic acid), HETE (hydroxyeicosatetraenoic acids), DHETE (dihydroxyepoxyeicosatrienoic acid), NO (nitric oxide), ROS (reactive oxygen species) and CO (carbon monoxide).

Conclusion

The nature of BK channels is not fully understood. Recent studieshave elucidated the details of the open-close structure of BK channels (Yuan et al., 2012), novel regulation systems (Gonzalez-Perez et al., 2012) and novel auxiliary proteinsofthe α subunits (Yan and Aldrich, 2010). The growing understanding of the properties of microglial BK channels may contribute to the development of BK channel inhibitors as novel neuroprotective agents.

References

Andrei, C., Margiocco, P., Poggi, A., Lotti, L. V., Torrisi, M. R., Rubartelli, A. (2004). Phospholipases C and A_2 control lysosome-mediated IL-1b secretion: Implications for inflammatory processes. *Proc. Natl. Acad. Sci. U S.A.* 101, 9745-9750.

Borbouse, L., Dick, G. M., Asano, S., Bender, S. B., Dincer, U. D., Payne, G. A., Neeb, Z. P., Bratz, I. N., Sturek, M., Tune, J. D. (2009). Impaired function of coronary BK_{Ca} channels in metabolic syndrome. *Am. J. Physiol. Heart Circ. Physiol.* 297, H1629-1637.

Bordey, A., Spencer, D. D. (2003). Chemokine modulation of high-conductance Ca^{2+}-sensitive K^{+} currents in microglia from human hippocampi. *Eur. J. Neurosci.* 18, 2893-2898.

Bouhy, D., Ghasemlou, N., Lively, S., Redensek, A., Rathore, K. I., Schlichter, L. C., David, S. (2011). Inhibition of the Ca^{2+}-dependent K^{+} channel, KCNN4/KCa3.1, improves tissue protection and locomotor recovery after spinal cord injury. *J. Neurosci.* 31, 16298-16308.

Brenner, R., Chen, Q. H., Vilaythong, A., Toney, G. M., Noebels, J. L., Aldrich, R. W. (2005). BK channel b4 subunit reduces dentate gyrus excitability and protects against temporal lobe seizures. *Nat. Neurosci.* 8, 1752-1759.

Colomar, A., Marty, V., Medina, C., Combe, C., Parnet, P., Amedee, T. (2003). Maturation and release of interleukin-1b by lipopolysaccharide-primed mouse Schwann cells require the stimulation of $P2X_7$ receptors. *J. Biol. Chem.* 278, 30732-30740.

Denson, D. D., Eaton, D. C. (1994). Ketamine inhibition of large conductance Ca^{2+}-activated K^{+} channels is modulated by intracellular Ca^{2+}. *Am. J. Physiol.* 267, C1452-1458.

DiChiara, T. J., Reinhart, P. H. (1997). Redox modulation of hslo Ca^{2+}-activated K^{+} channels. *J. Neurosci.* 17, 4942-4955.

Du, W., Bautista, J. F., Yang, H., Diez-Sampedro, A., You, S. A., Wang, L., Kotagal, P., Luders, H. O., Shi, J., Cui, J., Richerson, G. B., Wang, Q. K. (2005). Calcium-sensitive potassium channelopathy in human epilepsy and paroxysmal movement disorder. *Nat. Genet.* 37, 733-738.

Eder, C. (2005). Regulation of microglial behavior by ion channel activity. *J. Neurosci. Res.* 81, 314-321.

Franciosi, S., Choi, H. B., Kim, S. U., McLarnon, J. G. (2002). Interferon-g acutely induces calcium influx in human microglia. *J. Neurosci. Res.* 69, 607-613.

Girouard, H., Bonev, A. D., Hannah, R. M., Meredith, A., Aldrich, R. W., Nelson, M. T. (2010). Astrocytic endfoot Ca^{2+} and BK channels determine both arteriolar dilation and constriction. *Proc. Natl. Acad. Sci. U. S. A.* 107, 3811-3816.

Gonzalez-Perez, V., Zeng, X. H., Henzler-Wildman, K., Lingle, C. J. (2012). Stereospecific binding of a disordered peptide segment mediates BK channel inactivation. *Nature* 485, 133-136.

Gribkoff, V. K. et al. (2001). Targeting acute ischemic stroke with a calcium-sensitive opener of maxi-K potassium channels. *Nat. Med.* 7, 471-477.

Hayashi, Y., Kawaji, K., Sun, L., Zhang, X., Koyano, K., Yokoyama, T., Kohsaka, S., Inoue, K., Nakanishi, H. (2011). Microglial Ca^{2+}-activated K^+ channels are possible molecular targets for the analgesic effects of S-ketamine on neuropathic pain. *J. Neurosci.* 31, 17370-17382.

Hou, S., Xu, R., Heinemann, S. H., Hoshi, T. (2008a). Reciprocal regulation of the Ca^{2+} and H^+ sensitivity in the SLO1 BK channel conferred by the RCK1 domain. *Nat. Struct. Mol. Biol.* 15, 403-410.

Hou, S., Xu, R., Heinemann, S. H., Hoshi, T. (2008b). The RCK1 high-affinity Ca^{2+} sensor confers carbon monoxide sensitivity to Slo1 BK channels. *Proc. Natl. Acad. Sci. U. S. A.* 105, 4039-4043.

Ifuku, M., Farber, K., Okuno, Y., Yamakawa, Y., Miyamoto, T., Nolte, C., Merrino, V. F., Kita, S., Iwamoto, T., Komuro, I., Wang, B., Cheung, G., Ishikawa, E., Ooboshi, H., Bader, M., Wada, K., Kettenmann, H., Noda, M. (2007). Bradykinin-induced microglial migration mediated by B_1-bradykinin receptors depends on Ca^{2+} influx via reverse-mode activity of the Na^+/Ca^{2+} exchanger. *J. Neurosci.* 27, 13065-13073.

Kaushal, V., Koeberle, P. D., Wang, Y., Schlichter, L. C. (2007). The Ca^{2+}-activated K^+ channel KCNN4/KCa3.1 contributes to microglia activation and nitric oxide-dependent neurodegeneration. *J. Neurosci.* 27, 234-244.

Kettenmann, H., Hanisch, U. K., Noda, M., Verkhratsky, A. (2011). Physiology of microglia. *Physiol. Rev.* 91, 461-553.

Khanna, R., Roy, L., Zhu, X., Schlichter, L. C. (2001). K^+ channels and the microglial respiratory burst. *Am. J. Physiol. Cell Physiol.* 280, C796-806.

Kraft, R., Krause, P., Jung, S., Basrai, D., Liebmann, L., Bolz, J., Patt, S. (2003). BK channel openers inhibit migration of human glioma cells. *Pflugers Arch.* 446, 248-255.

Lee, U. S., Cui, J. (2009). b subunit-specific modulations of BK channel function by a mutation associated with epilepsy and dyskinesia. *J. Physiol.* 587, 1481-1498.

Lesuffleur, A., Lim, K. S., Lindquist, N. C., Im, H., Warrington, A. E., Rodriguez, M., Oh, S. H. (2009). Plasmonic nanohole arrays for label-free kinetic biosensing in a lipid membrane environment. *Conf. Proc. IEEE Eng. Med. Biol. Soc.* 1481-1484.

Liu, B. S., Ferreira, R., Lively, S., Schlichter, L. C. (2012). Microglial SK3 and SK4 Currents and Activation State are Modulated by the Neuroprotective Drug, Riluzole. *J. Neuroimmune Pharmacol.*(DOI: 10.1007/s11481-012-9365-0)

Lorenz, S., Heils, A., Kasper, J. M., Sander, T. (2007). Allelic association of a truncation mutation of the KCNMB3 gene with idiopathic generalized epilepsy. *Am. J. Med. Genet. B Neuropsychiatr. Genet.* 144B, 10-13.

Martin, G. E., Hendrickson, L. M., Penta, K. L., Friesen, R. M., Pietrzykowski, A. Z., Tapper, A. R., Treistman, S. N. (2008). Identification of a BK channel auxiliary protein controlling molecular and behavioral tolerance to alcohol. *Proc. Natl. Acad. Sci. U. S. A.* 105, 17543-17548.

Moller, T., Contos, J. J., Musante, D. B., Chun, J., Ransom, B. R. (2001). Expression and function of lysophosphatidic acid receptors in cultured rodent microglial cells. *J. Biol. Chem.* 276, 25946-25952.

Orio, P., Rojas, P., Ferreira, G., Latorre, R. (2002). New disguises for an old channel: MaxiK channel beta-subunits. *News Physiol. Sci.* 17, 156-161.

Runden-Pran, E., Haug, F. M., Storm, J. F., Ottersen, O. P. (2002). BK channel activity determines the extent of cell degeneration after oxygen and glucose deprivation: a study in organotypical hippocampal slice cultures. *Neuroscience* 112, 277-288.

Salkoff, L., Butler, A., Ferreira, G., Santi, C., Wei, A. (2006). High-conductance potassium channels of the SLO family. *Nat. Rev. Neurosci.* 7, 921-931.

Sausbier, M., Hu, H., Arntz, C., Feil, S., Kamm, S., Adelsberger, H., Sausbier, U., Sailer, C. A., Feil, R., Hofmann, F., Korth, M., Shipston, M. J., Knaus, H. G., Wolfer, D. P., Pedroarena, C. M., Storm, J. F., Ruth, P. (2004). Cerebellar ataxia and Purkinje cell dysfunction caused by Ca^{2+}-activated K^{+} channel deficiency. *Proc. Natl. Acad. Sci. U. S. A.* 101, 9474-9478.

Schilling, T., Eder, C. (2007). Ion channel expression in resting and activated microglia of hippocampal slices from juvenile mice. *Brain Res.* 1186, 21-28.

Schilling, T., Lehmann, F., Ruckert, B., Eder, C. (2004a). Physiological mechanisms of lysophosphatidylcholine-induced de-ramification of murine microglia. *J. Physiol.* 557, 105-120.

Schilling, T., Stock, C., Schwab, A., Eder, C. (2004b). Functional importance of Ca^{2+}-activated K^{+} channels for lysophosphatidic acid-induced microglial migration. *Eur. J. Neurosci.* 19, 1469-1474.

Schlichter, L. C., Kaushal, V., Moxon-Emre, I., Sivagnanam, V., Vincent, C. (2010). The Ca^{2+} activated SK3 channel is expressed in microglia in the rat striatum and contributes to microglia-mediated neurotoxicity in vitro. *J. Neuroinflammation* 7:4.

Soroceanu, L., Manning, T. J., Jr., Sontheimer, H. (1999). Modulation of glioma cell migration and invasion using Cl^{-} and K^{+} ion channel blockers. *J. Neurosci.* 19, 5942-5954.

Sun, X., Zhou, D., Zhang, P., Moczydlowski, E. G., Haddad, G. G. (2007). b-subunit-dependent modulation of hSlo BK current by arachidonic acid. *J. Neurophysiol.* 97, 62-69.

Tang, X. D., Xu, R., Reynolds, M. F., Garcia, M. L., Heinemann, S. H., Hoshi, T. (2003). Haem can bind to and inhibit mammalian calcium-dependent Slo1 BK channels. *Nature* 425, 531-535.

Turnheim, K., Costantin, J., Chan, S., Schultz, S. G. (1989). Reconstitution of a calcium-activated potassium channel in basolateral membranes of rabbit colonocytes into planar lipid bilayers. *J. Membr. Biol.* 112, 247-254.

Wiecha, J., Munz, B., Wu, Y., Noll, T., Tillmanns, H., Waldecker, B. (1998). Blockade of Ca^{2+}-activated K^{+} channels inhibits proliferation of human endothelial cells induced by basic fibroblast growth factor. *J. Vasc. Res.* 35, 363-371.

Williams, S. E., Wootton, P., Mason, H. S., Bould, J., Iles, D. E., Riccardi, D., Peers, C., Kemp, P. J. (2004). Hemoxygenase-2 is an oxygen sensor for a calcium-sensitive potassium channel. *Science* 306, 2093-2097.

Yamamura, H., Ohi, Y., Muraki, K., Watanabe, M., Imaizumi, Y. (2001). BK channel activation by NS-1619 is partially mediated by intracellular Ca^{2+} release in smooth muscle cells of porcine coronary artery. *Br. J. Pharmacol.* 132, 828-834.

Yan, J., Aldrich, R. W. (2010). LRRC26 auxiliary protein allows BK channel activation at resting voltage without calcium. *Nature* 466, 513-516.

Yuan, P., Leonetti, M. D., Hsiung, Y., MacKinnon, R. (2012). Open structure of the Ca^{2+} gating ring in the high-conductance Ca^{2+}-activated K^+ channel. *Nature* 481, 94-97.

In: Glial Cells
Editors: Charanjit Kaur and Eng-Ang Ling
ISBN: 978-1-62618-448-0
© 2013 Nova Science Publishers, Inc.

Chapter 9

PHYSIOLOGICAL INTERACTIONS BETWEEN NEURONS AND GLIA: ROLES OF TRANSPORTERS IN THE CONTROL OF INTERSYNAPTIC CROSSTALK

Shiro Konishi[1*] and Shin'Ichiro Satake[2,3]
[1]Department of Neurophysiology, Kagawa School of Pharmaceutical Sciences and Institute of Neuroscience, Tokushima Bunri University, Sanuki, Japan
[2]Department of Information Physiology, National Institute of Physiological Sciences (NIPS), Myodaiji-cho, Okazaki, Japan
[3]School of Life Science, The Graduate University for Advanced Studies (SOKENDAI), Myodaiji-cho, Okazaki, Japan

ABSTRACT

Since the pioneering work by Stephen Kuffler and his colleagues on physiology of glial cells in 1960s, there had been a considerable delay until recent extensive efforts to recognize and understand the physiological significance of glial cells. In the vertebrate nervous system, glia outnumber neurons by over fivefold, but they had been considered as an element that would play only a supportive role for maintaining neurons. A number of studies during the past decade have provided a line of evidence that the major subtype of glial cells, astrocytes, not only sense the electrical activity within neuronal circuits but also they can control the gain of synaptic transmission and neural plasticity in the brain. Consequently, we are now on the cusp of a new understanding of the brain that forms a century of conventional thinking about the role of the brain's neurons (Fields, 2009).

In this chapter, we focus on the physiological significance of neuron-astrocyte interactions in the control of brain function. Particular attention is also placed on the differential roles of glial and neuronal glutamate transporters in the control of synaptic transmission as well as intersynaptic diffusion of an excitatory neurotransmitter that could regulate neurotransmission at nearby synapses.

[*] Correspondence to: Shiro Konishi, skonishi@kph.bunri-u.ac.jp.

INTRODUCTION

The central nervous system (CNS) contains two main populations of cells: neurons and glial cells. In fact, only 15 percent of the cells in our brain are neurons, and the rest of our brain cells are glia (Fields, 2009; Kuffler, 1967). Previously glial cells were presumed to play a supportive and housekeeping role in the CNS to help the neuron's function of information processing in the brain and spinal cord.

Over the past decade, however, glial cells, and especially astrocytes, have been proposed to serve as a conductor in orchestrating a variety of brain functions that include synaptic plasticity associated with learning and memory (Dityatev and Rusakov, 2011), magnocellular neuroendcrine control of pituitary hormones (Tasker et al., 2012) and sleep and circadian rhythm control (Blutstein and Haydon, 2013).

Accumulating evidence has suggested that neurons and astrocytes communicate via chemical transmitters in reciprocal manners. Much focus of recent studies in neuroscience has been placed on roles of neuron-astrocyte interactions in the control of brain functions. In response to neuronal activity and neurotransmitters, astrocytes can release the gliotransmitters glutamate, D-serine and ATP, which act on nearby neurons and modulate the gain of synaptic transmission in diverse temporal and spatial domains (Halassa and Haydon, 2010). For instance, glutamate liberated by astrocytes targets neuronal NMDA receptors and results in two forms of modulation, slow-inward currents and a tonic change of synaptic transmission in the hippocampus (Fellin et al., 2006).

Another intriguing example of astrocyte-neuron interactions has been provided in the hypothalamus where D-serine secreted by astrocytes in the supraoptic nucleus co-activates NMDA receptors and modulates the state of synaptic plasticity in the neuroendocrine system (Tasker et al., 2012).

ATP can also be released by astrocytes and has been proposed to serve as the signal mediating propagation of Ca^{2+} wave through the coupled glial network as well as communicating to neurons for modulation of synaptic transmission. Indeed, ATP released from glial cells in response to noradrenaline stimulation has been shown to enhance glutamatergic excitatory transmission at the paraventricular nucleus of hypothalamus (Gordon et al., 2005). Moreover, ATP released into the cerebellar cortex has also been reported to induce long-term facilitation of GABAergic inhibitory transmission at cerebellar interneuron-Purkinje cell synapses through an increase in the postsynaptic $GABA_A$ receptor sensitivity (Saitow et al., 2005b, see also Figure 3).

Thus, glial cells can actively participate in synaptic transmission by clearing neurotransmitters from the synaptic cleft, receiving signals from adjacent neurons and, in turn, liberating gliotransmitters that can modulate signal transfer within neuronal circuits. This chapter will focus on some aspects of neuron-glia interactions involved in clearing neurotransmitters released into the synaptic cleft.

In particular, we will discuss about differential roles of glial and neuronal glutamate transporters that participate in the clearance of glutamate released by excitatory synaptic inputs to the cerebellar neural circuits mainly based on results of recent studies from our and other laboratories. Some features of astrocyte-mediated modulation of neurotransmission at central synapses will also be reviewed.

Table 1. The high-affinity glutamate transporters (SLC1 family)

Gene name	Protein name	Gene locus	Tissue distribution
SLC1A1	EAAT3, EAAC1	Mouse 19C1 Human 9p24	Brain (neurons), intestine, kidney, liver, heart
SLC1A2	EAAT2, GLT-1	Mouse 2E2 Human 11p13-p12	Brain (astrocytes), liver
SLC1A3	EAAT1, GLAST	Mouse 15A2 Human 5p13	Brain (astrocytes), heart, placenta skeletal muscle
SLC1A6	EAAT4	Mouse 10C1 Human 19p13.12	Cerebellum (Purkinje cells)
SLC1A7	EAAT5	Mouse 4C7 Human 1p32.3	Retina (photoreceptor cells, bipolar cells)

EAAT protein transports glutamate depending on the electrochemical gradients of cotransported three sodium ions and one proton, and counter-transports one potassium ion. In addition, EAAT displays a glutamate-activated chloride conductance that is not thermodynamically coupled to the substrate translocation (for reviews, Danbolt, 2001; Tzingounis and Wadiche, 2007).

Differential Roles of Glial and Neuronal Transporters in the Control of Glutamatergic Neurotransmission

Glutamate transporters clear synaptically released glutamate and function to maintain extracellular glutamate concentrations below excitotoxic levels (for reviews, Danbolt, 2001; Kanai and Hediger et al., 2004; Tzingounis and Wadiche, 2007). Five structurally related glutamate transporters have so far been identified (GLAST/EAAT1, GLT-1/EAAT2, EAAC1/EAAT3, EAAT4, and EAAT5), and they are included in the solute carrier 1 (SLC1) gene family (Table 1).

Transport of glutamate into brain cells is an energy-consuming process. Glutamate taken up by cells is recycled not only for its neurotransmitter role, but also utilized for metabolic purposes, such as protein synthesis, energy production and ammonia fixation (Figure 1; for a review, McKenna, 2007).

In glial cells (astrocytes), glutamate taken up from the extracellular space is converted to glutamine. Glial glutamine is released again to the extracellular fluid and taken up by neurons (that is, glutamate-glutamine cycle, for reviews, Mackenzie and Erickson, 2004; McKenna, 2007).

In neurons, reuse of glutamate for a neurotransmitter seems to be straightforward. Namely, glutamate is transported into synaptic vesicles through vesicular transporters and subsequently released by exocytosis. For removal of the inhibitory neurotransmitter GABA, reuptake into the presynaptic terminal is thought as a prominent mechanism (Schousboe, 2003; Kristensen et al., 2011).

As neuronal glutamate transporters are accumulated at perisyanptic regions of postsynaptic dendrites (Furuta et al., 1997; Dehnes et al., 1998), it is not known whether these neuronal transporters are able to contribute to glutamate recycling. Glutamate taken up by neurons is metabolized to a large extent through transamination. For example, in cerebellar granule cells, glutamate is preferentially metabolized for energy production, rather than to glutamine (Olstad et al., 2007).

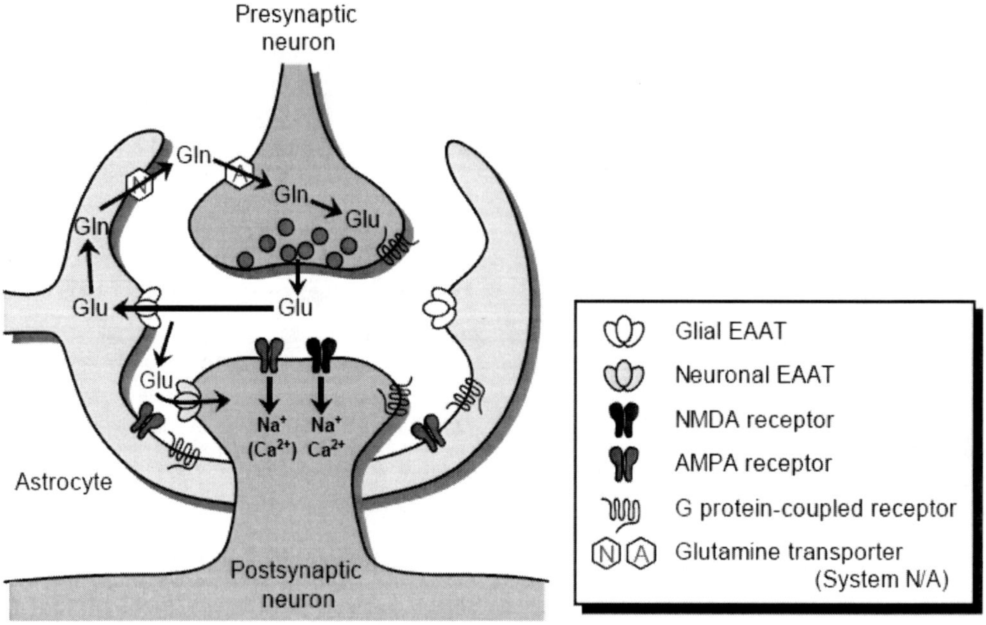

Figure 1. Schematic representation of transmitter uptake (EAAT) and recycling system (Gln-Glu cycle) around the glutamatergic synapse.

Exogenous glutamate taken up from the extracellular space and endogenous glutamate produced from glutamine via glutaminase can be distinguished by glial and neuronal cells. Formation of the neurotransmitter glutamate involves both transamination and its entry into mitochondria. Endogenous glutamate formed by glutaminase from glutamine enters the tricarboxylic acid (TCA) cycle, and energy derived from glycolysis is used for packaging glutamate into synaptic vesicles.

The transporter-mediated rapid clearance is indispensable for ensuring a high signal-to-noise ratio for glutamatergic neurotransmission, and it exerts a marked effect on the peak amplitude and kinetics of excitatory postsynaptic currents (EPSCs) at various synapses in the CNS (Takahashi et al., 1995; Takayasu et al., 2004, 2005; Tsukada et al., 2005).

Glutamate transporters are expressed in both neurons and glial cells, the glial transporters clearly outnumber the neuronal transporters (Danbolt, 2001). As discuss below, electrophysiological experiments using EAAT (excitatory amino acid transporter) mutant mice have provided evidence that glial and neuronal transporters mediate differential roles at different excitatory synapses converging onto cerebellar Purkinje cells (PCs) (Takayasu et al., 2009).

Roles of Glial Transporter in Cerebellar Synaptic Transmission

The glial transporters (GLAST and GLT-1) are expressed on the lamellate processes of Bergmann glia (BG, astrocytes in the cerebellum) that surround excitatory synapses on dendritic spines of PCs, but they are located remotely from the synaptic cleft (Chaudhry et al., 1995; Yamada et al., 2000). GLAST plays a major role in clearing glutamate that spills out of the synaptic cleft immediately after the release from climbing fibers (CFs) and parallel fibers (PFs). In the presence of cyclothiazide, which reduces the desensitization of AMPA receptors and increases the affinity of glutamate to these receptors, there were clear increases in the amplitude and decay time constant of CF- or PF-mediated EPSCs in GLAST$^{-/-}$ mice as compared to CF- or PF-EPSCs in wild-type mice, respectively (Takayasu et al., 2005). Such changes in the EPSC amplitude and kinetics were not observed in the absence of cyclothiazide, suggesting that the clearance of glutamate at PC synapses is impaired in GLAST$^{-/-}$ mice but the transporter activity is largely masked by rapid and strong desensitization of AMPA receptors under physiological conditions.

This GLAST-mediated uptake can allow a one-to-one (point-to-point) synaptic transmission at the CF-PC synapse and prevent escape of the CF transmitter glutamate from the synaptic cleft to extrasynaptic sites (Takayasu et al., 2006). The dendritic arbors of PCs spread widely in the molecular layer to the transverse plane of the folium within a restricted longitudinal plane, and fine lamellate processes of BG segregate dendritic arbors of individual PCs (Müller and Kettenmann, 1995). Thus, flat dendritic sheets of PCs are compactly arranged in parallel with the transverse plane. In association with this morphological arrangement and the GLAST-mediated glutamate uptake, BG can prevent longitudinal interactions of glutamate that might diffuse from synaptic sites between the dendritic sheets of adjacent PCs.

Not only GLAST, but also GLT-1 is involved in the glutamate uptake at cerebellar synapses. The impact of GLT-1 on the uptake appears to be less effective than that of GLAST, because of roughly one-sixth less amount of GLT-1 proteins in BG (Lehre and Danbolt, 1998). Moreover, deletion of GLT-1 has been reported to have no significant influences on morphological development of the cerebellum and cause no signs of cerebellar ataxia (Tanaka et al., 1997).

However, the deletion of the GLT-1 gene resulted in lethal spontaneous seizures and enhanced susceptibility to acute cortical injury (Tanaka et al., 1997; Mitani and Tanaka, 2003). These phenotypes appear to originate from elevated extracellular glutamate concentrations in forebrain regions (Tanaka et al., 1997; Tsukada et al., 2005).

Deletion of both GLAST and GLT-1 genes causes severe developmental defects in the CNS, which include disorganization of the cortex, hippocampus and olfactory bulb, thereby resulting in perinatal death. By contrast, deletion of either GLAST or GLT-1 does not affect the gross development of the cerebellum, suggesting that the presence of either GLAST or GLT-1 is sufficient for clearing glutamate from the extrasynaptic space and preventing its neurotoxicity to allow the normal development of the cerebellum. Although GLT-1 is a less abundant glutamate transporter compared to GLAST (Lehre and Danbolt, 1998), this molecule is capable of maintaining normal morphogenesis of the cerebellum in the absence of GLAST. The findings thus indicate that the two distinct types of glial glutamate transporters GLAST and GLT-1 can secure clearing of glutamate from the extracellular space for normal development of the cerebellum.

Neuronal Transporter Controls Extrasynaptic Diffusion of Synaptically Released Glutamate

In contrast to the glial transporters, the neuronal transporter EAAT4 in PCs has been implicated in the removal of residual glutamate that escapes from the uptake mechanism mediated by glial transporters during the late phase of EPSCs. Thus, EAAT4 appears to limit residual glutamate reaching to adjacent synapses via intersynaptic diffusion (Takayasu et al., 2005). EAAT4 proteins are specifically and predominantly expressed in the extra-junctional membranes of dendritic spines of PCs (Furuta et al., 1997). Type 1 metabotropic glutamate receptors, mGluR1, also occur at perisynaptic sites, namely the edge of postsynaptic densities, of PF-PC synapses and play an important role in mediating synapse formation, synaptic plasticity (long-term depression, LTD), and motor coordination associated with the cerebellum (Ichise et al., 2000). Repetitive activation of PFs elicits an mGluR1-mediated slow synaptic excitation in PCs (Batchelor et al., 1994; Hirono et al., 1998). Subsequently, Kim et al. (2003) reported that this slow synaptic response is produced by activation of mGluR1 coupled to non-specific cation channels, TRPC1. Then, Wadiche and Jahr (2005) found that there is a reverse correlation between the amplitude of this mGluR1/TRPC1-mediated synaptic current and the density of the glutamate transporter EAAT4 in PCs, and demonstrated that regional differences in glutamate transporter expression affect the degree of mGluR activation at perisynaptic sites.

EAAT4 in PCs has been shown to exhibit different expression patterns throughout the cerebellar cortex (Dehnes et al., 1998). The amplitude of mGluR1/TRPC1-mediated synaptic currents produced by PF stimulation is significantly larger in $EAAT4^{-/-}$ mice than that in wild-type mice (Nikkuni et al., 2007). Pharmacological blockade of neuronal glutamate transporters in PCs has been shown not only to increase the mGluR1/TRPC1-mediated synaptic response but also to enhance a form of mGluR-mediated synaptic plasticity, LTD (long-term depression) (Brasnjo and Otis, 2001). These findings suggest that the regional difference in the neuronal glutamate transporter EAAT4 expression is critical for mGluR1-mediated slow synaptic excitation that could be induced in a neural circuit specific manner, namely particular PCs being controlled by mGluR-mediated slow EPSPs in the cerebellar cortex.

In summary, glial and neuronal transporters in the cerebellar cortex play differential roles in clearing glutamate from the extracellular space. The glial glutamate transporter GLAST and GLT-1 appear to clear a large portion of synaptically released glutamate spreading over glial processes that surround the synaptic cleft. By contrast, the neuronal transporter EAAT4 appears to mediate the removal of less abundant glutamate escaping from the GLAST-mediated uptake and remaining in the extrasynaptic space at a later phase after synaptic release. Because the affinity of EAAT4 to glutamate is ten-fold higher than that of GLAST (Arriza et al., 1994; Fairman et al., 1995), each of these transporters would mediate different roles in glutamatergic synaptic signaling within the cerebellar cortex.

Regulation of Glutamate-Mediated Intersynaptic Modification by Neuronal Transporter

Neurotransmitters act not only on postsynaptic receptors, but also spill out of the synaptic cleft and reach neighbouring receptors to modulate the gain and synaptic plasticity of neurotransmission at nearby synapses. Glutamate exerts a variety of synaptic modulation by acting on either autoreceptors within single synaptic connections or heteroreceptors in neighbouring synapses (for a review, Frerking and Wondolowski, 2008). Glutamate-induced presynaptic modification of neurotransmission is mediated by either metabotropic or ionotropic receptors (for reviews, Pinheiro and Mulle, 2008; Dorostkar and Boehm, 2008; Upreti et al., 2013).

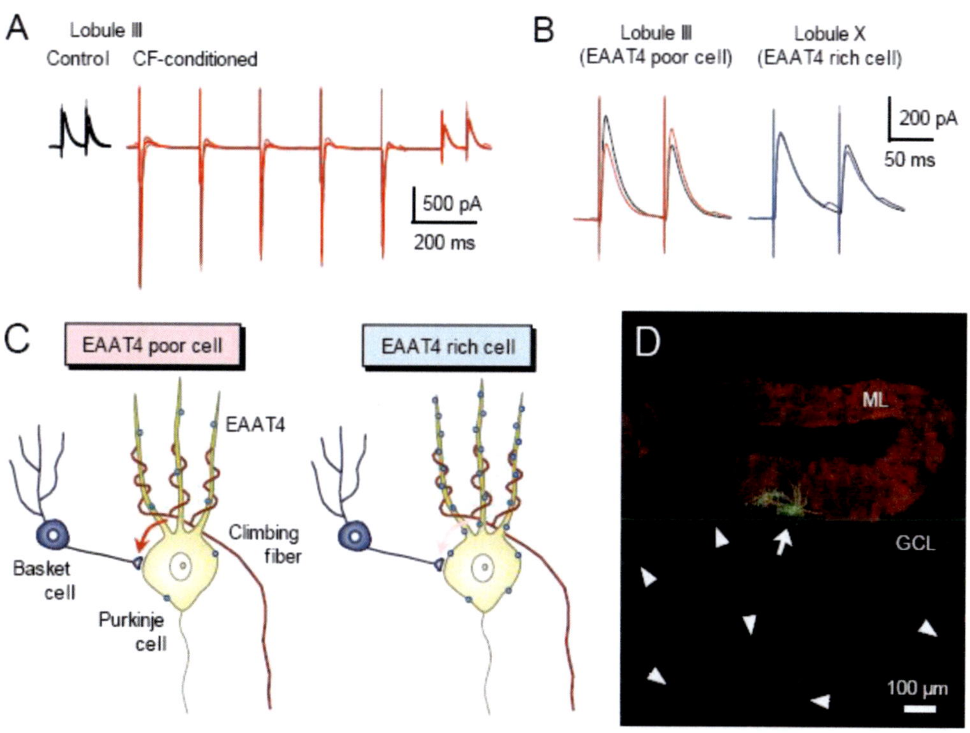

Figure 2. Regional differences in EAAT4 expression and intersynaptic modification in the cerebellar cortex. (A) Inhibition of GABA release at basket cell (BC)-Purkinje cell (PC) synapses induced in response to conditioning stimulation of climbing fibers (CF) (5 Hz for 1 s). Five successive traces recorded every 15 s were superimposed. Upward and downward deflections are BC stimulation-induced test IPSCs and EPSCs produced in a PC by CF-conditioning stimulation, respectively. (B) Averaged traces of IPSCs in PCs at lobules III and X examined before (*black*) and after the conditioning stimulation (*red* and *blue*, respectively). (C) Schematic drawing illustrating the relationship between the density of EAAT4 expression in PCs and the degree of intersynaptic glutamate diffusion from CFs to BC terminals. (D) Double-immunofluorescence staining of EAAT4 (*red*) and biocytin (*green*) injected into a single BC in a parasagittal cerebellar section derived from the cerebellum of 2 week-old rat. Note that EAAT4 immunoreactivity preferentially distributes to discrete regions. This labeled basket cell indicated by an arrow is located in an EAAT4 rich region. PCs with poor EAAT4 expression are also shown by arrowheads. ML, molecular layer; GCL, granule cell layer.

In the cerebellar cortex, activation of CFs elicits a powerful postsynaptic excitation of PCs. When repeatedly activated, the CF causes another action, depression of GABA release at interneuron basket cell (BC)-PC synapses (Figure 2A; Satake et al., 2000). A line of evidence has suggested that the latter CF-mediated modification of GABA release is produced by intersynaptic diffusion of the CF transmitter glutamate and activation of AMPA receptors expressed on the BC axon terminals (Satake et al., 2004, 2006). Indeed, application of AMPA suppresses Ca^{2+} transients into BC axon terminals produced in response to activation of the BC soma (Satake et al., 2004; Rusakov et al., 2005). Therefore, the CF input causes not only excitation of the PC by the direct postsynaptic action on the PC but also inhibition of GABAergic transmission from BCs converging onto the same PC (namely, disinhibition) by the indirect action of intersynaptic diffusion of the CF transmitter (Figure 2 and 3).

The neuronal glutamate transporter EAAT4 in PCs has been implicated in the regulation of the intersynaptic diffusion of CF-derived glutamate that can underlie heterosynaptic depression of GABA release (Satake et al., 2010). EAAT4 displays a unique expression pattern that is closely analogous to a parasagittal band pattern of PCs positive to a specific protein, zebrin II/aldolase C (Dehnes et al., 1998; Welsh et al., 2002).

There is a close relationship between the magnitude of the CF-induced depression of GABAergic transmission and the extent of EAAT4 expression in PC populations. The inhibitory action of CF on GABA release is profound in lobule III, where the EAAT4 expression level was low, whereas the action is marginal in lobule X, where EAAT4 was abundant (Figure 2B–D; see also Satake et al., 2010). The olivocerebellar projection is organized into a parasagittally oriented band of PCs and, in turn, the PCs in this particular band project to a circumscribed region in the cerebellar deep nuclei. In this way, this loop results in forming discrete olivo-cortico-nuclear complexes in association with discrete densities of EAAT4 bands in the PC layer. Thus, the regional difference in the anatomical and chemical architectures within the parasagittal bands of the cerebellar cortex likely underlies decision of the strength for individual neural pathways.

In addition to this role of neuronal glutamate transporter, tetanic stimulation given to CF-PC synapses results in long-term potentiation (LTP) of a CF-evoked glutamate transporter current, possibly mediated by EAAT4 in PCs. This LTP is postsynaptically expressed and requires activation of mGluR1–protein kinase C cascade (Shen and Linden, 2005). In consistent with this finding, the magnitude of CF-induced heterosynaptic depression of GABA release is reduced by inducing this use-dependent enhancement of the glutamate transporter activity in PCs (Satake et al., 2010). Collectively, it is highly likely that the glutamate uptake mechanism mediated by the neuronal transporter EAAT4 in the postsynaptic PC serves as a crucial element for retrograde and dynamic regulation of intersynaptic diffusion of glutamate that could mediate the crosstalk between CFs and BCs in the cerebellar cortex.

Glial Regulation of Synaptic Transmission: Gliotransmitter Release and Morphological Plasticity

It has become increasingly clear that glial cells, in particular astrocytes, are active and dynamic participants along with neuronal cells in generating, coordinating and sustaining electrical activity in the neuronal network. A single astrocyte closely apposes their processes to more than tens of thousands of synapses, though individual astrocytes occupy distinct and non-overlapping domains in the brain (Halassa and Haydon, 2010).

Thus, astroglia respond to changes in the activity of their adjacent neurons by the use of ion channels, receptors, and transporters expressed on their surface, and using this set of molecular machinery they can identify the activity of individual neurons. For example, when particular G protein-coupled receptors on astrocytes are activated, this signal stimulates phospholipase C and production of inositol 1,4,5-triphosphate (IP3), thereby leading to increase in the intracellular Ca^{2+} concentration through the release of Ca^{2+} from intracellular stores (Guček et al., 2012). Moreover, astrocytes are implicated in regulation of synaptic information flow through their contacting volume domains. This has led to the concept of tripartite synapses, in which glial cells share integral elements with pre- and post-synaptic neurons.

Astrocytes release active signaling molecules, which includes glutamate, ATP (and the metabolite, adenosine), D-serine, neuropeptides, neurotrophins and lipid mediators, to modulate neighboring neuron activity (Tasker et al., 2012; Guček et al., 2012). In particular, D-serine plays a prominent role as an endogenous co-agonist at the glycine site of NMDA receptors. Intriguingly, a recent study by Papouin et al. (2012) has demonstrated that astrocyte-derived D-serine and glycine are both endogenous coagonists for neuronal NMDA receptors but act at distinct population of receptors, with D-serine present at synaptic NMDA receptors and glycine at their extrasynaptic counterparts. Thus, it would be of interest to further ask what differential physiological and pathological roles could be played by D-serine and glycine derived from glial cells through activation of synaptic and extrasynaptic NMDA receptors.

The neuronal network activity, when it is intense and sustained, recruits Ca^{2+} increases in subpopulations of astrocytes not only through glutamate spillover but also via point-to-point signaling from neurons to astrocytes (Panatier et al., 2011). The occurrence of glial processes on the postsynaptic side is 3-4-fold higher than that on the presynaptic side (Figure 1; see also Lehre and Rusakov, 2002). This postsynaptically asymmetric distribution appears to be suitable for astroglia to track synaptic activity efficiently. Astrocytes can detect local neurotransmitter release both at synaptic and ectopic sites (Matsui and Jahr, 2003). Calcium elevation in astroglia is associated with a release of gliotransmitters. Several different mechanisms appear to underlie gliotransmitter release, including exocytosis, reverse operation of transporters, and hemichannel (Guček et al., 2012). Each of gliotransmitters has different synaptic targets in influencing the synaptic activity. In the hippocampal CA1 area, astrocytic glutamate release elicits various effects on neuronal activity depending on the kinetics of Ca^{2+} elevations in the astrocyte.

A slow Ca^{2+} elevation in astrocytes triggers a slow inward current in CA1 neurons through activation of extrasynaptic NMDA receptors (Fellin et al., 2004). By contrast, a faster Ca^{2+} elevation elicits presynaptic modulation of neurotransmitter release through activation of A_{2A} receptors by the gliotransmitter adenosine (Panatier et al., 2011). In addition, depending on the intensity, timing of coincidence, and pattern of synaptic activity, these local modifications spread out to the whole astrocyte bodies through propagation of the Ca^{2+} waves (Verkhratsky et al., 2012). Glial cells therefore can integrate and adapt the neuronal network activity in accord with the activity history of the synapse.

In addition to gliotransmission leading to modulation of electrical signaling at synapses, morphological change of glial processes in the vicinity of synapses also has a profound impact on the concentration and the degree of neurotransmitter diffusion. A striking example of glial cell–mediated regulation of neuronal activity in association with anatomical remodeling has been provided in the magnocellular neuroendocrine system of the hypothalamic paraventricular and supraoptic nuclei (for a review, Tasker et al., 2012). The supraoptic nucleus (SON) is a homogenous neuronal center composed of oxytocin and vasopressin neurons projecting to the posterior lobe of the pituitary gland, and known to undergo an extensive withdrawal of astrocytic coverage on neurons and synapses under conditions like lactation (Oliet et al., 2001). This anatomical change of astrocytic processes leads to modification of the action range of signaling molecules.

Synaptically released glutamate diffuses away from its release site to extrasynaptic regions and heterosynaptically acts on group III-mGluRs expressed in neighboring GABAergic axon terminals, thereby causing inhibition of GABA release. First, this heterosynaptic inhibition is enhanced when astroglial ensheathing of SON neurons is reduced in lactating animals (Oliet et al., 2001; Piet et al., 2004).

Second, the anatomical remodeling of the SON dramatically affects gliotransmission as well. When glial coverage of magnocellular neurons is retracted during lactation, NMDA receptor-mediated processes, such as synaptic plasticity, are impaired as a result of a diminished concentration of the gliotransmitter D-serine within the synaptic cleft (Panatier et al., 2006). Therefore, under basal conditions (i.e., in virgin animals), uptake of ambient glutamate by astrocytic coverage restrains the activity, namely the excitability, of SON neurons, whereas during lactation, as a consequence of an activity-dependent remodeling of the local neuronal-glial microenvironment, a decrease in the capability of glial glutamate uptake mechanism enhances the synchronization of SON neuron bursting. The function of astrocytes and gliotransmission revealed at this anatomical locus would be extended to other central synapses.

CONCLUSION

One population of glial cells, astrocytes, surround synapses and serve as the structural substrate for reciprocal chemical signaling between neurons and glia. Astrocytes can detect the neuronal activity by sensing neurotransmitters released by neurons via a plethora of receptors expressed in astrocytes and, in turn, release gliotransmitters that can influence information processing and plasticity at excitatory and inhibitory synapses within the CNS. The gliotransmitters glutamate, D-serine and ATP likely play crucial roles in modulation of excitatory and inhibitory transmission with the short- and long-term ranges at various anatomical loci in the brain (see Figure 3). Thus, perturbations of neuron-glia interactions could underlie pathogenesis of numerous neurological disorders. Further studies on neuron-glia interactions in normal and disease model animals therefore will not only provide more detailed information about their effects on the relationship between the activity of particular brain pathways and behavioral responses, and also their influences on disorders of brain functions that include psychiatric diseases and neurodegenerative diseases.

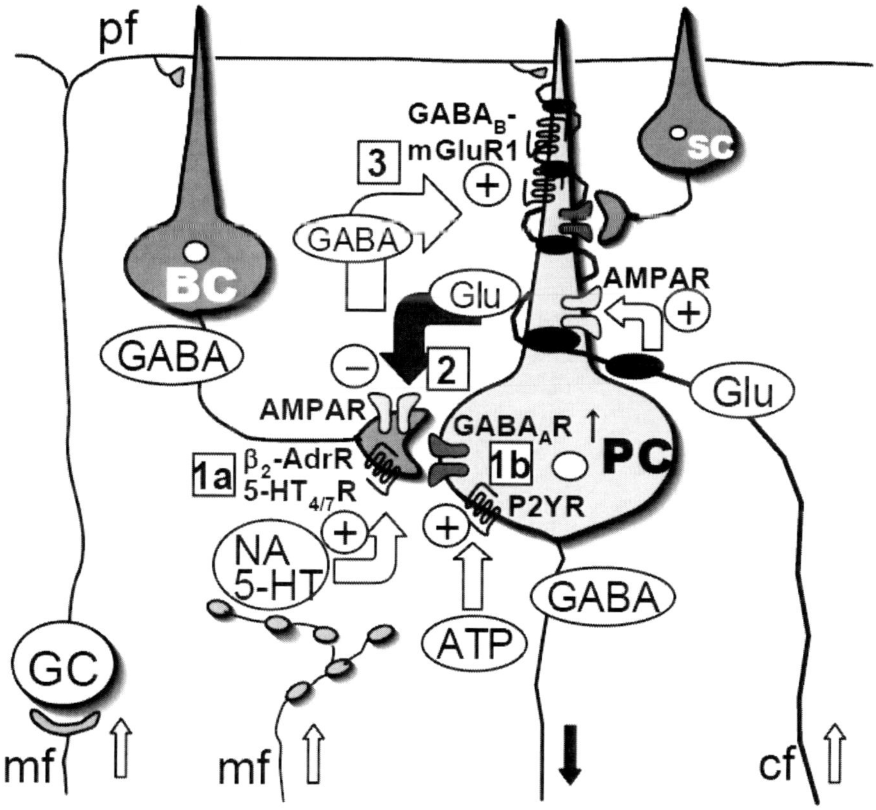

Figure 3. Positive and negative regulation of inhibitory GABAergic transmission, and crosstalk between $GABA_B$ receptors and metabotropic glutamate receptors in the cerebellar cortex. (1a) Monoamines, noradrenaline and serotonin, causes long-lasting facilitation of GABA release from cerebellar interneurons, BCs (Saitow et al., 2005a). (1b) ATP causes long-term potentiation of GABAergic transmission on to Purkinje cells through an increase in the postsynaptic $GABA_A$ receptor sensitivity (Saitow et al., 2005b). (2) The climbing fiber transmitter, possibly glutamate, elicits not only powerful excitation in Purkinje cells, but also profound inhibition of GABA release from basket cells via activation of AMPA receptors in basket cell terminals (Satake et al., 2010). (3) GABA released from basket cells acts on nearby $GABA_B$ receptors located at peripheral regions of excitatory PF-PC synapses and enhances via receptor crosstalk the slow synaptic excitation mediated by mGluR1-type metabotropic glutamate receptors in PCs (Hirono et al., 2001, 2012).

REFERENCES

Arriza, J.L., Fairman, W.A., Wadiche, J.I., Murdoch, G.H., Kavanaugh, M.P. and Amara, S.G. (1994) Functional comparisons of three glutamate transporter subtypes cloned from human motor cortex. *J. Neurosci.* 14, 5559–5569.

Batchelor, A.M., Madge, D.J., Garthwaite, J. (1994) Synaptic activation of metabotropic glutamate receptors in the parallel fibre-Purkinje cell pathway in rat cerebellar slices. *Neuroscience* 63, 911–915.

Blutstein, T. and Haydon, P.G. (2013) The importance of astrocyte-derived purines in the modulation of sleep. *Glia* 61, 129–139.

Brasnjo, G. and Otis, T.S. (2001) Neuronal glutamate transporters control activation of postsynaptic metabotropic glutamate receptors and influence cerebellar long-term depression. *Neuron* 31, 607–616.

Chaudhry, F.A., Lehre, K.P., van Lookeren Campagne, M., Ottersen, O.P., Danbolt, N.C. and Storm-Mathisen, J. (1995) Glutamate transporters in glial plasma membranes: highly differentiated localizations revealed by quantitative ultrastructural immunocytochemistry. *Neuron* 15, 711–720.

Danbolt, N.C. (2001) Glutamate uptake. *Prog. Neurobiol.* 65, 1–105.

Dehnes, Y., Chaudhry, F.A., Ullensvang, K., Lehre, K.P., Storm-Mathisen, J. and Danbolt, N.C. (1998) The glutamate transporter EAAT4 in rat cerebellar Purkinje cells: a glutamate-gated chloride channel concentrated near the synapse in parts of the dendritic membrane facing astroglia. *J. Neurosci.* 18, 3606–3619.

Dityatev, A. and Rusakov, D.A. (2011) Molecular signals of plasticity at the tetrapartite synapse. *Curr. Opin. Neurobiol.* 21, 353–359.

Dorostkar, M.M. and Boehm, S. (2008) Presynaptic ionotropic receptors. In *Pharmacology of Neurotransmitter Release*, ed. Südhof, T.C. and Starke, K., *Handb. Exp. Pharmacol.* 184, 479–527.

Fairman, W.A., Vandenberg, R.J., Arriza, J.L., Kavanaugh, M.P. and Amara, S.G. (1995) An excitatory amino-acid transporter with properties of a ligand-gated chloride channel. *Nature* 375, 599–603.

Fellin, T., Pascual, O., Gobbo, S., Pozzan, T., Haydon, P.G. and Carmignoto, G. (2004) Neuronal synchrony mediated by astrocytic glutamate through activation of extrasynaptic NMDA receptors. *Neuron* 43, 729–743.

Fields, R.D. (2009) *The Other Brain: From Dementia to Schizophrenia, How New Discoveries about the Brain Are Revolutionizing Medicine and Science.* Simon and Schuster, New York, USA.

Frerking, M. and Wondolowski, J. (2008) Regulation of neurotransmitter release by presynaptic receptor. In *Molecular Mechanisms of Neurotransmitter Release*, ed. Wang, Z.W., pp. 297–314. Humana Press, Totowa, NJ, USA.

Furuta, A., Martin, L.J., Lin, C.-L.G., Dykes-Hoberg, M. and Rothstein, J.D. (1997) Cellular and synaptic localization of the neuronal glutamate transporters excitatory amino acid transporter 3 and 4. *Neuroscience* 81, 1031–1042.

Gordon, G.R., Baimoukhametova, D.V., Hewitt, S.A., Rajapaksha, W.R., Fisher, T.E. and Bains, J.S. (2005) Norepinephrine triggers release of glial ATP to increase postsynaptic efficacy. *Nat. Neurosci.* 8, 1078–1086.

Guček, A., Vardjan, N. and Zorec, R. (2012) Exocytosis in astrocytes: transmitter release and membrane signal regulation. *Neurochem. Res.* 37, 2351–2367.

Halassa, M.M. and Haydon P.G. (2010) Integrated brain circuits: astrocytic networks modulate neuronal activity and behavior. *Annu. Rev. Physiol.* 72, 335–355.

Hirono, M., Konishi, S. and Yoshioka, T. (1998) Phospholipase C-independent group I metabotropic glutamate receptor-mediated inward current in mouse Purkinje cells. *Biochem. Biophys. Res. Commun.* 251,753–758.

Hirono, M., Yoshioka, T. and Konishi, S. (2001) $GABA_B$ receptor activation enhances mGluR-mediated responses at cerebellar excitatory synapses. *Nat. Neurosci.* 4, 1207–1216.

Hirono, M., Saitow, F., Kudo, M., Suzuki, H., Yanagawa, Y., Yamada, M., Nagao, S., Konishi, S. and Obata, K. (2012) Cerebellar globular cells receive monoaminergic excitation and monosynaptic inhibition from Purkinje cells. *PLoS One* 7, e29663.

Ichise, T., Kano, M., Hashimoto, K., Yanagihara, D., Nakao, K., Shigemoto, R., Katsuki, M., Aiba, A. (2000) mGluR1 in cerebellar Purkinje cells essential for long-term depression, synapse elimination, and motor coordination. *Science* 288, 1832–1835.

Kanai, Y. and Hediger, M.A. (2004) The glutamate/neutral amino acid transporter family SLC1: molecular, physiological and pharmacological aspects. *Pflügers Arch.* 447, 469–479.

Kim, S.J., Kim, Y.S., Yuan, J.P., Petraliam, R.S., Worley, P.F., Linden, D.J. (2003) Activation of the TRPC1 cation channel by metabotropic glutamate receptor mGluR1. *Nature* 426, 285–291.

Kristensen, A.S., Andersen, J., Jørgensen, T.N., Sørensen, L., Eriksen, J., Loland, C.J., Strømgaard, K., and Gether U. (2011) SLC6 neurotransmitter transporters: structure, function, and regulation. *Pharmacol. Rev.* 63, 585–640.

Kuffler, S.W. (1967) Neuroglia cells: physiological properties and a potassium mediated effect of neuronal activity on the glial membrane potential. *Proc. Roy. Soc. Lond. B* 168, 1–21.

Lehre, K.P. and Danbolt, N.C. (1998) The number of glutamate transporter subtype molecules at glutamatergic synapses: chemical and stereological quantification in young adult rat brain. *J. Neurosci.* 18, 8751–8757.

Lehre, K.P. and Rusakov, D.A. (2002) Asymmetry of glia near central synapses favors presynaptically directed glutamate escape. *Biophys. J.* 83, 125–134.

Mackenzie, B. and Erickson, J.D. (2004) Sodium-coupled neutral amino acid (system N/A) transporters of the SLC38 gene family. *Pflügers Arch.* 447, 784–795.

Matsui, K. and Jahr, C.E. (2003) Ectopic release of synaptic vesicles. *Neuron* 40, 1173–1183.

McKenna, M.C. (2007) The glutamate-glutamine cycle is not stoichiometric: fates of glutamate in brain. J. Neurosci. Res. 85, 3347–3358.

Mitani, A. and Tanaka, K. (2003) Functional changes of glial glutamate transporter GLT-1 during ischemia: an *in vivo* study in the hippocampal CA1 of normal mice and mutant mice lacking GLT-1. *J. Neurosci.* 23, 7176–7182.

Müller, T. and Kettenmann, H. (1995) Physiology of Bergmann glial cells. *Int. Rev. Neurobiol.* 38, 341–359.

Nikkuni, O., Takayasu, Y., Iino, M., Tanaka, K. and Ozawa, S. (2007) Facilitated activation of metabotropic glutamate receptors in cerebellar Purkinje cells in glutamate transporter EAAT4-deficient mice. *Neurosci. Res.* 59, 296–303.

Oliet, S.H.R., Piet, R., Poulain, D.A. (2001) Control of glutamate clearance and synaptic efficacy by glial coverage of neurons. Science 292, 923–926.

Olstad, E., Qu, H. and Sonnewald, U. (2007) Glutamate is preferred over glutamine for intermediary metabolism in cultured cerebellar neurons. *J. Cereb. Blood Flow Metab.* 27, 811–820.

Panatier, A., Theodosis, D.T., Mothet, J.-P., Touquet, B., Pollegioni, L., Poulain, D.A. and Oliet, S.H.R. (2006) Glia-derived D-serine controls NMDA receptor activity and synaptic memory. *Cell* 125, 775–784.

Piet, R., Vargová, L., Syková, E., Poulain, D.A., and Oliet, S.H.R. (2004) Physiological contribution of the astrocytic environment of neurons to intersynaptic crosstalk. *Proc. Natl. Acad. Sci. USA* 101, 2151–2155.

Pinheiro, P.S. and Mulle, C. (2008) Presynaptic glutamate receptors: physiological functions and mechanisms of action. *Nat. Rev. Neurosci.* 9, 423–436.

Papouin, T., Ladepeche, L., Ruel, J., Sacchi, S., Labasque, M., Hanini, M., Groc, L., Pollegioni L., Mothet, J.P. and Oliet, S.H. (2012) Synaptic and extrasynaptic NMDA receptors are gated by different endogenous coagonists. *Cell* 150, 633–646.

Rusakov, D.A., Saitow, F., Lehere, K.P. and Konishi, S. (2005) Modulation of presynaptic Ca^{2+} entry by AMPA receptors at individual GABAergic synapses in the cerebellum. *J. Neurosci.* 25, 4930–4940.

Saitow, F., Suzuki, H. and Konishi, S. (2005a) β-Adrenoceptor-mediated long-term up-regulation of the release machinery at rat cerebellar GABAergic synapses. *J. Physiol.* 565, 487–502.

Saitow, F., Murakoshi, T., Suzuki, H. and Konishi, S. (2005b) Metabotropic P2Y purinoceptor-mediated presynaptic and postsynaptic enhancement of cerebellar GABAergic transmission. *J. Neurosci.* 25, 2108–2116.

Satake, S., Saitow, F., Yamada, J. and Konishi, S. (2000) Synaptic activation of AMPA receptors inhibits GABA release from cerebellar interneurons. *Nat. Neurosci.* 3, 551–558.

Satake, S., Saitow, F., Rusakov, D. and Konishi, S. (2004) AMPA receptor-mediated presynaptic inhibition at cerebellar GABAergic synapses: a characterization of molecular mechanisms. *Eur. J. Neurosci.* 19, 2464–2474.

Satake, S., Song, S.-Y., Cao, Q., Satoh, H., Rusakov, D.A., Yanagawa, Y., Ling, E.-A., Imoto, K. and Konishi, S. (2006) Characterization of AMPA receptors targeted by the climbing fiber transmitter mediating presynaptic inhibition of GABAergic transmission at cerebellar interneuron-Purkinje cell synapses. *J. Neurosci.* 26, 2278–2289.

Satake, S., Song, S.-Y., Konishi, S. and Imoto, K. (2010) Glutamate transporter EAAT4 in Purkinje cells controls intersynaptic diffusion of climbing fiber transmitter mediating inhibition of GABA release from interneurons. *Eur. J. Neurosci.* 32, 1843–1853.

Schousboe, A. (2003) Role of astrocytes in the maintenance and modulation of glutamatergic and GABAergic neurotransmission. *Neurochem. Res.* 28, 347–352.

Shen, Y. and Linden, D.J. (2005) Long-term potentiation of neuronal glutamate transporters. *Neuron* 46, 715–722.

Takahashi, M., Kovalchuk, Y. and Attwell, D. (1995) Pre- and postsynaptic determinants of EPSC waveform at cerebellar climbing fiber and parallel fiber to Purkinje cell synapses. *J. Neurosci.* 15, 5693–5702.

Takayasu, Y., Iino, M. and Ozawa, S. (2004) Roles of glutamate transporters in shaping excitatory synaptic currents in cerebellar Purkinje cells. *Eur. J. Neurosci.* 19, 1285–1295.

Takayasu, Y., Iino, M., Kakegawa, W., Maeno, H., Watase, K., Wada, K., Yanagihara, D., Miyazaki, T., Komine, O., Watanabe, M., Tanaka, K. and Ozawa, S. (2005) Differential roles of glial and neuronal glutamate transporters in Purkinje cell synapses. *J. Neurosci.* 25, 8788–8793.

Takayasu, Y., Iino, M., Shimamoto, K., Tanaka, K. and Ozawa, S. (2006) Glial glutamate transporters maintain one-to-one relationship at the climbing fiber-Purkinje cell synapse by preventing glutamate spillover. *J. Neurosci.* 26, 6563–6572.

Takayasu, Y., Iino M., Takatsuru, Y., Tanaka, K. and Ozawa, S. (2009) Functions of glutamate transporters in cerebellar Purkinje cell synapses. *Acta Physiol.* 197, 1–12.

Tanaka, K., Watase, K., Manabe, T., Yamada, K., Watanabe, M., Takahashi, K., Iwama, H., Nishikawa, T., Ichihara, N., Kikuchi, T., Okuyama, S., Kawashima, N., Hori, S., Takimoto, M. and Wada, K. (1997) Epilepsy and exacerbation of brain injury in mice lacking the glutamate transporter GLT-1. *Science* 276, 1699–1702.

Tasker, J.G., Oliet, S.H.R., Bains, J.S., Brown, C.H. and Stern, J.E. (2012) Glial regulation of neuronal function: from synapse to systems physiology. J. Neuroendocrinol. 24, 566–576.

Tsukada, S., Iino, M., Takayasu, Y., Shimamoto, K. and Ozawa, S. (2005) Effects of a novel glutamate transporter blocker, (2S,3S)-3-{3-[4-(trifluoromethyl)benzoylamino] benzyloxy}aspartate (TFB-TBOA), on activities of hippocampal neurons. *Neuropharmacology* 48, 479–491.

Tzingounis, A.V. and Wadiche, J.I. (2007) Glutamate transporters: confining runaway excitation by shaping synaptic transmission. *Nat. Rev. Neurosci.* 8, 935–947.

Upreti, C., Zhang, X.-L., Alford, S. and Stanton, P.K. (2013) Role of presynaptic metabotropic glutamate receptors in the induction of long-term synaptic plasticity of vesicular release. *Neuropharmacology* 66, 31–39.

Yamada, K., Fukaya, M., Shibata, T., Kurihara, H., Tanaka, K., Inoue, Y. and Watanabe, M. (2000) Dynamic transformation of Bergmann glial fibers proceeds in correlation with dendritic outgrowth and synapse formation of cerebellar Purkinje cells. *J. Comp. Neurol.* 418, 106–120.

Verkhratsky, A., Rodríguez, J. and Parpura, V. (2012) Calcium signaling in astroglia. *Mol. Cell. Endocrinol.* 353, 45–56.

Wadiche, J.I., Jahr, C.E. (2005) Patterned expression of Purkinje cell glutamate transporters controls synaptic plasticity. *Nat. Neurosci.* 8, 1329–1334.

Welsh, J.P., Yuen, G., Placantonakis, D.G., Vu, T.Q., Haiss, F., O'Hearn, E., Molliver, M.E. and Aicher, S.A. (2002) Why do Purkinje cells die so easily after global brain ischemia? Aldolase C, EAAT4, and the cerebellar contribution to posthypoxic myoclonus. *Adv. Neurol.* 89, 331–359.

List of Contributors

Kasra Ahmadinia
Department of Orthopedic Surgery, Rush University Medical Center, Chicago, IL, US

Richard A. Armstrong
Vision Sciences, Aston University, Birmingham B4 7ET, UK

Manpreet Bahniwal,
Department of Biology, University of British Columbia Okanagan Campus, Kelowna, BC, Canada

Anna K. Bal-Price
Institute for Health and Consumer Protection, European Commission Joint Research Centre, via E. Fermi 2749, 21027 Ispra (VA), Italy

Marcos R. Costa
Brain Institute, Federal University of Rio Grande do Norte, 59072-970 Natal, Brazil

Masaharu Hayashi
Department of Brain Development and Neural Regeneration, Tokyo Metropolitan Institute of Medical Science, Tokyo, Japan

Yoshinori Hayashi
Department of Aging Science and Pharmacology, Faculty of Dental Sciences, Kyushu University, Fukuoka, 812-8582, Japan

Hee-Jeong Im
Department of Biochemistry, Department of Orthopedic Surgery, Department of Internal Medicine (Rheumatology), Rush University Medical Center, Chicago, IL, US

Charanjit Kaur
Department of Anatomy, MD10, 4 Medical Drive, Yong Loo Lin School of Medicine, National University of Singapore, Singapore-117597

Agnieszka Kinsner-Ovaskainen
Institute for Health and Consumer Protection, European Commission Joint Research Centre, via E. Fermi 2749, 21027 Ispra (VA), Italy

Andis Klegeris
Department of Biology, University of British Columbia Okanagan Campus, Kelowna, BC, Canada

Shiro Konishi
Department of Neurophysiology, Kagawa School of Pharmaceutical Sciences and Institute of Neuroscience, Tokushima Bunri University, 1314-1 Shido, Sanuki 769-2193, Japan

Eng-Ang Ling
Department of Anatomy, MD10, 4 Medical Drive, Yong Loo Lin School of Medicine, National University of Singapore, Singapore-117597

Jonathan P. Little
Department of Biology, University of British Columbia Okanagan Campus, Kelowna, BC, Canada

Rie Miyata
Department of Brain Development and Neural Regeneration, Tokyo Metropolitan Institute of MedicalScience, Tokyo, Japan

Shuki Mizutani
Department of Pediatrics, Tokyo Medical and Dental University, Tokyo, Japan

Madhuvika Murugan
Department of Anatomy, MD10, 4 Medical Drive, Yong Loo Lin School of Medicine, National University of Singapore, Singapore-117597

Keisuke Nakajima
Department of Pediatrics, Tokyo Medical and Dental University, Tokyo, Japan

Hiroshi Nakanishi
Department of Aging Science and Pharmacology, Faculty of Dental Sciences, Kyushu University, Fukuoka, 812-8582, Japan
Japan Science and Technology Agency, Core Research for Evolutional Science and Technology, Tokyo 102-0075, Japan

Luciana Nogaroli
Institute of Biophysics Carlos Chagas Filho, Federal University of Rio de Janeiro, 21941-902 Rio de Janeiro, Brazil

Gurugirijha Rathnasamy
Department of Anatomy, MD10, 4 Medical Drive, Yong Loo Lin School of Medicine, National University of Singapore, Singapore-117597

Bryan M. Saltzman
Department of Orthopedic Surgery, Rush University Medical Center, Chicago, IL, US

Shin'Ichiro Satake
Department of Information Physiology, National Institute of Physiological Sciences (NIPS), 5-1 Higashiyama, Myodaiji-cho, Okazaki 444-8787, Japan
School of Life Science, The Graduate University for Advanced Studies (SOKENDAI), 5-1 Higashiyama, Myodaiji-cho, Okazaki 444-8787, Japan

Naoyuki Tanuma
Department of Brain Development and Neural Regeneration, Tokyo Metropolitan Institute of Medical Science, Tokyo, Japan

Frank B. Wydra
Department of Biochemistry, Department of Orthopedic Surgery, Rush University Medical Center, Chicago, IL, US

INDEX

#

A

B

C

D

I

J

K

L

M

N

O

P

Q

R

S

T

U